AF334406

MECHANISMS OF DRUG RESISTANCE IN EPILEPSY:
LESSONS FROM ONCOLOGY

Novartis Foundation Symposium 243

MECHANISMS OF DRUG RESISTANCE IN EPILEPSY:
LESSONS FROM ONCOLOGY

2002

JOHN WILEY & SONS, LTD

Other Wiley Editorial Offices

John Wiley & Sons, Inc., 605 Third Avenue,
New York, NY 10158-0012, USA

WILEY-VCH Verlag GmbH, Pappelallee 3,
D-69469 Weinheim, Germany

Jacaranda Wiley Ltd, 33 Park Road, Milton,
Queensland 4064, Australia

John Wiley & Sons (Asia) Pte Ltd, 2 Clementi Loop #02-01,
Jin Xing Distripark, Singapore 129809

John Wiley & Sons (Canada) Ltd, 22 Worcester Road,
Rexdale, Ontario M9W 1L1, Canada

Novartis Foundation Symposium 243
viii+246 pages, 28 figures, 27 tables

British Library Cataloguing in Publication Data

A catalogue record for this book is available from the British Library

ISBN 0 470 84146 X

Typeset in $10\frac{1}{2}$ on $12\frac{1}{2}$ pt Garamond by Dobbie Typesetting Limited, Tavistock, Devon.
Printed and bound in Great Britain by Biddles Ltd, Guildford and King's Lynn.
This book is printed on acid-free paper responsibly manufactured from sustainable forestry,
in which at least two trees are planted for each one used for paper production.

Contents

Participants

N. Joan Abbott   Blood–Brain Barrier Research Group, Centre for Neuroscience Research, King's College London, London SE1 1UL, UK

Fred Andermann   Department of Neurology and Neurosurgery, Montreal Neurological Institute, 3801 University Street, Montréal, QC, Canada H3A 2B4

Peter Atadja   Functional Genomics, Novartis Pharmaceuticals Corporation, 556 Morris Avenue, Summit, New Jersey 07901, USA

Susan Bates   Molecular Therapeutics Section, Medicine Branch, National Cancer Institute, Bldg 10, 9000 Rockville Pike, Bethesda, MD 20892, USA

Ulrich Brinkmann   Epidauros Biotechnology, Pharmacogenetics Laboratory, Am Neuland 1, 82347 Bernried, Germany

Rudolf Deisz   Department of Cell and Neurobiology, Institute of Anatomy, Charité, Philippstrasse 10, D-10098 Berlin, Germany

Harry Hendrikse   PET center, University Hospital of Groningen, PO Box 30.001, 9700 RB Groningen, The Netherlands

Patrick Kwan (*Novartis Foundation Bursar*)   Department of Medicine & Geriatrics, United Christian Hospital, Kwun Tong, Hong Kong

Victor Ling (*Chair*)   BC Cancer Agency, 601 West 10th Avenue, Vancouver, BC, Canada V5Z 1E6

Wolfgang Löscher   Department of Pharmacology, Toxicology & Pharmacy, School of Veterinary Medicine, Bünteweg 17, D-30559 Hanover, Germany

Brian Meldrum   GKT School of Biomedical Sciences, Henriette Raphael House, Guy's Campus, London SE1 1UL, UK

Michael J. Newman   Ontogen Corporation, 6451 El Camino Real, Carlsbad, CA 92009, USA

Amit M. Oza   Princess Margaret Hospital, 610 University Avenue, Toronto, Ontario, Canada M5G 2M9

Munir Pirmohamed   Department of Pharmacology & Therapeutics, University of Liverpool, Ashton Street Medical School, Ashton Street, Liverpool L69 3GE, UK

Stephan Ruetz   Novartis Pharma Inc., Department of Oncology, CH-4002 Basel, Switzerland

J.W. Sander   University College London, Institute of Neurology, Queen Square, London WC1N 3BG, UK

Rik J. Scheper   Vrije Universiteit Medical Center, de Boelelaan 1117, 1081 HV, Amsterdam, The Netherlands

Markus Schmutz   Nervous System Research, Novartis Pharma AG, WKL-125.11.10, CH-4002 Basel, Switzerland

S. D. Shorvon   University College London, Institute of Neurology, Queen Square, London WC1N 3BG, UK

Graeme Sills   Epilepsy Unit, Department of Medicine and Therapeutics, Western Infirmary, 44 Church Street, Glasgow G11 6NT, UK

Sanjay Sisodiya   Epilepsy Research Group, Institute of Neurology, University College London, Queen Square, London WC1N 3BG, UK

András Váradi   Active Transport Proteins Group, Institute of Enzymology, Hungarian Academy of Sciences, Karolina ut. 29, Budapest H-1113, Hungary

Annamaria Vezzani   Istituto di Ricerche Farmacologiche Mario Negri, via Eritrea 62, I-20147 Milano, Italy

Jan Wijnholds   The Netherlands Ophthalmic Research Institute, Koninklijke Nederlandse Akademie van Wetenschappen, Meibergdreef 47, 1105 BA Amsterdam, The Netherlands

Alastair Wood   Vanderbilt University Medical Center, Departments of Medicine and Pharmacology, Medical Research Building I, Room 552A, 1211 22nd Ave S, Nashville, TN 37232-6602, USA

Chair's introduction

Victor Ling

BC Cancer Agency, 600 West 10th Avenue, Vancouver, BC, Canada V5Z 4E6

In this introduction I'll try to set the tone for this meeting and raise some issues that I hope we will address over the next few days. I would like to create an inventory of some of the key issues that we should aim to cover during the discussion sessions. Unusually, this meeting is bringing together two scientific fields: the multidrug resistance field from oncology and the epilepsy field from brain biology. The purpose of this meeting is to see whether there are lessons that can be learned from drug resistance in oncology that may have parallels in drug-resistant epilepsy. This reminds me of a favourite story of mine. An eminent professor once set his class a three hour exam, with 300 questions which they had to answer with either 'true' or 'false'. He handed out the paper and told the students to begin. Immediately, one of the students at the back of the class began flipping a coin and marking his answers down. The professor was offended by this affront to intellectual integrity, but he thought, well, this is a drug transporter exam and we don't know what is going on anyway, so this is as good an approach as any. Towards the end of the exam the professor announced that there were 10 minutes left to go. The person at the back was by now flipping the coin very rapidly. The professor said, 'What are you doing now?'. The student replied, 'I'm checking my answers!' Sometimes in our field we create a consistent set of assumptions and paradigms. It may take someone completely outside the field to look in and realize that there is some fatally flawed assumption. Or perhaps it just requires a naïve question to bring to light these mistaken assumptions. This is what I hope will happen in this meeting. In bringing the two groups together, I hope we will lay aside our assumptions and try to use logical reasoning and ask each other questions in an intense but non-personal way, thus challenging each of us to examine our own particular paradigm.

I would like to tell you a bit about where I think the history of drug resistance comes in. This is rooted a long time ago in the treatments of microbial diseases. Erlich, the great German physiologist/chemist, was working in the dye industry. He realized that certain chemicals adhered better to different materials than others. He speculated that such chemistry can also be specific for microorganisms. He said that what was needed was a 'chemotherapia specifica': agents that on the one hand are able to kill certain parasites and on the other hand are not going to cause too much harm to the host organism when applied in effective doses. This is a paradigm that has driven both antibiotic development and also the concept of cancer chemotherapy. Many years later Erlich lamented that drug resistance has followed the development of new drugs 'like a faithful shadow'.

I want to give a brief history of the development of P glycoprotein (Pgp) and the mechanism of drug resistance. Drug resistant clones of cells were derived, and these all turned out to be multidrug resistant (MDR). We identified Pgp as a highly over-expressed protein that was the causative mechanism of resistance by cloning the gene, transfecting it into a naïve cell and showing that it caused a similar MDR phenotype. We found where it was localized and we purified and characterized it. We looked for expression in human cancers and normal tissues, and looked for correlation of expression and clinical outcome. We modulated Pgp function using different compounds *in vitro* and in clinical studies. For those of you who don't work on molecular biology or cell genetics, I'll describe an old experiment in which a cell line is taken and treated with a chemotherapeutic drug. The few cells that survive form drug resistant clones. As an example, a clone selected for adriamycin could be about 80 times more resistant to adriamycin than the parental cells. Yet the same cells might be 500 times more resistant to an unrelated drug, vinblastine, which they have never seen before, and 2000 times more resistant to vincristine and 6000 times more resistant to gramicidin. At the same time, another cell line selected by the same drug can have a different phenotype: even though it is 50 times more resistant to adriamycin than the parent cell line, it is 5000 times more resistant to colchicine and only six times more resistant to gramicidin. Both these cell lines are MDR cell lines, and are the result of MDR molecules that are related to each other but are different.

One way in which cancer is a little different from epilepsy is that cancer is a progressive disease in which it is believed that clonal selections occur: the original cells divide and evolve into a preneoplastic lesion and then evolve into a localized tumour. This then metastasizes and becomes resistant to anticancerous agents. There is a continuous selection during which time numerous genomic changes occur. Pgp is expressed in normal tissue, but molecules such as Pgp can be modulated by various factors such as drugs, radiation and growth factors. One of the issues is whether something like Pgp when found in tissue is a cause of the non-response, or whether it is be a side effect of differentiation, for example.

Finally, I would like to say something about more recent profiling studies. We have used a quantitative PCR technique with which we have profiled about 40 ABC transporters. These belong to the Pgp family and MDR family. In the mammary gland these ABC transporters are expressed around mid to low levels. TAP_1, which is involved in the transport of antigenic peptides, is at a high level. In this discussion, the organ of interest is the brain. Most of the ABC transporters are expressed at fairly high levels in the brain. MDR1 is high, and MRP1 is very high. The challenge for us is to work out which cell types these transporters are expressed in and what role they play.

Another major challenge is to apply effectively the findings from experimental systems into the clinic. From an oncology perspective, we work on cell lines and experimental tumours, and our experimental system is fairly homogeneous: it can be manipulated with a fairly uniform response. Many mechanisms of resistance have been identified at the molecular level and specific probes have been generated. Then the experimental system can be manipulated to confirm studies of everything above that. The other side of the coin is of course the patient. Patients are non-uniform and the tumour cell (or in epilepsy the brain cell) population involved may be quite heterogeneous. There may be a wide range of responses from the cells themselves or from the patients. Functional assays of the tumour cells correlating with the patient responses are often quite variable. Correlation studies involve getting the right people to do clinical studies, which is logistically often very difficult. These are some of the challenges ahead of us.

The problem of the drug-resistant epilepsies

J. W. Sander

Institute of Neurology, University College London, Queen Square, London WC1N 3BG, UK

Abstract. For the majority of patients with epilepsy, the prognosis for seizure control is very good; however, refractory epilepsy develops in about 20–30% of patients and represents a significant challenge for both clinical management and for research. Physicians treating epilepsy are often asked to predict prognosis and make decisions about commencing and withdrawing treatment. Practice can be guided by epidemiological studies of prognosis. It seems that prognosis depends largely on the aetiology of the seizures and the clinical background of the patient rather than on the seizures themselves or the treatment prescribed. Aetiologies are, however, not the sole determinant of outcome and response to treatment and unknown factors must exit. It is likely that some of these unknown factors are genetically determined but this needs confirmation. The search for these unknown factors that may determine intractability in epilepsy is a very exciting prospect, which may prove to be multifactorial. In some patients, epilepsy may indeed become resistant to treatment whilst in others the propensity for intractability to the drugs currently available may be part and parcel of the condition. Further research is urgently needed to elucidate the full range of mechanisms that lead to drug resistant epilepsy.

2002 Mechanisms of drug resistance in epilepsy: lessons from oncology. Wiley, Chichester (Novartis Foundation Symposium 243) p 4–18

The epilepsies overall carry a good prognosis with over 70% of patients developing a seizure disorder achieving long-term remission, usually in response to the first or second anti-epileptic drug (AED) utilized (Sander 1993). Up to 30% of patients, however, do not respond to the usual AEDs and these patients pose a major management problem for the clinicians involved in their care. These patients have increased psychosocial and physical morbidity and their mortality is greatly increased over that of the general population as a result of their continuing liability to seizures (Cockerell et al 1994, Sander 1995, Nashef et al 1995). Only a small number of these patients are amenable to surgical treatment for their epilepsy and therefore novel therapeutic approaches are urgently needed to improve this picture (Sander 1998).

Physicians managing patients with epilepsy are often asked to predict the prognosis and response to treatment. Although precise individual prognostication is difficult, syndrome classification may help to guide practice.

Prognosis seems to depend largely on the background aetiology rather than on the seizures themselves or the treatment prescribed, although unknown factors are likely to play a role (Hauser & Hesdorffer 1990, Sander & Shorvon 1996, Sander & Pal 2000). This chapter considers, from an epidemiological point of view, the prognosis of different epileptic syndromes in terms of seizure remission, the influence of AED treatment on prognosis and other factors that may determine drug resistance and lead to intractability.

Syndromic approach

Different conditions may express themselves solely by the occurrence of recurrent unprovoked epileptic seizures, thus qualifying for the label of 'epilepsy' (Sander & Sillampaa 1998). Once the diagnosis of epilepsy is established, a syndromic diagnosis should be attempted. A syndrome is a group of symptoms and signs which, when taken together, form the description of an illness. In the case of epilepsy the features that usually define the syndrome are the types of seizures that occur, the presence of characteristic structural lesions, the age at onset, the presence of a family history, the natural history and characteristic changes in the EEG (Commission on classification and terminology 1989). It is often possible to infer prognosis from the syndromic classification (Sander & Pal 2000) as distinctions can be made between benign epilepsy syndromes with good outcome, and intractable syndromes that have a gloomy outcome. Epilepsy is also a common feature of acute and chronic brain syndromes, in which the underlying pathology may be static or progressive. (Hauser & Hesdorffer 1990, Hart et al 1990, Sander 1993, Sander & Pal 2000).

Benign syndromes

The benign syndromes are usually age-limited, stereotyped, often provoked and occur in otherwise normal children, adolescents or young adults. Genetic predisposition is common. Many of these seizure disorders do not fit neatly into the syndrome classification, but some prognostic features are useful in predicting a good outcome (Sander & Pal 2000). These include single seizure type, seizures of a short duration, an overall low number of seizures and good initial response to AEDs (McDonald et al 2000, Kwan & Brodie 2000).

Febrile convulsions

Febrile convulsions are seizures triggered by fever of extracranial origin and occur in at least 3% of children, mainly between the ages of 6 months and 5 years (Hauser & Hesdorffer 1990, McDonald et al 1999, Sander & Pal 2000). The seizures are usually brief tonic–clonic convulsions. However about 10% of these children have complex, focal, or prolonged seizures requiring emergency treatment. Overall, 2–7% of children with febrile convulsions go on to have an unprovoked seizure in childhood or early adult life, a risk which is at least four times that of the rest of the population (McDonald et al 1999). A family history of epilepsy, complex febrile convulsions and prior neurological abnormality are risk factors for the subsequent development of epilepsy which usually takes the form of mesial temporal lobe epilepsy associated with hippocampal sclerosis and is usually resistant to drug therapy. Continuous treatment for recurrent febrile convulsions is not recommended as overall it is a benign condition and the risks of treatment probably outweigh the benefits. There is also no evidence to suggest that treating febrile convulsions with AEDs prevents the onset of subsequent mesial temporal lobe epilepsy (Hauser & Hesdorffer 1990, McDonald et al 1999, Sander & Pal 2000).

Rolandic epilepsy

Benign epilepsy with centro-temporal (Rolandic area) interictal discharges usually starts between 2 and 12 years, most commonly between 7 and 10 years, and will have stopped by the age of 14 years (Sander & Sillampa 1998, Sander & Pal 2000). About 30% have a family history of epilepsy. Children with the condition are free of major impairments but may have some neuropsychological deficits (Sander & Pal 2000). Less than 2% of patients with benign partial epilepsies develop chronic epilepsy.

Occipital epilepsy

The majority of children with partial seizures with occipital discharges accompanied by visual phenomena, postictal headache, and migrainous characteristics have a benign prognosis, but some have a poor cognitive and seizure outcome. The latter usually have lesions, particularly cortical malformations (Hauser & Hesdorffer 1990, Sander & Sillampa 1998, Sander & Pal 2000).

Absence epilepsy

The absence epilepsies are uncommon in the general population, representing only 1–2% of all epilepsies (Hauser & Hesdorffer 1990, Sander 1993, 1994, Sander & Pal 2000). Up to 80% of children with absence epilepsy will go into terminal remission with treatment. The most favourable prognosis is for those who do not have generalized tonic–clonic seizures as part of their condition. The risk of tonic–clonic seizures in adult life can be predicted from a past history of tonic–clonic seizures, a lower IQ, and a family history of seizures. 10% of those with either one or no adverse features continue to have absence seizures, with all of those with three adverse features going on to have generalized tonic–clonic seizures (Sander 1994).

Intractable or drug-resistant syndromes

Developmental arrest and regression as a consequence of intractable syndromes are common; it is, however, essential to rule out metabolic, degenerative and structural brain diseases (Hauser & Hesdorffer 1990, Sander & Sillampa 1998, Sander & Pal 2000). Cerebral malformations are particularly associated with a poor prognosis for seizure control, except in cases where surgical options are available. Metabolic causes of epilepsy are often fatal, and seizures may be intractable. Progressive myoclonic epilepsies include Lafora's disease, Unverricht–Lundeborg disease, and mitochondrial disorders, which have a uniformly poor prognosis for seizure control, and variable pace of degeneration.

Infantile spasms

West syndrome is symptomatic of many static cortical diseases, particularly cortical malformations, with less than a quarter being cryptogenic (Hauser & Hesdorffer 1990, Sander & Sillampa 1998, Sander & Pal 2000). The overall mortality of treated West syndrome is 20%, with 30–50% of the remaining patients developing cerebral palsy, and up to 85% having cognitive impairment. The outcome varies according to pathology but most survivors will develop learning disabilities. Infantile spasms due to hypoxic–ischaemic damage and cortical malformations are also associated with poor developmental and seizure prognosis. In contrast, up to 50% of those patients with cryptogenic West syndrome may go on to have normal development. Most infants with unprovoked seizure disorders in the first year of life, whether they have West syndrome or not, have a poor developmental outcome (Hauser & Hesdorffer 1990, Sander & Sillampa 1998, Sander & Pal 2000).

Severe myoclonic epilepsy of childhood

This syndrome usually begins at 4–10 months, often with a prolonged partial clonic seizure associated with moderate fever. Later attacks may have multiple seizure types, including complex absences, myoclonias, complex partial seizures and apnoeic attacks, and developmental regression accompanies this phase (Hauser & Hesdorffer 1990, Sander & Sillampa 1998, Sander & Pal 2000).

Lennox–Gastaut syndrome

It is likely that Lennox–Gastaut syndrome (LGS) represents a final common pathway for several diverse pathologies. Prognoses for seizure control and development are generally poor, although slightly better in idiopathic cases (Hauser & Hesdorffer 1990, Sander & Sillampa 1998, Sander & Pal 2000). Half of affected children have primary developmental delay, and all have learning difficulties after five or more years of the condition. Only about 10% have a reasonable outcome. Preceding infantile spasms or abnormalities on neuroimaging are associated with poorer prognosis (Hauser & Hesdorffer 1990, Sander & Sillampa 1998, Sander & Pal 2000). Episodes of non-convulsive status complicate the clinical course.

Partial seizures of lesional origin

Partial seizures of lesional origin may be static or progressive. Static disorders include cortical malformations, vascular and traumatic pathologies and benign tumours. Cavernous angiomas and arterio–venous malformations respond well to surgical removal, but major lesions may be associated with motor impairment and intractable partial seizures. The long-term prognosis of lesional partial epilepsy is of one third achieving remission, one third having continuing functional impairments, and one third becoming completely dependent (Hauser & Hesdorffer 1990, Sander & Sillampa 1998, Sander & Pal 2000). A mortality of 0.5% per annum occurs. Adverse prognostic features can be identified early and justify surgery in childhood. Young children with developmental tumours of the temporal lobe may present with cognitive and autistic regression, which may respond to surgery (Sander & Pal 2000).

Rasmussen's encephalitis

Rasmussen's syndrome is a progressive intractable partial epilepsy syndrome with cognitive deterioration, aphasia and hemiplegia, for which medical treatment with immunoglobulins or steroids is disappointing and early surgery as the only treatment modality leading to a chance of long-term seizure freedom (Sander & Pal 2000).

Landau–Kleffner syndrome

This is a rare condition. Typically, partial or generalized seizures begin and language comprehension and speech are lost, after two or more years of normal development. The condition may cause behavioural disorders and global cognitive, motor and social regression often with autistic features, sometimes without clinical seizures. AEDs may reduce seizures and EEG abnormalities, but prognosis for cognitive functioning is more pessimistic. Sometimes a dramatic response to steroids can be seen but side effects and long-term dependency may limit their use. Multiple subpial transections may occasionally be helpful (Sander & Sillampa 1998, Sander & Pal 2000).

AED treatment and intractability

There are few placebo-controlled trials to justify much of the use of AEDs in epilepsy (Sander & Sillampa 1998, Sander & Pal 2000). Thus arguments about whether to start treatment after the first, second, or third seizure are based on convention rather than evidence. Two studies have shown an increased risk of recurrence in patients not treated after the first seizure compared to those treated (Camfield et al 1989, First Seizure Trial Group 1993). In one trial, the risk was 2.5 times greater in the untreated group (95% CI: 1.9–4.2). In the other, respective recurrence rates were 78% versus 56% at 36 months. There is no evidence, however, that early treatment improves prognosis (Sander 1993, Musico et al 1994, Sander & Pal 2000). AEDs can prevent seizures in acute encephalopathies, prevent the recurrence of febrile convulsions and control epilepsy, but there is no evidence that they prevent the development of chronic epilepsy. They may however, improve cognitive function in certain epileptic syndromes, change the quality of life of people with epilepsy and reduce morbidity and mortality.

Natural history of treated epilepsy

Most studies of the treatment of newly diagnosed epilepsy have reported one-year remission rates of 65–80%. The prognosis for seizure remission is not as good for pure partial seizures (16–43% at one year) as it is for secondarily generalized seizures (48–53%). Similarly, seizure remission is less likely in patients with multiple seizure types or associated neurological impairments. The most important predictors of remission are aetiology and syndrome type, although many studies of remission have not used syndromic classification (Hauser & Hesdorffer 1990, Sander & Sillampa 1998, Sander & Pal 2000). Large population-based studies have shown that the likelihood of remission is greatest in the first two years, and thereafter the probability diminishes. A further large scale study has shown that age and seizure type have little effect on the chance of five year remission, although patients with symptomatic epilepsies were more likely to die prematurely (Cockerell et al 1994).

There is no evidence that any one particular first-line AED monotherapy is associated with a superior seizure outcome. In a Canadian population-based study, about 17% of children treated with a first-line AED monotherapy had inadequate seizure control, and 42% of them successfully achieved control with a second AED (Camfield et al 1997). Complex partial seizures and neurological impairments were associated with a less favourable response to the first AED. It would seem logical therefore to use the natural history of the epileptic syndrome, or the presence of adverse clinical features, to guide the decision to commence and finally to withdraw treatment (Sander & Sillampa 1998, Sander & Pal 2000).

Risk of relapse after AED withdrawal

Most people with epilepsy treated with AEDs eventually become seizure free, and it is common clinical practice to consider discontinuing drugs after a substantial remission period. Withdrawal in itself carries a risk of relapse, which is reportedly lower in children than in adults. Large studies of AED withdrawal indicate that the risk of relapse is greatest in the first two years after discontinuing medication. Relapse is actually greatest in those continuing medication in the period after that, although this may be due to voluntary withdrawal of medication. Risk factors for seizure recurrence after discontinuing therapy include a long history of seizures before remission, occurrence of more than one seizure type, presence of cerebral impairment, past history of remission on relapse, and diagnosis of Juvenile Myoclonic Epilepsy. Patients with remote symptomatic seizures or an abnormal EEG pattern were also more likely to relapse. Reinstituting previously effective treatment usually easily controls relapse in the majority of patients. In a small minority, however, this is not the case and remission is never achieved again. (Sander & Sillampa 1998, Sander & Pal 2000.)

Predictors of intractability

About 20–30% of patients with epilepsy do not enter remission and are not candidates for surgical treatment. Only a small fraction of these patients with intractable epilepsy will be rendered seizure free by adjunctive treatment with new AEDs. The strongest predictor for intractability seems to be syndromic classification or background aetiology, although the understanding of this is still patchy. For instance, the inherently poor prognosis for remission in infantile spasms, Lennox–Gastaut syndrome and polymorphic epilepsy of infancy are recognized. Other well-recognized risk factors for intractability include early age at onset, remote symptomatic epilepsy, cortical malformations and a history of status epilepticus either before or after a diagnosis of epilepsy has been made (Sander 1993, Sander & Sillampa 1998, Sander & Pal 2000).

One difficulty with this syndromic approach to prognosis is that other factors may be involved which we still do not fully understand; for instance, the reason why, in pathologically well-defined syndromes, the response to treatment and final outcome is not always the same (Sander & Shorvon 1996). This seems to indicate that factors other than pathology influence outcome. Some patients respond to drug treatment whereas others who have the same aetiology develop intractable epilepsy. For instance, some people with mesial temporal lobe epilepsy associated with hippocampal sclerosis seem to respond favourably to certain AEDs whereas the majority do not respond to any drug. Thus aetiologies and syndromes are not the sole determinant of response to treatment and outcome, and unknown factors must exist. It is interesting to speculate about the nature of these factors. The concept that intractability may develop if seizures are left unchecked has long been discussed (Sander 1993, Shinnar & Berg 1994). Epidemiological data, however, does not support this, at least in the large scale; in population terms neither the duration of epilepsy or number of seizures are predictors of outcome (Feksi et al 1991). A genetic predisposition to intractability is a more tantalizing prospect although the exact manner in which this would operate is unknown at this stage (Johnson & Sander 2001). Recently, suggestions have been made of a possible role of a multidrug-resistance protein in the development of intractability in certain forms of epilepsy that could be genetically determined (Sisodiya et al 2001). It is possible that more than one mechanism is involved and further research in this area is urgently required if we are ever to conquer the drug-resistant epilepsies.

References

Camfield PR, Camfield CS, Dooley JM, Smith EB, Garner B 1989 A randomised study of carbamazepine versus no medication after a first unprovoked seizure in childhood. Neurology 39:851–852

Camfield PR, Camfield CS, Gordon K, Dooley JM 1997 If a first antiepileptic drug fails to control a child's epilepsy, what are the chances of success with the next drug? J Pediatr 131:821–824

Cockerell OC, Johnson AL, Sander JW, Hart YM, Goodridge DM, Shorvon SD 1994 Mortality from epilepsy: results from a prospective population-based study. Lancet 344:918–921

Commission on classification and terminology of the International League of epilepsy 1989 Proposal for revised classification of epilepsies and epileptic syndromes. Epilepsia 30:389–399

Feksi AT, Kaamugisha J, Gatiti S, Sander JW, Shorvon SD 1991 Comprehensive primary health care antiepileptic drug treatment programme in rural and semi-rural Kenya ICBERG (International Community-based Epilepsy Research Group). Lancet 337:406–409

First Seizure Trial Group 1993 Randomised clinical trial on the efficacy of antiepileptic drugs in reducing the risk of relapse after a first unprovoked tonic-clonic seizure. Neurology 43:478–483

Hart YM, Sander JW, Johnson AL, Shorvon SD 1990 National General Practice Study of Epilepsy: recurrence after a first seizure. Lancet 336:1271–1274

Hauser WA, Hesdorffer DC 1990 Epilepsy. Demos Publications, Maryland

Johnson M, Sander JW 2001 The clinical implications of the genetics of epilepsy. J Neurol Neurosurg Psychiatry 70:428–430

Kwan P, Brodie MJ 2000 Early identification of refractory epilepsy. N Engl J Med 342:314–319

MacDonald BK, Johnson AL, Sander JW, Shorvon SD 1999 Febrile convulsions in 220 children—neurological sequelae at 12 years follow-up. Eur Neurol 41:179–186

MacDonald BK, Johnson AL, Goodridge DM, Cockerell OC, Sander JW, Shorvon SD 2000 Factors predicting prognosis of epilepsy after presentation with seizures. Ann Neurol 48: 833–841

Musicco M, Berghi E, Solari A et al 1994 Effects of antiepileptic treatment initiated after the first unprovoked seizure in long term prognosis of epilepsy. Neurology 44:A337–A338

Nashef L, Fish D, Sander JW, Shorvon SD 1995 Incidence of sudden unexpected death in an adult out patient cohort with epilepsy at a tertiary referral centre. J Neurol Neurosurg Psychiatry 58:462–464

Sander JW 1993 Some aspects of prognosis in the epilepsies: a review. Epilepsia 34:1007–1016

Sander JW 1994 The epidemiology and prognosis of typical absence seizures. In: Duncan JS, Panayiotopoulos CP (eds) The typical absences and related epileptic syndromes. Churchill Livingstone, Edinburgh, p 135–141

Sander JW 1995 The prognosis, prevention, morbidity and mortality of epilepsy. In: Duncan JS, Shorvon SD, Fish DR (eds) Clinical epilepsy. Churchill Livingstone, Edinburgh, p 299–320

Sander JW 1998 New treatments for epilepsy. Curr Opin Neurol 11:141–148

Sander JW, Pal D 2000 Long term prognosis of epilepsy. In: Schachter S, Schmidt D (eds) Epilepsy: problem solving in clinical practice. Martin Dunitz, London, p 367–380

Sander JW, Shorvon SD 1996 Epidemiology of the epilepsies. J Neurol Neurosurg Psychiatry 61:433–443

Sander JW, Sillampaa M 1998 The natural history and prognosis of the epilepsies. In: Engel J, Pedley TA (eds) Epilepsy: a comprehensive textbook. Raven Press, New York p 69–86

Shinnar S, Berg AT 1994 Does antiepileptic drug therapy alter the prognosis of childhood seizures and prevent the development of chronic epilepsy? Semin Pediatr Neurol 1:111–117

Sisodiya SM, Lin WR, Squier MV, Thom M 2001 Multidrug-resistance protein 1 in focal cortical dysplasia. Lancet 357:42–43

DISCUSSION

Ling: A critical issue is the question of heterogeneity. The term 'epilepsy' appears to encompass many diseases. The classification may not be completely clear. When you talk about drug-resistant epilepsy (DRE), is this fundamentally a different disease from epilepsy that has a good prognosis? One possibility is that DRE is a good-prognosis epilepsy that has drug resistance mechanisms on top of it. This is a fundamental issue. If DRE is actually a different disease, perhaps we just haven't found a good drug for it yet.

Sander: You are right; that is the major issue. Until we sort out the full spectrum of epilepsies, we will not be able to advance the cause. It is only with the advent of high-resolution brain imaging and neurogenetics in the last 10 years that we are getting a handle on many of the different syndromes. I could list 10–15 syndromes that have been described in the last 5 years. The whole spectrum has not yet been defined, and this is an area we need to work on with urgency.

Andermann: There are very few epidemiologists working in the field of epilepsy. We have heard here an excellent survey of the problems this field faces. Before one begins to address specific issues one has to hear what the whole spectrum represents. But lest we give up at this point, one still has to identify some specific issues that are particularly relevant for this meeting. A common experience of anyone who treats epilepsy is meeting the parent who reports that when you change the medication the child is seizure free for a couple of months, and then the seizures return. This is something we hear all the time. It is extremely likely that this intractability develops in some way, not only in response to drugs, but also in response to certain surgical interventions. For example, we see this with patients who have had a callosal section (a section of the band that unites the two hemispheres). They will often improve for a period of time and then, over some years, their seizures will return, and the pattern will return to the level it was previously, as if new pathways had been created. There are, however, other situations where the change is long lasting, which indicates that intractability does develop. Another interesting example is that of people who have what is generally a fairly benign epilepsy. This often represents idiopathic generalized epilepsy, in which there is not supposed to be any evidence for an obvious brain lesion. These people's disease may be well controlled by anti-epileptic medication, and then, for one reason or another, they stop their medication. When they resume the medication, they may not respond as well as they had initially and the reason for this later intractability remains unclear.

Meldrum: When we start from the data that Ley Sander has presented, giving these four prognostic groups, the obvious interpretation of the results in the drug-resistant group is that it is a complex network phenomenon. In the good-prognostic group, we already know that some of those epilepsies are single-gene defects involving one ion channel, and these somehow get better spontaneously or are easier to treat. All the epilepsies of the patients in the bad prognosis group are self-evidently complex disorders in terms of formation of incorrect connections, either developmentally, or following injury or prolonged febrile convulsions. This is a long-term process in which we know there is a multiplicity of different molecular changes involving ion channels, transporters and receptors. In the animal models of kindling and hippocampal sclerosis, we know that there are dozens of changes occurring diffusely throughout the brain (Mody 1993). We also know that new connections have developed that provide incorrect pathways or patterns of feedback (Babb et al 1992). The simple interpretation, therefore, is that DRE is a result of a multiplicity of changes including faulty connections. It is a complex network phenomenon, and you can't expect to correct it just by hitting one ion channel or GABA receptor. This hypothesis doesn't exclude the role of P glycoprotein or other drug transporter molecules, but it certainly challenges that view.

Bates: Could you clarify your current understanding of the molecular basis of epilepsy?

Meldrum: This is one of the other things about drug resistance. Maybe it is because all the drugs we use have two main mechanisms of action: they either act on ion channels (principally on Na^+ channels), or on inhibitory transmission mediated by GABA. Because we have used such peculiar screening procedures, we have selected only these two classes of drugs. It is because we didn't have screening procedures that involved epileptic animals or chronic drug administration that we now have a limited group of AEDs.

Bates: What is known about the cell types that trigger the epileptic activity?

Scheper: I'd also be interested to hear more on the cell types involved and the potential drug targets.

Meldrum: It is a complex topic. The molecular defects that are known in the different models cover a broad spectrum. There is a whole range of changes in Na^+ channels, K^+ channels and Ca^{2+} channels that can produce epilepsy. In humans we now know of a variety of single-gene defects that cause epilepsy (Prasad et al 1999). In mice there is a large range of single-gene defects, particularly involving Ca^{2+} channels. Ley Sander mentioned benign familial neonatal convulsions: this involves K^+ channels. This defect is lifelong and yet it gives rise to seizures solely from 3 days of life to 3 months of life. So ion channels are one cause of epilepsy. Another cause is changes in receptors. If certain subunits of the $GABA_A$ receptor are lost (as shown for the $\beta3$ subunit in knockout mice), this causes seizures. There can also be changes in enzymes, such as the one responsible for GABA synthesis, GAD, that contribute to epilepsy. There is an enormous number of molecular changes that have a potential for causing epilepsy. These can occur secondarily following lesions. In kindling or lesion studies, a whole range of changes in ion channels, receptors and transporters can be seen. This occurs spontaneously in humans. Similar changes occur in temporal lobe epilepsy with hippocampal sclerosis.

Scheper: Are these changes principally located in the brain?

Meldrum: These are neuronal changes. There are some changes in transporters in glia, but primarily we are talking about changes in the neuronal membrane. These are changes in ion channels in the membrane, or receptors or transporters.

Löscher: A week ago I attended a meeting at the US National Institutes of Health (NIH), who invited most of the well known basic scientists working in the USA on epilepsy. There is a very simple answer to Susan Bates' earlier question about the molecular basis of epilepsy: we don't know. This was the outcome of that meeting. People have studied for many years the consequences of epilepsy, for instance looking at tissue samples from patients. There are a variety of consequences of seizures in epilepsy, but no one knows what changes a normal brain into an epileptic brain. There are some familial epilepsies with known gene defects, but these are very rare. The NIH set one benchmark for the next few years, which is that we have to concentrate more on what is happening in the transition from a normal brain to an epileptic brain. There are several models for this. Various patients with epilepsy have an initial pathological event such as a stroke, head trauma or status epilepticus, and this can be reproduced in animal models. In these there is a latent 'silent' period, between the initial event and the development of epilepsy.

I have a comment on Brian Meldrum's hypothesis that pharmacoresistance in epilepsy is a network phenomenon. If you take 10 patients with temporal lobe epilepsy, which is one of the most common types of epilepsy, normally five of them respond to AEDs and five don't. Despite this, the 10 patients may have almost identical seizures, with the same frequency and severity: no difference can be seen. For me this is an interesting challenge. Are there any data that a temporal lobe epilepsy developing for example after stroke has a different prognosis to a temporal lobe epilepsy developing after head trauma?

Sander: Yes, there are some data on this. Epilepsy caused by stroke is independent of the location. If it is in an elderly person a sniff of any drug seems to do the trick. However, if you have head injury and temporal lobe epilepsy, probably only about 50% will respond to teatment. Different drugs can be tried and about 50% will respond. I don't think we have the whole picture yet. Very interestingly, there is one thing that really changes the equation and pushes up the odds of developing epilepsy: this is the presence of family history. If someone has prolonged febrile convulsions we know their risk of developing temporal lobe epilepsy. The risk is increased if there is a family history, regardless of the type. If someone has head injury, the risk goes up. If they have a family history of epilepsy, this is telling us something which we haven't yet worked out. We have to make clear to the non-epileptologists here that AED treatment is not rational, it is empirical. We shoot in the dark and hope that we will get it right. It works about half the time. The first drug we try, if people do not have a problem with tolerance they do well. It doesn't seem to matter much which drug we use. AEDs have been around for 100 years and in population terms they all seem to work with the same success.

Atadja: With the genomics revolution and the advent of pharmacogenomics, people are trying to identify single-nucleotide polymorphisms in genes. Do you think it is worth looking for any such polymorphisms that might be the underlying factors in drug-resistant epilepsy?

Sander: Yes. People are doing this.

Varadi: Could the cause of resistance be that the drug never actually reaches the target, like in cancer therapy? Or are we dealing with such a heterogeneous disease that even if the drug does reach its target, the target is different in that special case? In this event, we would not be dealing with drug resistance but just the problem that we don't have the right drug.

Sander: Absolutely.

Andermann: The fact that there is no simple answer to the question of what causes epilepsy should not discourage this audience. There are situations where intractability develops under our eyes. No matter what the causes of the epilepsies in general may be, we should address and attempt to define this issue. If we accomplish this in the next two days we will have come a long way.

Newman: I want to get back to the question of the mechanisms of resistance. Professor Andermann focused on the situations where there is an initial response and then resistance. Professor Meldrum spoke about the situations where resistance exists from the beginning and many factors are probably involved. I wonder whether it might be useful to go back to something we do in oncology, that is, to distinguish between intrinsic and acquired resistance. Both can be caused by Pgp, but I wonder if, in the case of epilepsy, we may say that intrinsic resistance could be multifactorial, whereas the acquired form may be a bit closer to something that may involve an oncology-type of resistance. This might be a useful distinction.

Ling: This could be a working definition as we progress in our discussions.

Ruetz: I would say that in oncology there is a physiological resistance, and then there is the disease- and drug-induced resistance. I think many people are mixing these three resistance types together.

Deisz: I want to make a more general statement concerning the drug resistance in epilepsy. Most of the anticonvulsant drugs are successfully getting into the CNS and most likely reach the appropriate target sites. I am also quite confident that clinicians find the best anticonvulsant drug for a given patient. When these drugs do not achieve a satisfactory control of seizure activity, is it possible that the concepts behind these drugs are not adequate? There is a considerable increase in the percentage of patients responding to the modern AEDs compared to the old AEDs, yet even with the modern AEDs, in an embarrassing percentage of patients the epilepsy fails to respond satisfactorily. As far as drugs such as tiagabine are concerned, the concept of prolonging the action of GABA by reducing re-uptake may cause problems. It could alter the spatiotemporal pattern of inhibition because it would augment the negative feedback of GABA on its own release (Deisz & Prince 1989). This may relate to the established side-effects of tiagabine such as inducing absence status. The failure of some of these drugs may be due to a limited benefit through epiphenomena rather than by aiming at the crucial target mechanisms.

Sills: I agree to a certain extent that the drugs we have available for epilepsy have limited mechanisms of action. As Professor Meldrum said, we are essentially restricted to using drugs which either block voltage-gated ion channels or potentiate inhibitory neurotransmission in the brain. However, we forget that up to 70% of people with epilepsy do respond to these drugs.

Sander: The epidemiological evidence from the developing countries is quite overwhelming. There should be a much higher prevalence, but this isn't the case.

There are studies from India and Ecuador, there is even a study from Finland that shows that 35% of people go into spontaneous remission. When we treat newly diagnosed epilepsy with our drugs, we are treating those that will do well. We don't really yet know the role of AEDs. We might know it in individual patients, but in population terms we haven't a clue.

Wood: The logical extension of that is that there is no such thing as drug resistance in epilepsy. If people are not responding to drugs in the first place, and therefore they can't be becoming resistant to these drugs.

Sander: That is a possible explanation.

Wood: If you really believe that, it is a self-defeating kind of argument in terms of drug resistance.

Schmutz: A second extension of that argument would be that placebo treatment would be as good as treatment with AEDs. The 50% seizure freedom of the new drugs and the old drugs is always against placebo when add-on treatment was used. Under monotherapy conditions a number of the new AEDs were also tested in specific study designs against placebo. In many of these add-on and monotherapy studies treatment with AEDs was significantly superior to placebo treatment.

Sander: I am not saying that this is always the case; what I am saying is that the disease will go into spontaneous remission in 30–40% of patients. In about 30% of people AEDs seem to make a difference. In another 20%, you have to find the right drug. Then there are 20% of people in whom none of our drugs work. In this latter 20% it might not be drug resistance that is the problem but rather something else. In the 50% that respond to any drug, some of them would respond to herbal tea or placebo. There has never been a proper study of placebo against new drugs, because this is not ethical. It is as simple as that. There was a study from Finland, where people didn't get treatment after the diagnosis of epilepsy for a number of reasons (Keranen & Riekkinen 1993). They looked at outcome in quite a large group and found that 50% became spontaneously seizure free, most of them with less than 2 years' duration. There are studies from India where they report 36% spontaneous remission, and a study from Ecuador that gives a figure of about 40%. In population terms we don't really know. In individual patients, it is very different. In those patients where you have to struggle you try to find a drug that will work.

Schmutz: I agree with most of what you say. However, there are of course proper, controlled clinical trials of AEDs against placebo that have passed numerous ethical committees and are globally recognized by health authorities. These also include monotherapy studies. The placebo-controlled monotherapy studies mostly use the 'presurgical' design. In addition, there are longer-term monotherapy studies where the new AED is given at a high (=supposedly effective) and a very low (=placebo-like) dose. In both of these monotherapy designs the efficacy of at least some of the AEDs used was clearly and significantly superior to placebo.

Sander: But these are extremely selected, unnatural circumstances.

Oza: What is the precision with which you can define response and resistance in epilepsy? One of the things that we struggle with in oncology is trying to correlate clinical drug resistance with other objective parameters of resistance. In oncology it is a lot easier: you can correlate clinical resistance with objective parameters from radiology and other studies. How precisely can you define clinical resistance, and how precisely can you define response to treatment?

Sander: We could spend the rest of the day discussing this; we don't have a precise answer. Everyone seems to have a different opinion on this. How many drugs should we use before we say that epilepsy is resistant? If you are in a tertiary referral centre, the notion of resistance and response will be different. The other problem we have is that until recently, most people would be happy with the regulatory outcome, which is 50% seizure reduction, which doesn't make a big difference. Neurologists and epileptologists have to move out of this paradigm that 50% seizure reduction is a response, which it is not. The new drugs in this sort of population at the extreme end of the spectrum have not really made a big difference.

Oza: Is there a spectrum from 50% reduction to the complete resolution of convulsions?

Sander: When we talk about good prognosis, we are talking about complete resolution of the seizures. This is what we are aiming for, and we will only settle for less if we have to.

Oza: Do you have some statistics on people who have incomplete resolution of their convulsions and then have second-line treatment?

Sander: The first drug works in about 50% of cases. About 20–30% do not tolerate the drug, and so you try the next one. With the second drug you get about another 50% seizure free. After this the numbers start to fall dramatically. If you have to go to the fourth or fifth drug, it is surprising to see a response. The new drugs have not lived up to expectations. One of the reasons is the regulatory outcome we have been using.

References

Babb TL, Pretorius JK, Mello LE, Mathern GW, Levesque MF 1992 Synaptic reorganizations in epileptic human and rat kainate hippocampus may contribute to feedback and feedforward excitation. Epilepsy Res Suppl 9:193–202

Deisz RA, Prince DA 1989 Frequency-dependent depression of inhibition in guinea pig neocortex in vitro by $GABA_B$ receptor feedback on GABA release. J Physiol 412:513–541

Keranen T, Riekkinen PJ 1993 Remission of seizures in untreated epilepsy. Br Med J 307:483

Mody I 1993 The molecular basis of kindling. Brain Pathol 3:395–403

Prasad AN, Prasad C, Stafstrom CE 1999 Recent advances in the genetics of epilepsy: insights from human and animal studies. Epilepsia 40:1329–1352

Drug resistance molecules: lessons from oncology

George L. Scheffer and Rik J. Scheper[1]

Department of Pathology, Free University Medical Center, de Boelelaan 1117, 1081 HV, Amsterdam, The Netherlands

Abstract. Tumour cell insensitivity to anticancer drugs frequently appears as multidrug resistance (MDR), associated with overexpression of one or more of a set of at least 10 different molecules, causing reduced drug levels at the intracellular target sites. They include transmembrane transporter proteins such as P glycoprotein, MRP1–9 and BCRP. In addition, the lung-resistance protein, recently identified as the major vault protein, has been associated with MDR. We have generated monoclonal antibodies that specifically recognize most of these proteins, which we are using to try to identify their roles in clinical drug resistance, and also to explore their occurrence in normal human tissues and physiology. Both types of studies will also provide further insights into the molecular features of drugs associated with distinct MDR transporters.

2002 Mechanisms of drug resistance in epilepsy: lessons from oncology. Wiley, Chichester (Novartis Foundation Symposium 243) p 19–37

Drug resistance

Drug resistance has recently received attention as an important impediment in the treatment of a range of diseases from rheumatoid arthritis to epilepsy. The phenomenon of multidrug resistance (MDR; reviewed in Moscow et al 1997) has been acknowledged for many years as a major obstacle in cancer therapies and is characterized by resistance to a broad range of structurally and functionally unrelated cytotoxic agents. Our immunology research group at the Free University Medical Centre in Amsterdam became involved in cancer MDR through the development of monoclonal antibodies detecting the causative molecules. In the late 1970s, Victor Ling presented his exciting data on the *MDR1*-encoded P glycoprotein (Pgp) at a scientific meeting. This inspired Bob Pinedo, chairman of our medical oncology department, to approach us about whether we could develop antibodies that would detect MDR1 Pgp in patient

---

[1]This paper was presented at the symposium by Rik J. Scheper, to whom correspondence should be addressed.

tumour samples. Then, after the successful development of the JSB-1 antibody, now widely used as a marker for Pgp, we began a broad range of studies on the mechanisms of MDR.

ABC transporters in MDR

Energy-dependent, active, transport processes neutralizing the therapeutic toxic effect of cytotoxic agents operate in MDR cells. Drugs are prevented from entering cells, or are exported outward from the cytoplasm, reducing levels at their intracellular targets. The prototypic transporter protein involved in MDR is MDR1 Pgp (symbol ABCB1, reviewed in Ambudkar et al 1999), discovered in 1976 by Victor Ling (Juliano & Ling 1976). This heavily glycosylated 170 kDa protein is a member of the ATP binding cassette (ABC) transporters (Higgins 1992) and transports a broad range of substrates, including several anticancer drugs (Gottesman & Pastan 1993). The ABC superfamily also comprises several subfamilies with members that are involved in MDR, in particular the ABCB (MDR/TAP subfamily), ABCC (CFTR/MRP subfamily) and ABCG (White subfamily) subfamilies (see Table 1).

As mentioned, the ABCB subfamily includes the classical MDR transporter MDR1 Pgp, but the contribution of the other members in this subfamily to MDR is much less clearly defined. The MDR3 Pgp protein (ABCB4) and sister of Pgp (sPgp; also known as the bile salt efflux pump [BSEP], ABCB11) are highly related to MDR1 Pgp but although transport of some cytotoxic agents has been reported for both of these proteins (Childs et al 1998, Smith et al 2000), no clear involvement in MDR has been shown. The two TAP molecules (ABCB2 and ABCB3) are very important molecules in the field of immunology as they act in concert as a heterodimer in transporting peptides for antigen recognition over the cell membrane. Interestingly, we have previously reported a (moderate) contribution to MDR for the TAP molecule (Izquierdo et al 1996). For the other members of the ABCB subfamily no involvement in MDR is known.

In the early 1990s Susan Cole in Canada (Cole et al 1992) cloned multidrug resistance protein 1 (MRP1; ABCC1) from a lung cancer cell line. This is a 190 kDa MDR-related ABC transporter from the ABCC subfamily. MRP1 was shown to confer a similar resistance phenotype to MDR1 Pgp, although these two proteins share only 14% amino acid identity (Grant et al 1994, Zaman et al 1994). Later on, several closely related family members were described (Borst et al 2000). Of this MRP subfamily, MRP1–3 (ABCC1–3) are particularly involved in the transport of chemotherapeutic agents in human cancer cells (Cole & Deeley 1998, Cui et al 1999, Kool et al 1999a), whereas for the other ABCC family members no clear involvement in MDR has yet been shown.

The latest (and, since the completion of the Human Genome Project has put a stop to discovering new ABC transporter proteins, most likely last) ABC transporter involved in MDR was cloned by Ross and Doyle in 1998 from a mitoxantrone-resistant subline of the breast cancer cell line MCF-7/Adr/Vp. This transporter was named breast cancer resistance protein (BCRP, MXR, ABCP; ABCG2) (Doyle et al 1998, Miyake et al 1999, Allikmets et al 1998) and belongs to the ABCG subfamily. The BCRP is a half-transporter that probably acts as a homo- or heterodimer in transporting cytotoxic agents. Transfection experiments with the BCRP cDNA result in a full blown MDR phenotype (Doyle et al 1998), and therefore it seems valid to conclude that the BCRP is capable of transporting MDR drugs as a homodimer. Also, as yet, no heterodimer partner for BCRP has been described. For the other members of the ABCG subfamily no involvement in MDR has been reported.

Structure, gene localization and
disease linkage of the ABC transporters

All of the above mentioned transporters belong to the superfamily of ABC transporters. The schematic representation of several family members in Fig. 1 shows that these proteins look very similar. In general, they all are composed of two core halves, each containing a nucleotide binding domain characterized by the consensus sequences of ABC transporters; Walker A and B motifs and the ABC signature, and a membrane-spanning domain with six transmembrane segments (TMs). In the MRP subfamily, the MRP1, -2, -3, -6 and -7 proteins have an extra N-terminal domain (MSD_0) which contains an extra set of five TMs.

Although some of the ABC transporter genes are localized in tandem per chromosome (e.g. MDR1 Pgp/MDR3 Pgp on chromosome 7, TAP1/ TAP2 on chromosome 6 and MRP1/MRP6 on chromosome 16), they generally seem to be localized quite randomly on diverse chromosomes (see Table 1).

For some transporters it has become clear that mutations in the gene or lack of expression can cause genetic diseases. Absence of the TAP2 molecule causes a bare lymphocyte syndrome (BLS) (de la Salle et al 1994), in which patients lack surface major histocompatibilty complex (MHC) class I molecules and are immunodeficient due to the resulting absence of $CD8^+$ T cells. Lack of expression of *MDR3* in the liver is responsible for type 3 progressive familial intrahepatic cholestasis (PFIC3) (de Vree et al 1998), whereas type 2 PFIC is caused by absence of sPgp. Mutations in the *MRP2* gene cause another liver disease, the Dubin–Johnson syndrome (Paulusma et al 1996). Recently, it was found that mutations in the *MRP6* gene are responsible for the connective tissue disorder pseudoxanthoma elasticum (PXE) (Ringpfeil et al 2000, Bergen et al 2000, Le Saux et al 2000).

Cystic fibrosis is the result of mutations in the *CFTR* gene. Mutations in the recently described *MRP8* and/or *MRP9* genes are positional candidates for paroxysmal kinesigenic choreoathetosis (Tammur et al 2001). None of the transporters in the ABCG subfamily has been linked to a genetic disease as yet.

For some of these transporters the contribution to the disease is direct, e.g. in PFIC3 patients the lack of translocation of bile salt neutralizing phosphatidylcholine across the canalicular membrane of the hepatocyte is the cause of the observed cholestasis in the liver. For other transporters, the exact role in the disease is unclear. Whether mutations in *MRP6* are directly responsible for PXE or contribute to this disease indirectly through deficient transport in liver and or kidney is still unclear.

Substrates of the ABC transporters

In general, the substrates of these transporters are rather diverse and range from salts to anionic conjugates and peptides (Table 1). Some transporters seem highly specialized in transporting just one substrate, such as phosphatidylcholine transport by the MDR3 Pgp. However, most transporters are capable of transporting a range of (un)related substrates that share some common features. The TAP molecule has a preference for peptides of a certain size, but the exact sequence of the peptides is less critical, since the TAP molecule can process peptides digested from many different foreign proteins. Pgp and the MRP1 transporter seem to pump substrates predominantly based on charge. Pgp mainly transports organic neutrals, including steroids, but also phenytoin-like anti-epileptic drugs (Tishler et al 1995), whereas MRP1 transports conjugates of organic anions. Glutathione is a negatively charged tripeptide that may also be co-transported. Of course, for both these proteins the substrate list also includes many cytotoxic agents, such as doxorubicin and vincristine. The substrate specificity of MRP2 is very similar to that of MRP1 (Keppler et al 1998, Jedlitschky et al 1997), whereas the transport range of MRP3 is rather limited compared to these two proteins. The MRP3 transporter is mainly involved in resistance to etoposide (Kool et al 1999a) and vincristine (Zeng et al 1999). For MRP4 (ABCC4) and MRP5 (ABCC5), no major changes were found in mRNA levels in doxorubicin- or cisplatin-resistant cells (Kool et al 1997). However, it was recently found that these transporters are able to transport nucleoside analogues used for antiviral therapies (Scheutz et al 1999, Wijnholds et al 2000). In addition, some low-level resistance against $CdCl_2$ and potassium antimonyl tartrate was found in *MRP5*-transfected cell lines (McAleer et al 1999). Overproduction of *MRP6* (*ABCC6*) mRNA in tumour cell lines was found to be invariably associated with the amplification of the adjacent *MRP1* gene, and MRP6 probably does not contribute to the resistance of these cell lines (Kool et al

1999b). However, a preliminary report has suggested that MRP6 may mediate modest resistance to anthracyclines and epipodophyllotoxins (Belinsky et al 2001).

The MRP7, -8 and -9 transporter proteins were only very recently discovered and not much is yet known about their substrate preferences. BCRP is capable of transporting many anticancer agents. Of these, mitoxantrone is probably the best substrate for BCRP. Thus BCRP is actually the long-sought mitoxantrone transporter.

Recently, the occurrence of single nucleotide polymorphisms (SNPs) in ABC transporters have attracted quite a bit of attention because they can be highly critical for the substrate specificity of the pump (Zhang et al 2001, Kerb et al 2001, Honjo et al 2001). The presence of a threonine or a glycine at position 482 in the BCRP transporter was found to be essential for rhodamine 123 efflux; cells with the wild-type arginine at that position were unable to transport this substrate (Honjo et al 2001).

Blockers: resistance-modifying agents

For several of the transporters, molecules have been identified that block transport activities. Most of these blocking agents, or resistance-modifying agents, are themselves substrates for the transporters. They block the activity of the transporter by competing with the toxic substrate. Some of these blockers specifically block one of the transporters, whereas others have a negative effect on the transport activities of two or more pumps.

More-or-less specific blockers for MDR1 Pgp are verapamil, bepridil and cyclosporin A. For MRP1, probenecid, indomethacin and MK571 may be considered to be specific blockers. PSC 833 has a blocking effect on both MDR1 Pgp and MRP1, whereas GF120918 blocks both MDR1 Pgp- and BCRP-mediated transport (Bart et a; 2000). Fumitremorgin C (FTC) is a BCRP-specific blocker (Rabindran et al 2000).

Monoclonal antibodies specifically detecting the MDR transporters

As mentioned above, specific monoclonal antibodies are essential for facilitating studies on transporter proteins in clinical material, to reveal their physiological functions and their possible contributions to MDR. In collaborative studies with our colleagues from the Department of Medical Oncology (Bob Pinedo, Henk Broxterman), the Dutch Cancer Center (NKI; Piet Borst, Jan Schellens), the Academic Medical Center (AMC; Ronald Oude Elferink) and The Netherlands Ophthalmic Research Institute (NORI; Arthur Bergen, Jan Wijnholds) we have produced monoclonal antibodies specifically detecting MDR1 Pgp, MDR3 Pgp, MRP1, -2, -3, -4, -5 and -6, and BCRP (Scheper et al 1988, Scheffer et al 2000a,b,

TABLE 1 Characteristics of selected ABC transporter molecules

Name	Symbol	Chromosome	RNA	AA	Disease link	Normal tissue distribution	Substrate	role in MDR
MDR1 Pgp	ABCB1	7q21	4.5	1279	n.k.	Many tissues, apical membranes	Many neutral hydrophobic compounds	yes
TAP1	ABCB2	6p21.3	2.5	808	n.k.	Most cells, ER	Peptides	possibly
TAP2	ABCB3	6p21.3	2.8	653	BLS	Most cells, ER	Peptides	possibly
MDR3 Pgp	ABCB4	7q21	4.5	1279	PFIC3	Hepatocyte, apical membranes	Phosphatidylcholine	no
Est422562	ABCB5	7p14	7.5	n.k.	n.k.	Ubiquitous	n.k.	no
ABCB6	ABCB6	2q33-q36	3.5	842	n.k.	Mitochondria	Iron	no
ABC7	ABCB7	Xq13.1-q13.3	2.4	752	Anaemia	Mitochondria	Iron?	no
M-ABC1	ABCB8	7q35-q36	2.4	718	n.k.	Mitochondria	n.k.	no
ABCB9	ABCB9	12q24	3.5	723	n.k.	Heart brain lysosomes	n.k.	no
M-ABC2	ABCB10	1q42	4.1	738	n.k.	Mitochondria	Peptides?	no
BSEP/sPgp	ABCB11	2q24	5.4	1321	PFIC2	Hepatocytes, apical membranes	Biles salts	no
MRP1	ABCC1	16p13.1	6.5	1531	n.k.	Ubiquitus, lateral membranes	Anionic conjugates glutathione	yes
MRP2/ cMOAT	ABCC2	10q24	5.5	1545	Dubin–Johnson	Liver kidney intestine apical membranes	Anionic conjugates glutathione, bilirubin	yes
MRP3	ABCC3	17q21.3	6.5	1527	n.k.	Kidney intestine lateral membranes	Anionic conjugates, bile salts	yes

MRP4	ABCC4	13q32	6.5	1325	n.k.	Many tissues	Cyclic nucleotides	no?
MRP5	ABCC5	3q27	6.6	1437	n.k.	Many tissues	Cyclic nucleotides	no?
MRP6	ABCC6	16p13.1	6.5	1503	PXE	Liver kidney lateral membranes	Peptides?	no?
CFTR	ABCC7	7q31.2	6.0	1480	Cystic fibrosis	Lung intestine cholangiocytes	Organic anions?	no
SUR1	ABCC8	11p15.1	5.0	1581	fPHHI	Pancreas	n.k.	no
SUR2	ABCC9	12p12.1	5.0	1549	n.k.	Skeletal muscle heart	n.k.	no
MRP7	ABCC10	6p21	5.5	1513	n.k.	Low in all tissues	n.k.	no?
MRP8	ABCC11	16q12.1	4.6	1382	PKC?	Low in all tissues	n.k.	no?
MRP9	ABCC12	16q12	5.0	1359	PKC?	Low in all tissues	n.k.	no?
ABC8/White	ABCG1	21q22.3	2.7	638	n.k.	Brain spleen lung	Sterols? lipids?	no
BCRP/MXR	ABCG2	4q22	2.4	655	n.k.	Breast liver intestine	Drugs	yes
White 2	ABCG4	11q23	n.k.	749?	n.k.	Liver	n.k.	no
White 3	ABCG5	2p21	2.3	651	Sitosterolemia	Liver small intestine	Plant sterols	no
White 4	ABCG8	2p21	2.0	673	Sitosterolemia	Liver small intestine	Plant sterols	no

AA, amino acids; BLS, bare lymphocyte syndrome; PFIC2, type 2 progressive intrahepatic cholestasis; PFIC3, type 3 progressive intrahepatic cholestasis; PXE, pseudoxanthoma elasticum; fPHHI, familial persistent hyperinsulinemic hypoglycemia of infancy; PKC, paroxysmal kinesigenic choreoathetosis; n.k., not known.

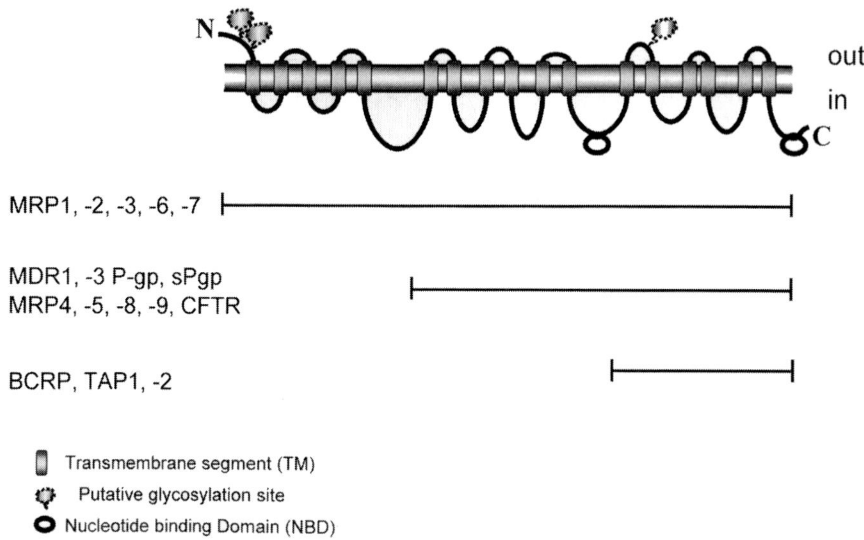

FIG. 1.   A schematic representation of the structure of some ABC transporters.

G. L. Scheffer, unpublished results). For the immunization and the selection of monoclonal antibodies (Mabs), most of the time we used fusion proteins of the *Escherichia coli* maltose binding protein (MBP) and fragments of the transporter protein of interest. Intriguingly, only for MDR1 Pgp have several Mabs been described that detect external epitopes (Mechetner & Roninson 1992, Hamada & Tsuruo 1986, Cianfriglia et al 1994). Mabs that detect external epitopes are widely used to detect the protein on viable cells that have not been altered by fixation. Those binding a functional epitope of the protein, as is the case with the UIC2 Mab (Mechetner & Roninson 1992), allow studies of the substrate specificity in blocking experiments. Despite many attempts by ourselves—employing methods ranging from peptide and DNA immunization to the use of knockout mice and the phage display method—and colleagues all over the world, it has not been possible to produce Mabs for any of the other MDR-related transporter molecules. Whether this is due to a lack of immunogenicity of the external regions or a limited exposure of protein at the external side, possibly because of glycosylation moieties, is unknown.

Normal tissue localization and function of the MDR transporters

The development of this broad panel of Mabs allowed us first to study the localization of several transporter molecules in normal tissues (Scheffer et al

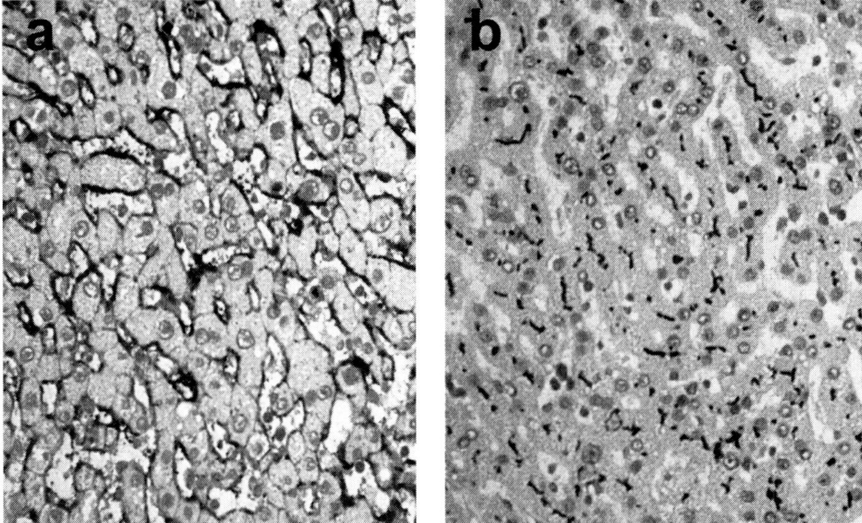

FIG. 2.   Immunostaining of normal human liver tissue for MRP6 and MRP2. MRP6 is present
at the basolateral membranes of the hepatocytes (a), whereas MRP2 is present at the apical site of
the hepatocyte, the canalicular membrane (b).

2000a, Maliepaard et al 2001, G. L. Scheffer, unpublished results). In general, the
transporters can be found at locations and tissues that are heavily exposed to toxic
materials, e.g. along the gastrointestinal tract and the lung mucosa. At these sites
there is a real need to protect the inside against potentially dangerous exogenous
compounds, toxic materials, microbial products, etc. Furthermore, the
transporters can be found in organs which are involved in secretion processes
such as liver and kidney. Some of the transporter molecules turned out to be
(almost) ubiquitously expressed (MDR1 Pgp, MRP1), whereas others have a
(much) more restricted normal tissue distribution. MDR3 Pgp is expressed
exclusively at the hepatocyte membrane and MRP2 is mainly present at the
canalicular membrane of the hepatocyte. Of the genuine MDR transporters,
MDR1 Pgp, BCRP and MRP1, only the first two are present at the apical
membrane sections of polarized cells. MRP1, like the other MRP family members
(except for MRP2), localizes laterally instead. As an example, in Fig. 2 normal
human liver tissue is immunostained for both MRP6 and MRP2. MRP6 is
present at the basolateral membranes of the hepatocytes (Fig. 2a), whereas MRP2
is present at the apical site of the hepatocyte, the canalicular membrane (Fig. 2b).
An important implication of the opposite localization of MRP1 is, that this
transporter protects the surrounding tissue in a different way than MDR1 Pgp
and BCRP. In drug transport, MRP1 is most likely involved in transport from

the exposed (epithelial) tissue to the bloodstream, rather than preventing the entry of toxic compounds by re-effluxing these xenobiotics from the tissue to the lumen.

The presence of all three of the most prominent MDR transporters on endothelial cells is very interesting and deserves further attention. Of course, functionally blocking these transporters would cause increased uptake of therapeutic drugs from the bloodstream. This may be particularly important for the treatment of diseases which require the drugs to cross the blood–brain barrier.

Many of the physiological functions of the transporters are still unknown. Very likely, the MDR transporter molecules function normally as xenobiotic pumps. Still, other functions have been attributed to both MDR1 Pgp and MRP1. Recently, Gwendolyn Randolph reported particularly intriguing immunological functions for these transporter proteins (Randolph et al 1998, Robbiani et al 2000). She noted a role for MDR1 Pgp in the migration of antigen-presenting dendritic cells (DC) from explants of cultured human skin into the culture medium via dermal lymphatic vessels, since only anti-MDR1 Pgp Mabs or antagonists inhibited this process. Because of MRP1's role in transporting the important inflammatory mediator leukotriene LTC4, it has an essential role in DC migration from skin to lymph nodes. DC mobilization from the epidermis and trafficking into lymphatic vessels was greatly reduced in MRP1$^{-/-}$ mice, while migration was restored by exogenous cysteinyl leukotrienes LTC4 or LTD4. Indeed, experiments in our own laboratory have shown a marked up-regulation of the expression of both MDR1 Pgp and MRP1 during DC maturation. Interestingly, strong up-regulation of another MDR marker, the major vault protein (MVP), was also observed during this maturation process (Schroeijers et al 2000). Of note, the MVP was originally described by us as the lung resistance protein (LRP) and subsequently found to be unrelated to the ABC superfamily of transporter proteins (Scheffer et al 1995). Experiments to further elucidate the precise roles of these molecules during DC maturation and in antigen-presentation are ongoing.

Concluding remarks

At least three ABC transporter molecules (MDR1 Pgp, MRP1 and BCRP) have been identified that act like genuine MDR transporters adversely affecting chemotherapeutic approaches in cancer treatment. Several drugs used in the treatment of a broad variety of other diseases, e.g. phenytoin-like drugs in epilepsy and the anti-malarial drug chloroquine in rheumatoid arthritis, have also been identified as substrates for these transporter molecules. Therefore, efficacy of treatments of these diseases is most likely to be influenced by the presence or, after extended periods of exposure to these drugs, increased expression of these transporter molecules on target cells. Extended analyses of critical tissues in these patients for the presence of these molecules therefore seem warranted.

Ackowledgements

This work was supported by the Dutch Cancer Society, grants VU95-923 and VU96-1256.

References

Allikmets R, Schriml LM, Hutchinson A, Romano-Spica V, Dean M 1998 A human placenta-specific ATP-binding cassette gene (ABCP) on chromosome 4q22 that is involved in multidrug resistance. Cancer Res 58:5337–5339

Ambudkar SV, Dey S, Hrycyna CA, Ramachandra M, Pastan I, Gottesman MM 1999 Biochemical, cellular, and pharmacological aspects of the multidrug transporter. Ann Rev Pharmacol Toxicol 39:361–398

Bart J, Groen HJ, Hendrikse NH, van der Graaf WT, Vaalburg W, de Vries EG 2000 The blood-brain barrier and oncology: new insights into function and modulation. Cancer Treat Rev 26:449–462

Belinsky MG, Shchaveleva I, Zeng H, Kruh GD 2001 Drug-resistance phenotype of multidrug-resistance protein-6-transfected chinese hamster ovary cells. Proc Am Assoc Cancer Res Annu Meet 92:1510

Bergen AA, Plomp AS, Schuurman EJ et al 2000 Mutations in ABCC6 cause pseudoxanthoma elasticum. Nat Genet 25:228–231

Borst P, Evers R, Kool M, Wijnholds J 2000 A family of drug transporters: the multidrug resistance-associated proteins. J Natl Cancer Inst 92:1295–1302

Childs S, Yeh RL, Hui D, Ling V 1998 Taxol resistance mediated by transfection of the liver-specific sister gene of P-glycoprotein. Cancer Res 58:4160–4167

Cianfriglia M, Willingham MC, Tombesi M, Scagliotti GV, Frasca G, Chersi A 1994 P-glycoprotein epitope mapping. I. Identification of a linear human-specific epitope in the fourth loop of the P-glycoprotein extracellular domain by MM4.17 murine monoclonal antibody to human multi-drug-resistant cells. Int J Cancer 56:153–160

Cole SP, Deeley RG 1998 Multidrug resistance mediated by the ATP-binding cassette transporter protein MRP. Bioessays 20:931–940

Cole SP, Bhardwaj G, Gerlach JH et al 1992 Overexpression of a transporter gene in a multidrug-resistant human lung cancer cell line. Science 258:1650–1654

Cui YH, Konig J, Buchholz U, Spring H, Leier I, Keppler D 1999 Drug resistance and ATP-dependent conjugate transport mediated by the apical multidrug resistance protein, MRP2, permanently expressed in human and canine cells. Mol Pharmacol 55:929–937

de la Salle H, Hanau D, Fricker D et al 1994 Homozygous human TAP peptide transporter mutation in HLA class I deficiency. Science 265:237–241

de Vree JM, Jacquemin E, Sturm E et al 1998 Mutations in the *MDR3* gene cause progressive familial intrahepatic cholestasis. Proc Natl Acad Sci USA 95:282–287

Doyle LA, Yang WD, Abruzzo LV et al 1998 A multidrug resistance transporter from human MCF-7 breast cancer cells. Proc Natl Acad Sci USA 95:15665–15670

Gottesman MM, Pastan I 1993 Biochemistry of multidrug resistance mediated by the multidrug transporter. Annu Rev Biochem 62:385–427

Grant CE, Valdimarsson G, Hipfner DR, Almquist KC, Cole SP, Deeley RG 1994 Overexpression of multidrug resistance-associated protein (MRP) increases resistance to natural product drugs. Cancer Res 54:357–361

Hamada H, Tsuruo T 1986 Functional role for the 170- to 180-kDa glycoprotein specific to drug-resistant tumor cells as revealed by monoclonal antibodies. Proc Natl Acad Sci USA 83: 7785–7789

Higgins CF 1992 ABC transporters: from microorganisms to man. Annu Rev Cell Biol 8: 67–113

Honjo Y, Hrycyna CA, Yan QW et al 2001 Acquired mutations in the *MXR/BCRP/ABCP* gene alter substrate specificity in MXR/BCRP/ABCP-overexpressing cells. Cancer Res 61:6635–6639

Izquierdo MA, Neefjes JJ, Mathari AE, Flens MJ, Scheffer GL, Scheper RJ 1996 Overexpression of the ABC transporter TAP in multidrug-resistant human cancer cell lines. Br J Cancer 74:1961–1967

Jedlitschky G, Leier I, Buchholz U, Hummel-Eisenbeiss J, Burchell B, Keppler D 1997 ATP-dependent transport of bilirubin glucuronides by the multidrug resistance protein MRP1 and its hepatocyte canalicular isoform MRP2. Biochem J 327:305–310

Juliano RL, Ling V 1976 A surface glycoprotein modulating drug permeability in Chinese hamster ovary cell mutants. Biochim Biophys Acta 455:152–162

Keppler D, Leier I, Jedlitschky G, Konig J 1998 ATP-dependent transport of glutathione S-conjugates by the multidrug resistance protein MRP1 and its apical isoform MRP2. Chem-Biol Interact 111:153–161

Kerb R, Hoffmeyer S, Brinkmann U 2001 ABC drug transporters: hereditary polymorphisms and pharmacological impact in MDR1, MRP1 and MRP2. Pharmacogenomics 2: 51–64

Kool M, de Haas M, Scheffer GL et al 1997 Analysis of expression of cMOAT (MRP2), MRP3, MRP4, and MRP5, homologues of the multidrug resistance-associated protein gene (MRP1), in human cancer cell lines. Cancer Res 57:3537–3547

Kool M, van der Linden M, de Haas M et al 1999a MRP3, an organic anion transporter able to transport anti-cancer drugs. Proc Natl Acad Sci USA 96:6914–6919

Kool M, van der Linden M, de Haas M, Baas F, Borst P 1999b Expression of human *MRP6*, a homologue of the multidrug resistance protein gene *MRP1*, in tissues and cancer cells. Cancer Res 59:175–182

Le Saux O, Urban Z, Tschuch C et al 2000 Mutations in a gene encoding an ABC transporter cause pseudoxanthoma elasticum. Nat Genet 25:223–227

Maliepaard M, Scheffer GL, Faneyte IF 2001 Subcellular localization and distribution of the breast cancer resistance protein transporter in normal human tissues. Cancer Res 61:3458–3464

McAleer MA, Breen MA, White NL, Matthews N 1999 pABC11 (also known as MOAT-C and MRP5), a member of the ABC family of proteins, has anion transporter activity but does not confer multidrug resistance when overexpressed in human embryonic kidney 293 cells. J Biol Chem 274:23541–23548

Mechetner EB, Roninson IB 1992 Efficient inhibition of P-glycoprotein-mediated multidrug resistance with a monoclonal antibody. Proc Natl Acad Sci USA 89:5824–5828

Miyake K, Mickley L, Litman T et al 1999 Molecular cloning of cDNAs which are highly overexpressed in mitoxantrone-resistant cells: demonstration of homology to ABC transport genes. Cancer Res 59:8–13

Moscow JA, Schneider E, Ivy SP, Cowan KH 1997 Multidrug resistance. Cancer Chemother Biol Response Modif 17:139–177

Paulusma CC, Bosma PJ, Zaman GJ et al 1996 Congenital jaundice in rats with a mutation in a multidrug resistance-associated protein gene. Science 271:1126–1128

Rabindran SK, Ross DD, Doyle LA, Yang W, Greenberger LM 2000 Fumitremorgin C reverses multidrug resistance in cells transfected with the breast cancer resistance protein. Cancer Res 60:47–50

Randolph G J, Beaulieu S, Pope M et al 1998 A physiologic function for p-glycoprotein (MDR-1) during the migration of dendritic cells from skin via afferent lymphatic vessels. Proc Natl Acad Sci USA 95:6924–6929

Ringpfeil F, Lebwohl MG, Christiano AM, Uitto J 2000 Pseudoxanthoma elasticum: mutations in the *MRP6* gene encoding a transmembrane ATP-binding cassette (ABC) transporter. Proc Natl Acad Sci USA 97: 6001–6006

Robbiani DF, Finch RA, Jager D, Muller WA, Sartorelli AC, Randolph G J 2000 The leukotriene C(4) transporter MRP1 regulates CCL19 (MIP-3beta, ELC)-dependent mobilization of dendritic cells to lymph nodes. Cell 103:757–768

Scheffer GL, Kool M, Heijn M et al 2000a Specific detection of multidrug resistance proteins MRP1, MRP2, MRP3, MRP5 and MDR3 P-glycoprotein with a panel of monoclonal antibodies. Cancer Res 60:5269–5277

Scheffer GL, Maliepaard M, Pijnenborg AC et al 2000b Breast cancer resistance protein is localized at the plasma membrane in mitoxantrone- and topotecan-resistant cell lines. Cancer Res 60:2589–2593

Scheffer GL, Wijngaard PL, Flens M J et al 1995 The drug resistance-related protein LRP is the human major vault protein. Nat Med 1:578–582

Scheper R J, Bulte JW, Brakkee JG et al 1988 Monoclonal antibody JSB-1 detects a highly conserved epitope on the P-glycoprotein associated with multi-drug-resistance. Int J Cancer 42:389–394

Schroeijers AB, Reurs AW, Stam AG et al 2000 Upregulation of vaults, Pgp and MRP1 during dendritic cell development: a physiological role for vaults in dendritic cell differentiation. Proc Am Assoc Cancer Res Annu Meet 91:1392

Schuetz JD, Connelly MC, Sun DX et al 1999 MRP4: A previously unidentified factor in resistance to nucleoside-based antiviral drugs. Nat Med 5:1048–1051

Smith A J, van Helvoort A, van Meer G et al 2000 MDR3 P-glycoprotein, a phosphatidylcholine translocase, transports several cytotoxic drugs and directly interacts with drugs as judged by interference with nucleotide trapping. J Biol Chem 275:23530–23539

Tammur J, Prades C, Arnould I et al 2001 Two new genes from the human ATP-binding cassette transporter superfamily, ABCC11 and ABCC12, tandemly duplicated on chromosome 16q12. Gene 273:89–96

Tishler DM, Weinberg KI, Hinton DR, Barbaro N, Annett GM, Raffel C 1995 MDR1 gene expression in brain of patients with medically intractable epilepsy. Epilepsia 36:1–6

Wijnholds J, Mol CA, van Deemter L et al 2000 Multidrug-resistance protein 5 is a multispecific organic anion transporter able to transport nucleotide analogs. Proc Natl Acad Sci USA 97:7476–7481

Zaman G J, Flens M J, van Leusden MR et al 1994 The human multidrug resistance-associated protein MRP is a plasma membrane drug-efflux pump. Proc Natl Acad Sci USA 91:8822–8826

Zeng H, Bain L J, Belinsky MG, Kruh GD 1999 Expression of multidrug resistance protein-3 (multispecific organic anion transporter-D) in human embryonic kidney 293 cells confers resistance to anticancer agents. Cancer Res 59:5964–5967

Zhang DW, Cole SP, Deeley RG 2001 Identification of an amino acid residue in multidrug resistance protein 1 critical for conferring resistance to anthracyclines. J Biol Chem 276:13231–13239

DISCUSSION

Ling: Your antibodies are an exciting tool. You introduced the concept that many different molecules could be involved in the transport of various anti-epileptic drugs (AEDs). Another concept you have raised is the possibility that different cell types, such as the dendritic cells (DC), could be producing something that could cause another effect. In other words, the expression of a drug-resistant molecule in the DCs could be secreting some regulatory signal that may affect the course of the disease.

Vezzani: I was interested in what you said about the possible functional interactions between Pgp proteins and molecules of the immune system. Using experimental models of epilepsy we have found that there is a strong immune response in the epileptic tissue. In particular, there is huge up-regulation of proinflammatory cytokines produced by glial cells. Interleukins are also up-regulated. Proinflammatory cytokines are proconvulsant in experimental models. There might be some functional relationship between phenotypic changes in neurons and glia in epileptic tissue that can somehow make molecules produced by these different cellular compartments available to their receptors. This may change the susceptibility of the tissue to excitability, for example. This could be another concept rather than, or in addition to, reducing drug activity. Thus, increased Pgp may actually extrude a molecule that is increasing epileptic activity.

Scheper: I agree. The drug-induced up-regulation of multidrug resistance molecules can lead to a higher inflammatory status. It could lead to epilepsy in an indirect way, and contribute to the intractability of this disease.

Atadja: How does the expression of the immune system molecules help the cancer cell? Does it participate in the defence of the cancer cell against the drug? I am having trouble seeing how this expression helps the cancer cell defend itself.

Scheper: In studying a number of cell lines we found a clear correlation between the expression of TAP and HLA class I molecules, and drug resistance. I am not aware of a careful analysis in haematological malignancies of the level of expression of class I levels and drug resistance. From the panel of cell lines we studied, I am convinced that the effects are small. I think that the TAP complex was designed by evolution to handle peptides and not organic drugs — they are substrates, but poor ones. In acute myeloid leukaemia associations with Pgp or MRP1 may occur, but in clinical oncology all associations seem to be controversial in one way or another.

Schmutz: You made one association with epilepsy: phenytoin is a preferred drug substrate for MDR1. It may be worth looking in patients that are refractory to phenytoin or in the kindled rats that are refractory to phenytoin, to see whether there is an up-regulation of MDR1, compared with patients who are not refractory to phenytoin. I don't know how important the effect of MDR1 is compared to diffusion of phenytoin through the blood–brain barrier. You also told us that these refractory molecules are distributed in many systems outside the nervous system. When one considers developing AEDs based on the inhibition of Pgp, for example, it would be important to have such inhibitors mainly concentrated in the nervous system, or even confined to specific subcompartments of the nervous system. Should one use such widely distributed molecules for AED therapy at all?

Scheper: You would need to collect a sizeable number of postmortem brains to study possible roles of MDR molecules. Anyhow, the antibodies are available now. We should look at the cells that show overexpression of certain molecules. With regard to chemosensitizers or antagonists, we should try as soon as possible to identify the most relevant target cells. Then, for example, if over-expression of Pgp, MRP1 and BCRP is confirmed, second-generation antagonists might be developed that block all three at the same time.

Sisodiya: People have looked at the expression of Pgp and MRP1 in human brain tissue. The paper that set this off for me was one by Tischler et al (1995). They looked at the expression of Pgp in surgical resection samples from patients with refractory epilepsy. They found Pgp in glia, which is not normally where it is found. We have also looked at Pgp and MRP1 expression in surgical resection samples. One problem is that it is very difficult to look at patients who have tractable epilepsy. But there are some ways around this: in patients who have had surgery we can look at the surrounding normal tissue that is not epileptogenic.

Wood: Most drugs that are Pgp substrates are excluded from the brain. One of the characteristics of a drug that is a potent Pgp substrate is that it would enter to the brain in low concentrations. What are the data that support phenytoin as being a Pgp substrate? It seems fundamentally improbable to me that most of the drugs we are talking about here are potent Pgp substrates. Almost by definition, they would not have been developed if they had failed to gain entry into the brain. There is a fundamental disconnect between all that we know about Pgp substrates, entry into the brain, and the direction we are thinking here.

Ling: We have a few related issues here. One is the transport of drugs across the blood–brain barrier. But before we get into that topic, have we finished this issue of the expression of various kinds of transporter molecules in the brain?

Bates: When I have looked at MDR1 expression in the brain, it is only in the capillary endothelium. Where else has expression been reported?

Sisodiya: You have been looking in normal brain. Obviously, the brain we have been looking at is not normal. It has epileptogenic pathology in it.

Bates: What is an epileptogenic pathology?

Sisodiya: It is something that is going to cause epilepsy. I am not sure that one can relate that to normal brain.

Bates: Where do you see the pumps, and which ones do you see?

Sisodiya: We have only looked at Pgp and MRP1. We have seen Pgp on glia within the areas where the pathology is, but we don't see it elsewhere.

Scheper: If in a subgroup of patients microglial cells were to have a genetically based increased tendency to up-regulate Pgp and MRP, you might be able to pick this up in the circulation by doing blood tests. You could take out the monocytes, feed them with cytokines, and look at the Pgp and MRP expression. This is one of the things we are exploring in other chronic diseases such as rheumatoid arthritis. There is a large heterogeneity in the inducibility of MDR pumps on monocytes in the circulation.

Pirmohamed: At a recent meeting of the American Society for Clinical Pharmacology, data were presented showing that normal microglia also express Pgp. We have done work on temporal lobe resection specimens. We also find Pgp expression in astrocyte foot processes, as well as capillary endothelial cells.

I want to pick up on Professor Woods' point. The crucial issue here is whether AEDs are substrates for these pumps. As far as I am aware, phenytoin is a very poor substrate for Pgp. This has been shown in cells and also transgenic animals. We have also done some studies with carbamazepine which show that it isn't a substrate for Pgp (Owen et al 2001).

Brinkmann: I disagree. We have found that phenytoin uptake is dependent on the MDR1 genotype, although the blood levels are to a much higher degree determined by the liver enzymes.

Pirmohamed: There is some transgenic work from The Netherlands showing that phenytoin entry to the brain is not Pgp dependent (Schinkel et al 1996).

Brinkmann: I am not talking about the brain. I am talking about transfer into the blood. Uptake through the intestinal wall is dependent on the level of Pgp expressed in a genotype-dependent manner.

Newman: We have some preliminary evidence for both phenytoin and carbamazepine acting as Pgp substrates.

Sills: Dr Kwan and I have performed some preliminary studies, using Pgp knockout mice, looking at the pharmacokinetics of AEDs. We have some interesting results suggesting that there are some mild substrates among the commonly used AEDs. Topiramate, which is a new anticonvulsant drug, is the strongest substrate we have identified thus far.

Bates: We have done a series of studies over the years with a variety of substrates for Pgp. We talk about drugs as being good or bad substrates, which relates to the affinity of the drug. It is currently thought that the drug binds to a high-affinity binding site, followed by hydrolysis of ATP which induces a conformational change in Pgp that moves the drug across the membrane to a low-affinity binding site where it is released (Sauna & Ambudkar 2001). It is not known what makes some drugs good substrates and others bad. It is clear, however, that the same amount of Pgp in the membrane of a cell can render the cell 20-fold resistant to one drug and 2000-fold resistant to another drug. This must be an enormous spectrum in terms of the on-rate and off-rate. Some inhibitors of Pgp probably do bind, but don't come off very well and are classified as non-compatible inhibitors. Then there are some substrates that don't bind as well to begin with but do manage to come off, and phenytoin could be in that category.

Abbott: Whether a drug gets into the brain will depend on how well it crosses the brain endothelium forming the blood–brain barrier. As the tight junctions of the endothelium restrict the paracellular pathway, most movement will be transcellular via diffusion through the lipid membranes or entry on specific carriers. Lipophilic drugs may be recognized and effluxed by Pgp in the luminal membrane. In the gut, some drugs that are Pgp substrates may still be well absorbed as they can bypass Pgp via the more permeable paracellular (junctional) pathway. Agents like phenytoin may get into the brain in a normal patient for effective epilepsy treatment, but any change in expression of Pgp and other efflux carriers (on the endothelium or other cell types) may affect the pharmacokinetic profile of the drug in the brain to the point where the concentration becomes too low to be effective. It will be interesting to establish whether this contributes to drug resistance in epilepsy.

Löscher: In terms of the pharmacology of AEDs, most of these drugs were optimized during development to be drugs that enter the brain. What might be important here is that patients who are refractory to AEDs do show certain brain-derived (central) side effects of these drugs. Many clinicians consider pharmacoresistance as when no anticonvulsant effect is seen at the maximum dose of the drug that can be tolerated by the patient. The side effects restrict the dose that can be given. This argues against the mechanism for resistance being simply an up-regulation of drug transporters, because then there would be no central side effects. There is another argument. There is a large epilepsy surgery centre in Bethel, Germany. Chemists working there looked at the level of anticonvulsant drugs in focal tissue removed from patients during epilepsy surgery, and compared this with concentrations in the perifocal tissue. They found no difference at all. The drug concentrations in the brain tissue of those patients were almost the same as in brain tissue of normal animals that have received the same doses of these drugs. This is another indication that there might be differences in terms of drug transport into the brain of epileptic patients, but they are probably quite moderate.

Sisodiya: The question of side effects is very important, but what this doesn't tell you about is the regional distribution of the overexpression. You may have overexpression that is limited to the site of the pathology generating the epilepsy. Overexpression may not be widespread, so that patients will still get cerebellar toxicity and not be able to manage higher doses. But this does not exclude the possibility of local overexpression.

Kwan: There could be a regional expression around the seizure focus. The studies that have looked at Pgp expression in epilepsy were done in patients with discrete lesions. This would fit in with the general epidemiological data which have consistently shown that symptomatic epilepsies do less well than idiopathic epilepsies (Kwan & Brodie 2000) which we assume to be due to more widespread abnormalities, as opposed to a discrete origin of epileptic activity.

There could be an up-regulation of transporters around the seizure focus stopping drugs getting in, even though they are still able to get into the normal parts of the brain to cause side effects. The other possibility is that there could be physiological differences in regional expression of Pgp or other transporters in brain that have not been looked at.

Vezzani: I would like to add a comment about measuring AED concentrations in brain. There was an early study by Claudio Munari showing that there is a gradient in the concentration of AEDs from the epileptic focus to the surrounding area in human epileptic tissue. In the epileptic focus, the drug concentration is lower than in surrounding areas. This would fit with the idea that there is some mechanism eliminating the drug from the active site. We have to be careful when we attempt to correlate the activity of Pgp and other transporters with the drug concentration in the tissue measured as a whole. We may find similar levels, but what is important is the access to the critical sites where the drug acts. We are measuring the tissue concentration. If there is a dynamic distribution of the drug between active sites and the extracellular compartment, we may lose this difference.

Newman: My understanding is that the therapeutic blood target levels for phenytoin and carbamazepine are in the range of 20–50 μM. This is 10–100 times higher than most therapeutics in terms of targeted blood levels. Is this just a coincidence of poor optimization against the target, or is it something related to needing a lot in the blood to get a little into the brain?

Andermann: The answer to this is that the seizures unfortunately can't read. This concept of a therapeutic range is in fact a figment of pharmacological imagination.

I would also like to comment on Professor Löscher's statement about the side effects. It is interesting that people who are intractable to the usual doses and levels of AEDs very often stop having seizures as they develop drug toxicity. In this situation there is a mechanism that would bear further investigation: higher levels often stop the seizures but the price in terms of side effects is much too high.

Schmutz: Both phenytoin and carbamazepine pass the blood–brain barrier very well. There are similar concentrations in the brain as in the blood, which are both in the micromolar range.

References

Kwan P, Brodie MJ 2000 Early identification of refractory epilepsy. N Engl J Med 342:314–319

Owen A, Pirmohamed M, Tettey JN, Morgan P, Chadwick D, Park BK 2001 Carbamazepine is not a substrate for P-glycoprotein. Br J Clin Pharmacol 51:345–359

Sauna ZE, Ambudkar SV 2001 Characterization of the catalytic cycle of ATP hydrolysis by human P-glycoprotein. The two ATP hydrolysis events in a single catalytic cycle are kinetically similar but affect different functional outcomes. J Biol Chem 276:11653–11661

Schinkel AH, Wagenaar E, Mol CA, van Deemter L 1996 P-glycoprotein in the blood–brain barrier of mice influences the brain penetration and pharmacological activity of many drugs. J Clin Invest 97:2517–2524
Tishler DM, Weinberg KI, Hinton DR, Barbaro N, Annett GM, Raffel C 1995 MDR1 gene expression in brain of patients with medically intractable epilepsy. Epilepsia 36:1–6

Drug resistance in epilepsy: the role of the blood–brain barrier

N. Joan Abbott, Ehsan U. Khan, Christopher M. S. Rollinson, Andreas Reichel, Damir Janigro*, Stephen M. Dombrowski*, Michael S. Dobbie and David J. Begley

*Blood–Brain Barrier Research Group, Centre for Neuroscience Research, King's College London, London SE1 1UL, UK and *Cerebrovascular Research, Cleveland Clinic Foundation, Cleveland, Ohio OH 44195, USA*

Abstract. The blood–brain barrier (BBB) is formed by the endothelial cells lining the brain microvessels. Complex tight junctions linking adjacent endothelial cells make brain capillaries around 100 times tighter than peripheral capillaries to small hydrophilic molecules. As a result, drugs required to act in the brain, including anti-epileptic drugs (AEDs), have generally been made lipophilic, and are thus able to cross the brain endothelium via the lipid membranes. However, such lipophilic drugs are potential substrates for efflux carriers of the BBB, particularly P glycoprotein (Pgp), predominantly located on the endothelial luminal membrane. It is estimated that up to 50% of drug candidates may be substrates for Pgp. The barrier phenotype of the brain endothelium is induced and maintained by chemical factors released by brain cells, particularly perivascular astrocytic end feet. In several neuropathological conditions, the BBB is disturbed, either as a result of pathology of the endothelium, or of the cells responsible for barrier induction and maintenance. During epileptic attacks, there may be transient BBB opening in the epileptogenic focus. There is evidence that under such pathological conditions, 'second line defence' mechanisms in perivascular glia may be up-regulated, including expression of Pgp and other drug efflux transporters. This complicates interpretation of drug resistance in epilepsy, and therapeutic strategies.

2002 Mechanisms of drug resistance in epilepsy: lessons from oncology. Wiley, Chichester (Novartis Foundation Symposium 243) p 38–53

Structure and function of brain endothelium in relation to drug delivery

The blood–brain barrier (BBB) is formed by the endothelial cells of the brain microvasculature (Abbott & Romero 1996). Compared with vessels in the periphery, the endothelium of brain capillaries shows a number of specializations related to its unique functions. The tight junctions linking adjacent cells are more complex and effectively seal the paracellular (junctional) pathway for diffusion of hydrophilic solutes, so that the major traffic of chemicals through the endothelium occurs transcellularly. A number of specialized transport mechanisms have been described, mediating the brain uptake of glucose, amino acids, nucleosides, choline, and other essential substances (Tsuji & Tamai 1999). For certain compounds capable of exerting toxic effects in the CNS such as glutamate, efflux mechanisms are present. Morphometric analysis shows that the mitochondrial volume fraction is higher in brain endothelium than peripheral endothelium, consistent with a higher metabolic activity and the requirements of transporter-mediated flux. The barrier phenotype of the brain endothelium is induced and maintained by chemical factors released by brain cells, particularly perivascular astrocytic end feet; there is evidence for up-regulation of not only the tight junctional tightness but also the function of transport proteins by glial factors (Abbott & Romero 1996).

Lipophilic compounds are generally able to penetrate the endothelium via the lipid membranes, and there is a reasonable correlation between the permeability at the BBB (permeability coefficient P) and lipophilicity (e.g. measured as $\text{LogP}_{octanol}$, the partition coefficient between water and octanol) (Bodor & Buchwald 1999). Hence drugs designed to work in the brain have generally be made lipophilic to exploit this delivery route. However, more complex features of molecular structure, including hydrogen bonding ability, also influence permeability and need to be taken into account in refining drug design (Habgood et al 2000).

Anomalous BBB permeability of certain lipophilic compounds: P glycoprotein

It was clear from the earliest quantitative studies that certain compounds were outliers in the plot of BBB permeability versus LogP_{oct}, being more restricted in permeability than expected from their lipid solubility (Bodor & Buchwald 1999). Initial attempts to explain this phenomenon suggested that the anomalous behaviour was due to size or charge effects. However, it is now known that many of these outliers are substrates for efflux carriers in the brain endothelium, particularly the multidrug resistance protein P glycoprotein, Pgp (*MDR1* gene in human, *Mdr1a* and *Mdr1b* in rodent). Pgp is a member of the ATP binding cassette (ABC) transporter superfamily, a large protein consisting of two similar halves, with 12 membrane spanning segments and two ATP binding domains. A variety of models for Pgp function have been proposed, including action as a 'hydrophobic vacuum cleaner' and 'flippase'; however, based on similarity with the LMR-A transporter of the bacterium *Lactococcus*, the most likely mechanism involves recognizing and effluxing compounds from the inner leaflet of the membrane (Borst et al 2000a).

Localization of Pgp at the BBB

The first indication of Pgp expression at the BBB came from immunocytochemical studies showing that several monoclonal antibodies recognizing Pgp specifically stained blood capillaries of the brain (and testis) in human and rat, but not capillaries in other tissues (Cordon-Cardo et al 1989, see also Schinkel 1999). Studies on cultured brain endothelium showed functional expression of Pgp, and a localization predominantly on the luminal (apical) membrane (Tatsuta et al 1992). Studies in *Mdr1a* knockout $(-/-)$ mice showed a dramatic increase in the brain distribution of compounds known to be Pgp substrates (Schinkel et al 1994). Other careful confocal and electron microscopic studies have confirmed the brain endothelial expression of Pgp, with little or no expression in other brain cell types (e.g. glia) under normal conditions (Stewart et al 1996, Begley et al 2000). Isolated membrane preparations enriched in brain endothelial luminal membrane also show strong Pgp staining (Beaulieu et al 1997). There is thus a general agreement that Pgp in brain endothelium is one of the mechanisms present for protecting the brain from xenobiotics (Tsuji & Tamai 1997), with additional protective mechanisms including a range of intracellular enzyme systems within the endothelium (Minn et al 2000).

An alternative view was proposed in an immunocytochemical study using human brain capillaries, in which Pardridge et al (1997) observed a discontinuous staining pattern with the Pgp antibodies MRK16 and C219 very similar to that for an antibody specific for glial fibrillary acidic protein (GFAP). In brain sections from rhesus and squirrel monkeys, MRK16 staining was found on both capillaries and astrocytes, and in a squirrel monkey there was no luminal labelling of brain capillaries following intravenous administration of ^{125}I-labelled MRK16. From this evidence Pardridge et al (1997) concluded that Pgp was predominantly present on the glial end feet rather than the endothelial luminal membrane — which if correct would indicate a difference in function of Pgp in rodent and primate brain. However, given the earlier electron microscope immunocyto-chemical studies showing MRK16 staining of the luminal endothelial membrane in human brain (Sugawara et al 1990), this is unlikely. It is known that artefacts associated with immunocytochemical techniques can lead to problems of interpretation; for example, heavy *N*-glycosylation of Pgp in some tissues can cause shielding of the extracellular epitope recognized by MRK16 (Schinkel 1999). On balance it is unlikely that there will prove to be major differences between human and rodent BBB in relation to Pgp expression and localization.

Molecular and functional study of further brain endothelial efflux transporters

In addition to the MDR family, other efflux carriers have been described at the BBB, particularly the family of multidrug resistance-associated proteins (MRPs, Borst et al 2000b) transporting organic anions, and glucuronide- and glutathione-conjugated compounds (Table 1). There is considerable overlap in

TABLE 1 Examples of substrates and inhibitors of principal CNS drug efflux transporters

	Substrates	*Inhibitors*
MDR1/MDR1a/MDR1b	*Amphiphilic, neutral or cationic substrates*	
	Colchicine	Verapamil
	Vincristine	PSC833
	Doxorubicin	GF120918
	Cyclosporin A	
	Ivermectin	
	Phenytoin	
	Tetracyclins	
	Rifampicin	
	Fluoroquinolones	
	Chloramphenicol	
MRP1	*Organic, anionic substrates, glutathione, glucuonate or sulphate conjugates*	
	Vincristine	Indomethacin
	3-α-sulfatolitho-cholyltaurine	Genestein
	Tetracyclins	
	Fluoroquinolones	
MRP2 (cMOAT)		
	Paraminohippuric acid	Probenecid[a]
	β-lactam antibiotics	
MRP5	*Anionic substrates, glutathione conjugates*	
	CAMP	
	CGMP	
	Fluorochrome	

[a]Probenecid may also inhibit other members of the MRP family. However, until their substrate preferences are fully determined the situation remains unclear.

the substrate specificity of MRP1 and Pgp, in spite of only $\sim 15\%$ amino acid sequence homology (Kusuhara & Sugiyama 2001). Initial characterization made use of relatively specific inhibitors: verapamil/PSC833 for Pgp, indomethacin/genistein for MRP1, probenecid for MRP2 (formerly known as cMOAT), and *in situ* experiments, including efflux measurements (Kusuhara & Sugiyama 2001). Western blot and RT-PCR analysis suggested that *MRP1* is expressed at low levels on isolated rat brain capillaries and cultured brain endothelium, although *MRP4*, *MRP6* and especially *MRP5* appear to predominate in bovine brain capillaries (Zhang et al 2000). However, no MRP1 was detected immunocytochemically in either human or rat brain capillaries *in situ*, suggesting a minor physiological role in the normal brain endothelium (Seetharaman et al 1998, Begley et al 2000). Recently, members of the OATP (organic anion-transporting polypeptide) family have been detected on brain endothelium, Oatp1 and Oatp2 in rat and OATP-A in human, and have also been shown able to transport opioid peptide analogues from blood to brain for an analgesic effect (Gao et al 2000). However, as these are bidirectional Na^+-independent transporters, they can also mediate efflux from the nervous system down a concentration gradient. Evidence for the presence of an efflux system transporting *p*-aminohippurate (PAH) could indicate presence of further organic acid transporters (OAT, Kusuhara & Sugiyama 2001).

The choroid plexus and the blood–CSF barrier

The choroid plexus epithelium is responsible for the secretion of cerebrospinal fluid (CSF), which circulates through the cerebral ventricles, into the sub-arachnoid space, and back into the venous circulation through arachnoid granulations and via lymphatics in the neck (Davson & Segal 1995). The choroid plexus epithelium shows similar barrier properties (blood–CSF barrier) to the brain capillary endothelium (BBB). A number of efflux carriers have been reported in the choroid plexus, including MRP1, Pgp, OATPs and OAT, but their localization and functional properties are not fully established (Kusuhara & Sugiyama 2001). Although the ependymal lining of the ventricles is relatively permeable to small solutes, the CSF is not a major route for drugs to access the brain, as diffusion is a relatively inefficient mechanism for delivery over distances greater than a few hundred micrometres; moreover, secretion and flow of brain interstitial fluid creates a bulk flow draining into the CSF and hence working against diffusive entry (Begley et al 2000).

Substrates and modulators of Pgp

Several experimental models have been used to identify compounds inter-acting with Pgp: these include use of *Mdr1a* knockout or gene deletion mice to identify substrates, and use of the ATPase activity of Pgp as a measure of drug binding (Borst et al 2000a). Two main classes of chemicals have been identified — substrates, which are generally lipophilic and cationic, with long dwell times in the membrane, and 'reversers', modulators or inhibitors, which are more permeant and are generally not transported (Eytan & Kuchel 1999).

Structure–activity relationship (SAR) studies have been attempted but have generally been unsuccessful (Ueda et al 1997) although for some recent small studies they appear to offer predictive value (Osterberg & Norinder 2000, Seelig & Landwojtowicz 2000).

It is still unclear how ABC transporters recognize and translocate substrates (Borst et al 2000a). Electron microscopy of Pgp protein arrays has indicated that the protein contains a central pore closed at the inner end; however, it is not known whether drugs pass through this pore, or enter from the inner membrane leaflet via a 'gap' in the protein ring. Pgp appears to have two drug binding sites that interact, but the parts of the protein responsible are not yet precisely known (Borst et al 2000a). Some information is available on the 3D structure of the ATP binding part of the molecule, and translocation involves the alternating action of the two ATP binding sites. There is evidence that the lipid membrane environment can influence Pgp function, so for the accurate prediction of BBB Pgp function, it is important to work with BBB models. Experiments on the Pgp-expressing RBE4 immortalized cell line of rat brain endothelial cells using a [^{3}H]colchicine uptake assay (Begley et al 1996) show that lipophilicity is important for drug/Pgp interaction, but the presence of more specific interactions for certain compounds is consistent with the presence of higher affinity and regulatory sites (Begley et al 2000, Chishty et al 2001).

BBB function in epilepsy

The early literature from animal studies showed increased BBB permeability in experimentally induced seizures (electrical stimulation), demonstrated by extravasation of horseradish peroxidase (HRP, Lorenzo et al 1975). It was subsequently found that if the seizure-induced blood pressure increase was abolished by spinal transection, HRP leakage was not observed (Bolwig et al 1977). The route for HRP permeability was unclear, although vesicular traffic was implicated (Westergaard et al 1978). More recently it has been shown that the metabolic and transport functions of the BBB are disturbed in human epilepsy, with evidence for changes in expression of the glucose carrier GLUT1 (Cornford & Hyman 1999).

Drug treatments in epilepsy in relation to BBB transporters

Anti-epileptic drugs (AEDs) are designed to reduce the simultaneous neuronal spiking underlying seizures, using agents acting via a number of different mechanisms. AEDs with clinical applications include ethosuximide, tri-methadione, phenytoin, albutoin, phenobarbitone, primidone, carbamazepine, diazepam, clonazepam, sodium valproate (dipropylacetate), lamotrigine, vigabatrin, gabapentin, topiramate, tiagabine, oxcarbazepine, benzodiazepines and levetiracetam. Some of these have been shown to be substrates for efflux transporters at the BBB, e.g. phenytoin, phenobarbitone and carbamazepine for Pgp (Tsuji & Tamai 1999), and valproate for a probenecid-sensitive transporter (Cornford & Hyman 1999), likely to be MRP2. Gabapentin and some tricyclic pyridophthalazinedione NMDA glycine(B) antagonist anti-convulsants (MRZ 2/570, 571, 576) also appear to be effluxed from brain by a probenecid-sensitive mechanism (Sawchuk & Elmquist 2000). However, the fact that $\sim 70\%$ patients can be effectively treated with AEDs means Pgp/MRP at the BBB are unlikely to constitute an absolute barrier to penetration under normal conditions. This focuses interest on the problems in the remaining $\sim 30\%$ of patients.

Changes in efflux transporter expression in epilepsy

Immunocytochemical methods have shown presence of both Pgp (MDR1) and MRP1 in epilepsy patients, in both brain endothelium and astrocytes (Tishler et al 1995, Sisodiya et al 1999, 2001), with evidence for up-regulation of Pgp. cDNA gene array analysis applied to brain endothelial cells from patients with medically intractable epilepsy showed overexpression of several multidrug resistance genes, with significant increases for *MDR1*, *MRP2* and the cisplatin resistance-associated alpha protein, but no significant change in the case of *MRP1* or *MDR2* (Dombrowski et al 2002). Change in transporter expression in both human and rat brain endothelium has been detected when comparing freshly isolated brain microvessels and cultured brain endothelium — the latter generally shows a down-regulation of Pgp and up-regulation of *MRP1* (Seetharaman et al 1998). Cultured astrocytes show low levels of Pgp expression but strong expression of *MRP1* (Declèves et al 2000a). Although astrocytic Pgp expression is generally undetectable in normal rat brain, up-regulation follows intracerebro-ventricular injection with neurotoxic concentrations of kainate (Zhang et al 1999). Taken together, these studies suggest that activation of brain endothelium and astrocytes by damage, isolation or stress can alter the transporter phenotype, leading to a condition in which the primary endothelial barrier is supported by a 'second line of defence', the astrocytes. There are clearly implications for the epileptic brain and for treatment with AEDs. Exposure to drugs may also itself lead to up-regulation or induction of Pgp/MRP — as with tumour cells. The net result may be that less drug reaches target neurons in epileptogenic sites. However, it is hard to model or predict the resulting changes in drug CNS pharmacokinetics (PK) in patients, since real-time measurements of drug concentrations in the brain extracellular compartment are unavailable.

Variability in human Pgp function and comparison with other mammals

Recently, polymorphisms have been detected in exons 2 and 26 of human *MDR1* (Declèves et al 2000b, Hoffmeyer et al 2000), but analysis of the functional consequences, for example in relation to drug specificity, is not yet available. It is possible that humans are more vulnerable to xenobiotics than rodents or pigs, since humans have a single Pgp isoform (*MDR1*) compared with two (*Mdr1a and 1b*) in rodents, while pigs may have multiple isoforms. So far there is no evidence for spontaneous *MDR1* deletions in humans equivalent to that found in the CF-1 mouse and in collie dogs (see Schinkel 1999). Such *MDR1* loss is unlikely, as the Pgp substrate ivermectin has been used to treat river blindness (Onchocerciasis) in large parts of world, with very few cases of CNS toxicity reported (Schinkel 1999).

Conclusion

This review has shown that the normal brain microenvironment is strongly protected by the BBB, as a result of close cooperation between the endothelium and perivascular astrocytes. AEDs are generally lipophilic agents that penetrate effectively across the barrier to reach neuronal sites of action. However, some AEDs are substrates for efflux transporters at the barrier layers, which may limit their efficacy and necessitate higher systemic doses. In certain cases of medically intractable epilepsy, changes in the transporter profile on both endothelium and astrocytes have been reported, which may play a role in the reduced efficacy of AEDs in these patients. It is not clear whether the changed expression is due to the primary pathology which may involve epilepsy-induced dysfunction of the BBB, or to up-regulation of transporters in response to the chronic treatment with AEDs. Improved understanding based on analysis of clinical material is expected to lead to improved treatments tailored to the affected individual.

Acknowledgements

The KCL BBB Consortium with Industry was supported by Lilly, Astra Zeneca, Glaxo Wellcome, Aventis and Mindset. Work at the Cleveland Clinic (S. Dombrowski, D. Janigro) was supported by NIH-2RO1 HL51614 and NIH-RO1 NS38195 to DJ.

References

Abbott NJ, Romero IA 1996 Transporting therapeutics across the blood–brain barrier. Mol Med Today 2:106–113

Beaulieu E, Demeule M, Ghitescu L, Beliveau R 1997 P-glycoprotein is strongly expressed in the luminal membranes of the endothelium of blood vessels in the brain. Biochem J 326:539–544

Begley DJ, Lechardeur D, Chen ZD et al 1996 Functional expression of P-glycoprotein in an immortalized cell line of rat brain endothelial cells, RBE4. J Neurochem 67:988–995

Begley DJ, Khan EU, Rollinson C, Abbott NJ, Regina A, Roux F 2000 The role of brain extracellular fluid production and efflux mechanisms in drug transport to the brain. In: Begley DJ, Bradbury MW, Kreuter J (eds) The blood–brain barrier and drug delivery to the CNS. Marcel Dekker, New York, p 93–108

Bodor N, Buchwald P 1999 Recent advances in the brain targeting of neuropharmaceuticals by chemical delivery systems. Adv Drug Deliv Rev 36:229–254

Bolwig TG, Hertz MM, Westergaard E 1977 Acute hypertension causing blood–brain barrier breakdown during epileptic seizures. Acta Neurol Scand 56:335–342

Borst P, Zelcer N, van Helvoort A 2000a ABC transporters in lipid transport. Biochim Biophys Acta 1486:128–144

Borst P, Evers R, Kool M, Wijnholds J 2000b A family of drug transporters: the multidrug resistance-associated proteins. J Natl Cancer Inst 92:1295–1302

Chishty M, Reichel A, Abbott NJ, Begley DJ 2001 Stimulation of P-glycoprotein mediated efflux by H_1- and adenosine receptor ligands in RBE4 cells, an in vitro model of the blood–brain barrier. J Physiol 531:209–110P

Cordon-Cardo C, O'Brien JP, Casals D et al 1989 Multidrug-resistance gene (P-glycoprotein) is expressed by endothelial cells at blood–brain barrier sites. Proc Natl Acad Sci USA 86:695–698

Cornford EM, Hyman S 1999 Blood–brain barrier permeability to small and large molecules. Adv Drug Deliv Rev 36:145–163

Davson H, Segal MB 1995 Physiology of the CSF and blood–brain barriers. CRC Press, Boca Raton

Declèves X, Regina A, Laplanche JL et al 2000a Functional expression of P-glycoprotein and multidrug resistance-associated protein (mrp1) in primary cultures of rat astrocytes. J Neurosci Res 60:594–610

Declèves X, Chevillard S, Charpentier C, Vielh P, Laplanche JL 2000b A new polymorphism (N21D) in the exon 2 of the human MDR1 gene encoding the P-glycoprotein. Hum Mut 15:486

Dombrowski SM, Desai SY, Marroni M et al 2002 Overexpression of multiple drug resistance genes in endothelial cells from patients with medically intractable epilepsy. Epilepsia, in press

Eytan GD, Kuchel PW 1999 Mechanism of action of P-glycoprotein in relation to passive membrane permeation. Int Rev Cytol 190:175–250

Gao B, Hagenbuch B, Kullak-Ublick GA, Benke D, Aguzzi A, Meier PJ 2000 Organic anion-transporting polypeptides mediate transport of opioid peptides across blood–brain barrier. J Pharmacol Exp Ther 294:73–79

Habgood MD, Begley DJ, Abbott NJ 2000 Determinants of passive drug entry into the central nervous system. Cell Mol Neurobiol 20:231–253

Hoffmeyer S, Burk O, von Richter O et al 2000 Functional polymorphisms of the human multidrug-resistance gene: multiple sequence variations and correlation of one allele with P-glycoprotein expression and activity in vivo. Proc Natl Acad Sci USA 97:3473–3478

Kusuhara H, Sugiyama Y 2001 Efflux transport systems for drugs at the blood–brain barrier and blood–cerebrospinal barrier (Part 1). Drug Discov Today 6:150–156

Lorenzo AV, Hedley-Whyte ET, Eisenberg HM, Hsu DW 1975 Increased penetration of horseradish peroxidase across the blood–brain barrier induce by Metrazol seizures. Brain Res 88: 136–140

Minn A, El-Bachá RS, Bayol-Denizot C, Lagrange P, Suleman FG, Gradinaru D 2000 Drug metabolism in the brain: benefits and risks. In: Begley DJ, Bradbury MW, Kreuter J (eds) The blood–brain barrier and drug delivery to the CNS. Marcel Dekker, New York, p 145–170

Osterberg T, Norinder U 2000 Theoretical calculations and prediction of P-glycoprotein-interacting drugs using MolSurf parametrization and PLS statistics. Eur J Pharm Sci 10:295–303

Pardridge WM, Golden PL, Kang YS, Bickel U 1997 Brain microvascular and astrocyte localization of P-glycoprotein. J Neurochem 68:1278–1285

Sawchuk R J, Elmquist WF 2000 Microdialysis in the study of drug transporters in the CNS. Adv Drug Deliv Rev 45:295–307

Seelig A, Landwojtowicz E 2000 Structure–activity relationship of P-glycoprotein substrates and modifiers. Eur J Pharm Sci 12:31–40

Schinkel AH, Smit LLM, van Tellingen O et al 1994 Disruption of the mouse mdr1a P-glycoprotein gene leads to deficiency in the blood–brain barrier and to increased sensitivity to drugs. Cell 77:491–502

Schinkel AH 1999 P-glycoprotein, a gatekeeper in the blood–brain barrier. Adv Drug Deliv Rev 36:179–194

Seetharaman S, Barrand MA, Maskell L, Scheper R J 1998 Multidrug resistance-related transport proteins in isolated human brain microvessels and in cells cultured from these isolates. J Neurochem 70:1151–1159

Sisodiya SM, Heffernan J, Squier MV 1999 Over-expression of P-glycoprotein in malformations of cortical development. Neuroreport 10:3437–3441

Sisodiya SM, Kin W-R, Squier MV, Thom M 2001 Multidrug-resistance protein 1 in focal cortical dysplasia. Lancet 357:42–43

Stewart PA, Béliveau R, Rogers KA 1996 Cellular localization of P-glycoprotein in brain versus gonadal capillaries. J Histochem Cytochem 44:679–685

Sugawara I, Hamada H, Tsuruo T, Mori S 1990 Specialized localization of P-glycoprotein recognized by MRK16 monoclonal antibody in endothelial cells of the brain and spinal cord. Jpn J Cancer Res 81:727–730

Tatsuta T, Naito M, Oh-hara T, Sugawara I, Tsuruo T 1992 Functional involvement of P-glycoprotein in blood–brain barrier. J Biol Chem 267:20383–20391

Tishler DM, Weinberg KI, Hinton DR, Barbaro N, Annett GM, Raffel C 1995 MDR1 gene expression in brain of patients with medically intractable epilepsy. Epilepsia 36:1–6

Tsuji A, Tamai I 1997 Blood–brain barrier function of P-glycoprotein. Adv Drug Deliv Rev 25:287–298

Tsuji A, Tamai I 1999 Carrier-mediated or specialized transport of drugs across the blood–brain barrier. Adv Drug Deliv Rev 36:277–290

Ueda K, Taguchi Y, Morishima M 1997 How does P-glycoprotein recognize its substrates? Semin Cancer Biol 8:151–159

Westergaard E, Hertz MM, Bolwig TG 1978 Increased permeability to horseradish peroxidase across cerebral vessels, evoked by electrically induced seizures in the rat. Acta Neuropathol 41:73–80

Zhang L, Ong WY, Lee T 1999 Induction of P-glycoprotein expression in astrocytes following intracerebroventricular kainate injections. Exp Brain Res 126:509–516

Zhang Y, Han H, Elmquist WF, Miller DW 2000 Expression of various multidrug resistance-associated protein (MRP) homologues in brain microvessel endothelial cells. Brain Res 876:148–153

DISCUSSION

Löscher: The interesting thing about the work on Pgp expression after kainate-induced seizures by the Japanese group (Zhang et al 1999) is that there was a transient increase, and the highest overexpression of Pgp occurred about 10 days after status epilepticus. It then went down to normal again. This is the reason they speculated that Pgp expression might be a stress response. If these results are similar in patients, it will be very important for all patient studies to look at the latency between getting the material and the previous seizure. No one has yet done this.

Abbott: I agree that human material poses problems, since we can only study what is available, and at present it is difficult to separate the effects of the seizures themselves from more chronic changes, or from changes due to drug regimes.

Löscher: Another point which might be important is the effect of the AED itself on Pgp expression. As you know, phenobarbitol increases Pgp in certain tissues. As far as I know, no study has investigated whether it also increases Pgp in the blood–brain barrier, but why not? Many patients with epilepsy are pretreated with well-known enzyme inducers, at least some of which may have effects on Pgp. This could be another explanation for differences between patients.

Ling: This may be a naïve question, but are we absolutely sure that the site of action of AEDs is in the glial cells, rather than on the BBB itself? Clearly, some drugs do get across, but how sure are we about the site of action of the AEDs?

Löscher: There are two categories. One set of AEDs operates from outside the neurons, on Na^+ channels in neuronal membranes, for example. The other category is acting from the inside of the neuron and has to enter the cells. There are interesting data showing that valproate has difficulty entering the neuron, suggesting that there may be drug transporters in the neuronal membrane involved. There is some dispute about whether multidrug transporters exist at all in the neuronal membranes.

Ling: I am trying to focus on this question of whether we know what the target is.

Sander: We think we might know, but it is probably fair to say that we don't really know how any of the AEDs work. We have some ideas.

Löscher: Our ideas about how these drugs work are probably too simplistic. All the drugs are very dirty. If you look in a textbook, it will probably say that phenytoin acts solely on the Na^+ channels. If you look at what is published about phenytoin, however, there are more than 100 mechanisms described in the literature.

Ling: Let's say for the sake of argument that the target is endothelial cells, and that the endothelial cells in turn produce some signal inside the brain which changes the BBB. This might be more relevant than anything else that goes on inside the brain. However, this is just pure speculation. Perhaps we have to keep an open mind as to the actual target of these drugs.

Meldrum: Of course, one can demonstrate effects of these AEDs on cell excitability in slice preparations of brain, and even on single-cell preparations. This must be assumed to be an effect on neuronal membranes. For gabapentin and valproate, they have an action from inside the neuron. They are doing something that has a delayed effect through action on metabolism in the neuron. But for most of the other AEDs there is clear evidence that they are having a direct effect on the neuronal membrane.

Löscher: I have a question for the Pgp experts. Is this pump always exporting drugs from the inside of the cells to the outside, or is there any evidence that this pump, like other pumps, can change its direction?

Varadi: I have never seen any evidence that it can. Pgp needs ATP to act, and ATP is always inside the cell.

Abbott: But it could be transporting into an organelle, for example.

Löscher: The reason I asked is that there are data from human tissue where researchers looked at the whole-tissue level at levels of AEDs in human epileptic foci and found no difference (Schnabel et al 1995, 1996). One possibility could be that there is a changed distribution within the tissue so that the concentration in the whole tissue is the same, but it has changed in different compartments. For instance, there could be an accumulation in glial cells. This would only be possible if these multidrug transporters can pump from the outside of the cell to the inside.

Abbott: Was the study you mentioned done by taking whole brain tissue and homogenizing?

Löscher: No, it was done with excised focal tissue.

Abbott: But was the concentration measured in the whole piece of tissue, with no attempt to find out what the local extracellular concentration was?

Löscher: That is almost impossible to do.

Bates: One new area of research was presented at the recent ABC meeting in Austria by Dietrich Keppler, who is working on hepatocytes. He presented the argument that, rather than passive diffusion, many more drugs enter the cell by active uptake than had been previously thought. Even the lipophilic drugs. He showed that it was necessary to transfect the OAT or OATP uptake pump into a cell in order to get adequate bilirubin export by MRP2 (Cui et al 2001). It is possible that as you begin to look at transporters in these cells, you need to look at the potential expression of OAT and OATP uptake systems that could be down-regulated in the presence of epileptic resistance.

Brinkmann: There are some strange effects observed in drug-resistant cells. If we look for doxorubicin resistance, sometimes we find cells that are highly resistant but which do not look like MDR1 cells. They have doxorubicin at high concentrations inside the cell, but it is not present in the nucleus and does not appear to be in the cytoplasm. Instead, it appears to be in the vesicles. Some transporter appears to be transporting the drug into vesicles rather than out of the cells. The drug is no longer active because the cells are alive and can proliferate. Immunohistochemistry shows that the tissue contains lots of drug, but still it is not active.

Ling: That is a good point. In essence, the drug is being sequestered away from the target site.

Scheper: This has to do with the localization of these pumps. Most of the members of this pump family are routed towards the outer membrane. Clearly the TAP pump is not on the outer membrane. Under certain circumstances some of the molecules can be exocytosed in vesicles.

Brinkmann: What I was explaining is something that has been acquired. If you take a normal cell line that is normally not doing this, colonies can be selected that are now doing this. Something has changed: perhaps a transporter that is normally in the membrane pumping to the outside has been mislocalized so that it is now pumping into a vesicle.

Bates: GLC4-Adr is a good example of an Adriamycin (doxorubicin)-resistant cell line that overexpresses MRP1 on both vesicular and plasma membranes (Van Luyn et al 1998). Adriamycin is sequestered into the vesicles.

Wijnholds: It is also known that if you have monolayers of cells and these become disrupted, then the apical membranes go inside the cell and produce vesicles (Low et al 2000, Vega-Salas et al 1987). In this way, the cell may end up with transporters pumping drugs into vesicles.

Sisodiya: With regard to the sequestering into vesicles, if you do immuno-histochemistry for the drug resistance protein in those cases, what do you see?

Brinkmann: I don't know that. I am describing something that is seen in cell culture, where a cell line becomes resistant. I would expect immunohisto-chemistry for the drug to look quite normal, but I wouldn't know about the protein.

Abbott: In the choroid plexus Pgp has been described as being 'subapical' (Rao et al 1999) rather than actually located on the apical membrane, which could indicate expression on vesicles. As the choroid plexus, like the brain endothelium, helps regulate the brain microenvironment, Pgp would not be expected on the apical (CSF-facing) choroid plexus membrane, because it would be transporting into the CSF. The major drug efflux transporter of the choroid plexus appears to be MRP on the basolateral (blood-facing) membrane, so perhaps vesicular Pgp is a second line of defence to deal with compounds that get past the MRP.

Ling: One important challenge is getting a map showing the localization of these molecules. One really needs to do electron microscopy to get clear localization, particularly in endothelial cells which are so thin. Such a map would be valuable to the entire community.

Hendrikse: I have a question about the relationship between the logP value (the lipophilicity) of the molecule and the facility to be transported by Pgp. I can imagine that the efflux is dependent on the lipophilicity determinative for passive transport and active Pgp transport. When a substrate is very lipophilic, what is the contribution of Pgp? I would guess that Pgp is less relevant in this situation.

Abbott: Eytan & Kuchel (1999) have attempted to establish the factors that determine drug interaction with Pgp. MDR-type drugs are hydrophobic and generally positively charged. There were no clear chemical features associated with the distinction between Pgp substrates and Pgp inhibitors or modulators, but the most significant factor was the dwell time in the membrane. Pgp substrates tend to have long residence times in the membrane, presumably because this increases the probability that Pgp will remove a drug from the cell, while drugs with low dwell time tended to be modulators or inhibitors rather than substrates.

Wood: Does this hold true even for drugs with minor structural changes? For instance, the difference between PSC 833 and cyclosporin.

Abbott: It would be worth comparing their lipophilicities; in some cases lipophilicity is radically changed by minor changes in the molecule. In the series we have studied, there is an overall relation between drug–Pgp interaction and lipophilicity, but with some outliers which are likely to represent compounds interacting with higher-affinity binding sites (Khan et al 1998).

Bates: I think there is always a general relationship in that Pgp substrates are typically large, cationic and hydrophobic molecules, but people who have tried to create specific models have found differences that probably relate to the core molecule under study. I don't think you can draw any specific rules about what makes a drug a substrate.

Wood: The same relationship holds true for CYP3A4 for instance. We have to be cautious before jumping from a relationship to an effect.

Abbott: These are attempts to look at the data and try to see some patterns. They are usually an aid to designing experiments to test hypotheses.

Newman: The gut–xenobiotic barrier contains a metabolism component. Is there any possibility that metabolism takes place in the BBB?

Abbott: The brain endothelium does indeed act as a metabolic barrier, with a number of Phase 1 and Phase 2 enzymes present (El-Bacha & Minn 1999). Of the cytochrome P450 family, CYP1A, 2B, 2D and 2E1 have been identified. The functional coupling between CYP3A4 and Pgp described for the gut does not seem to be present in the brain endothelium.

Newman: If these types of cytochromes are expressed, we should add this component to the discussion of AED access to the brain.

Scheper: Related to this, are the glutathione levels in these endothelial cells known?

Abbott: In culture, both brain endothelial cells and astrocytes contain glutathione (GSH), but there seems to be some mutual regulation of GSH and antioxidant enzymes, suggesting a division of labour in protecting the brain from oxidative stress (Schroeter et al 1999).

Sander: You mentioned that verapamil inhibits Pgp. Will the other drugs of this class, such as nifedipine, do the same thing?

Abbott: Yes, but not as strongly (Krishna & Mayer 2000).

Sander: Nifedipine is a last-ditch drug for epilepsy. I have come across patients in whom we have tried this as a last resort and they do well for two–three months and then revert to their previous state. I haven't tried verapamil.

Sills: We did some work in Glasgow about 10 years ago (Larkin et al 1991, 1992a) looking at add-on treatment with nimodipine and nifedipine for epilepsy. These drugs didn't seem to be particularly effective, although we couldn't push the doses as high as we would have liked without getting cardiovascular side effects. We also did some support studies in the laboratory and proved that both agents were anticonvulsant in animal models (Larkin et al 1992b, Sills et al 1994). However, following chronic treatment there was a down-regulation of the L-type Ca^{2+} channel (G. J. Sills, unpublished observations) which may be related to the tailing-off effect observed in patients.

Wood: Mibefridil, the AED that was withdrawn, was withdrawn because it was a potent CYP3A inhibitor, but it was also a potent Pgp inhibitor. This probably explains why it produced much more drug interaction than the other CYP3A inhibitors, of which there are many on the market. The problem with verapamil and these other drugs is that they are very dirty.

Newman: An additional problem with many of the first-generation inhibitors is that they are Pgp substrates. This makes it difficult to achieve and maintain blood levels sufficient for inhibition.

Wood: We have shown that Imodium (loperamide) plus potent Pgp inhibitors can produce analgesic effects in animals and probably human patients, when there is normally no analgesic effect of Imodium in humans. This is presumably due to the fact that although Imodium is a potent opiate, it doesn't cross the blood–brain barrier because of Pgp. If Pgp is inhibited, it produces dramatic central opiate effects.

References

Cui Y, König J, Keppler D 2001 Vectorial transport by double-transfected cells expressing the human uptake transporter SLC21A8 and the apical export pump ABCC2. Mol Pharmacol 60:934–943

El-Bacha RS, Minn A 1999 Drug metabolizing enzymes in cerebrovascular endothelial cells afford a metabolic protection to the brain. Cell Mol Biol 45:15–23

Eytan GD, Kuchel PW 1999 Mechanism of action of P-glycoprotein in relation to passive membrane permeation. Int Rev Cytol 190:175–250

Khan EU, Reichel A, Begley DJ, Roffey SJ, Jezequel SG, Abbott NJ 1998 The effect of drug lipophilicity on P-glycoprotein-mediated colchicine efflux at the blood-brain barrier. Int J Clin Pharm Ther 36:84–86

Krishna R, Mayer LD 2000 Multidrug resistance (MDR) in cancer. Mechanisms, reversal using modulators of MDR and the role of MDR modulators in influencing the pharmacokinetics of anticancer drugs. Eur J Pharm Sci 11:265–283

Larkin JG, McKee PJW, Blacklaw J, Thompson GG, Morgan IC, Brodie MJ 1991 Nimodipine in refractory epilepsy: a placebo-controlled, add-on study. Epilepsy Res 9:71–77

Larkin JG, Besag FMC, Cox A, Williams J, Brodie MJ 1992a Nifedipine for epilepsy? A double-blind, placebo-controlled trial. Epilepsia 33:346–352

Larkin JG, Thompson GG, Scobie G, Forrest G, Drennan JE, Brodie MJ 1992b Dihydropyridine calcium antagonists in mice: blood and brain pharmacokinetics and efficacy against pentylenetetrazol seizures. Epilepsia 33:760–769

Low SH, Miura M, Roche PA, Valdez AC, Mostov KE, Weimbs T 2000 Intracellular redirection of plasma membrane trafficking after loss of epithelial cell polarity. Mol Biol Cell 11:3045–3060

Rao VV, Dahlheimer JL, Bardgett ME et al 1999 Choroid plexus epithelial expression of MDR1 P glycoprotein and multidrug resistance-associated protein contribute to the blood-cerebrospinal-fluid drug-permeability barrier. Proc Natl Acad Sci USA 96:3900–3905

Schnabel R, Rambeck B, May TW, Jurgens U, Lahl R, Villagran R 1995 Lack of effect of histological lesions on the phenytoin and phenobarbital concentrations in the brain cortex of epileptic patients. J Neurol Sci 133:177–182

Schnabel R, Rambeck B, May T, Jurgens U, Lahl R, Fritsch W 1996 Lack of influence of histopathological changes on carbamazepine and carbamazepine-10, 11-epoxide concentrations in the brain cortex of epileptic patients. J Neurol Sci 141:87–94

Schroeter ML, Mertsch K, Giese H et al 1999 Astrocytes enhance radical defence in capillary endothelial cells constituting the blood-brain barrier. FEBS Lett 449:241–244

Sills GJ, Carswell A, Brodie MJ 1994 Dose-response relationships with nimodipine against electroshock seizures in mice. Epilepsia 35:437–442

Van Luyn MJ, Müller M, Renes J et al 1998 Transport of glutathione conjugates into secretory vesicles is mediated by the multidrug-resistance protein 1. Int J Cancer 76:55–62

Vega-Salas DE, Salas PJI, Rodriguez-Boulan E 1987 Modulation of an apical plasmamembrane protein of Madin–Darby canine kidney epithelial cells: cell–cell interactions control the appearance of a novel intracellular storage compartment. J Cell Biol 104:1249–1259

Zhang L, Ong WY, Lee T 1999 Induction of P-glycoprotein expression in astrocytes following intracerebroventricular kainate injections. Exp Brain Res 126:509–516

P glycoprotein and the mechanism of multidrug resistance

András Váradi*, Gergely Szakács†, Éva Bakos* and Balázs Sarkadi†

*Institute of Enzymology, Hungarian Academy of Sciences, Karolina ut 29, Budapest H-1113, and †National Institute of Hematology and Immunology, Membrane Research Group of SEB-Hungarian Academy of Science, Daróczi ut 24, Budapest H-1113, Hungary

Abstract. The human P glycoprotein (Pgp; MDR1) is an ATP-driven transporter for hydrophobic drugs and causes multidrug resistance in cancer. Our knowledge related to the mechanistic details of the ATP hydrolytic cycle of MDR1 has recently significantly progressed due to studies on the formation of a catalytic intermediate (occluded nucleotide state). According to the most accepted current model, both catalytic sites in MDR1 are active and ATP is hydrolysed alternatively within the two sites. ATP hydrolysis at one site triggers conformational changes within the protein resulting in drug transport, while hydrolysis of a second ATP molecule (at the other site) is required for resetting the initial ('high-affinity binding') conformation. The two active sites act in a cooperative manner and experiments support a model where the two ATP binding cassette (ABC) domains form a coupled catalytic machinery. Although no high resolution structure is available as yet, some relevant structural information can be deduced from crystal structures obtained for several bacterial ABC units, and the recently solved bacterial ABC–ABC dimer crystal structures may provide the basis for a better understanding of the intramolecular cross-talk between the two catalytic sites. As intramolecular interactions between various domains of Pgp/MDR1 are essential in regulating both the ATPase and transport activity, compounds perturbing these interactions may interfere with the function of the transporter. Such compounds, as well as various substrate analogues may be useful in modulating multidrug resistance in cancer.

2002 Mechanisms of drug resistance in epilepsy: lessons from oncology. Wiley, Chichester (Novartis Foundation Symposium 243) p 54–68

The MDR phenomenon: transporters involved

Chemotherapy is often ineffective in the treatment of cancer; the tumour cells of a large number of patients are either inherently drug-resistant or a drug-resistant phenotype may develop during the treatment. It is generally accepted that in the majority of the cases the molecular basis of multidrug resistance (MDR) is the overexpression of the so-called multidrug transporters. Elevated expression of these proteins was found in drug-resistant tumour cells of patients as well as in cell lines exposed to selection by increasing concentration of cytotoxic compounds. At the time of writing, it is well established that there are three major multidrug transporter proteins contributing to the MDR phenotype: P glycoprotein (Pgp; also known as multidrug resistance protein [MDR1] or ABCB1, according to the Gene Nomenclature Database (*http://www.gene.ucl.ac.uk/cgi-bin/nomenclature/searchgenes.pl*); the multidrug resistance-associated protein 1 (MRP1/ABCC1); and the breast cancer resistance protein (BCRP/ABCG2). The multidrug transporters belong to the ATP binding cassette (ABC) protein family, and other members of this family (MDR3/ABCB4, MRP2/ABCC2, MRP3/ABCC3 and MRP5/ABCC5) were also linked to multidrug resistance, though their role in conferring this phenotype remains to be clarified. (The lung resistance-related protein/major vault protein, which may be associated to multidrug resistance, is not an ABC transporter.)

ABC proteins form one of the largest families in each genome studied. ABC proteins are defined by the presence of the ABC unit, a 200–250 amino acid 'mini' protein, which harbours two short, conserved peptide motifs (Walker A and Walker B), both are involved in ATP binding, and are present in many other ATP-utilizing proteins (Walker et al 1982). A third conserved sequence, which is diagnostic to the entire family is located between the Walker A and B, and it is called the 'ABC signature'.

Most ABC proteins are active membrane transporters, and they transport various substrates to various compartments, explaining the wide spectrum of functions fulfilled by these proteins in different organisms. Although the majority of the known ABC proteins are active pumps (i.e. they perform transport against the concentration gradient of the substrate) there are exceptions: the cystic fibrosis transmembrane conductance regulator (CFTR) is a chloride channel that also regulates other membrane proteins. The sulfonyl urea receptors, SUR1/ABCC8 and SUR2/ABCC9, are best described as intracellular ATP sensors regulating the permeability of K^+ channels (with which they form transmembrane complexes).

Being membrane transporters also implies that this class of molecules contains membrane-embedded/transmembrane domains (TMDs). These TMDs are usually composed of six TM helices, and the minimal structural requirement of an active ABC transporter seems to be two TMDs and two ABC units. These may be within one polypeptide chain ('full transporters'), or in a membrane-bound multi-protein complex. Various arrangements of the TMD and ABC domains can be observed among the human ABC proteins, and the domain arrangements of MDR1, MRP1 and BCRP are shown in Fig. 1.

MDR1/Pgp

MDR1/Pgp, the first human ABC protein cloned (Chen et al 1986, Gros et al 1986) remains to be one of the most intensively studied proteins of the ABC family.

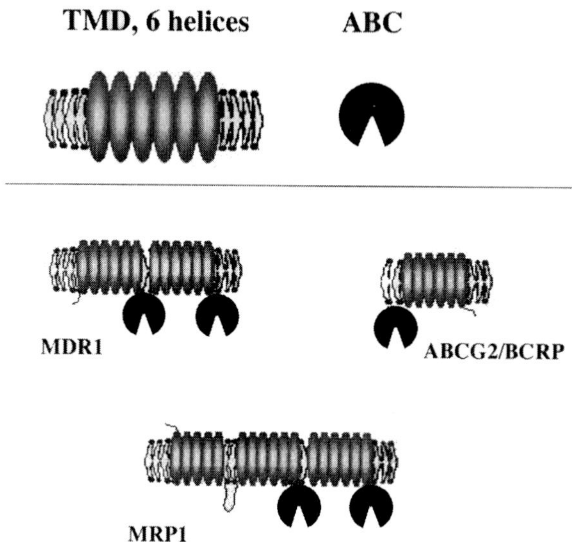

FIG. 1. Basic domains of the ABC transporters (upper panel) and the domain arrangements of MDR1, BCRP and MRP1 (lower panel). The membrane-embedded structures of the transporters are shown; extracellular is upwards.

MDR1 is localized in the plasma membrane, at the apical (or luminal) surface of polarized epithelial cells of the intestine and the proximal tubules of kidney, or in the biliary canalicular membrane of hepatocytes (Thiebaut et al 1987, van Helvoort et al 1996). MDR1 expression colocalizes with certain pharmacological barriers of the body, such as the blood–brain barrier (Cordon-Cardo et al 1989) and the choroid plexus (Rao et al 1999).

The MDR1 protein is a highly promiscuous transporter for a large variety of hydrophobic compounds, although with different affinities. The physiological function of MDR1 has been best studied in a knockout mouse model, after disrupting one or both of the *Mdr1* genes (Schinkel et al 1994, 1997). (Mice have two MDR1-like genes (*Mdr1a* and *Mdr1b*) with similar functions, and the expression of the two mice proteins covers the pattern of the single human MDR1). Although the *Mdr1a+b* knockout mice were viable and fertile with no obvious physiological abnormalities, careful analysis showed that mice lacking both MDR-like transporters were hypersensitive to xenobiotic compounds. On the basis of its localization and ability to mediate the vectorial transport of a range of toxic molecules, the general conclusion was that MDR1 is involved in the protection of the body against xenobiotic compounds.

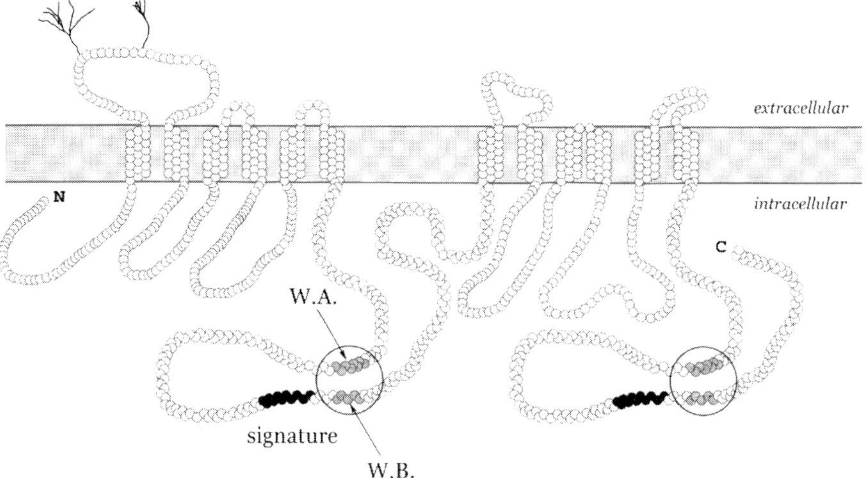

FIG. 2.   The membrane topology model of MDR1. The conserved motifs, Walker A (W.A.), Walker B (W.B.) and the ABC signature, as well as the N- (N) and C-termini (C) are indicated.

Structural considerations

Unfortunately, there is no high-resolution three-dimensional structure available for any of the mammalian ABC transporters, or for their separate transmembrane or ABC domains as yet. A low-resolution structure (2.5 nm) of MDR1, determined by electron microscopy and single particle image analysis, has been published (Rosenberg et al 1997). According to this model, MDR1 is embedded into the membrane as a 10×8 nm cylinder with a large central pore about 5 nm in diameter, which is closed at the inner (cytoplasmic) face of the membrane. The model also predicts an opening from this cylinder to the lipid phase (Fig. 2).

Drug-binding site

The site(s) in MDR1 interacting with the drug-substrates are presumably encoded in the transmembrane domains. It seems that several structural elements of the TMDs create the drug-substrate interacting region, which was shown to mediate drug binding even in the absence of ABC domains (Loo & Clarke 1999). Detailed mutagenesis as well as photochemical labelling with reactive drug-derivatives revealed that transmembrane helices 5 and 6 (in the N-proximal transmembrane domain) and helices 11 and 12 (in the C-proximal transmembrane domain), as well as the short cytoplasmic loops connecting these helices are involved in the formation of an extended drug-binding site.

Presently it is unknown how MDR1 can bind such a great variety of chemically dissimilar lipophilic cationic compounds. On the basis of the crystal structure of the multidrug-binding domain of BmrR, a transcription activator from *Bacillus subtilis*, a possible mechanism for the binding of cationic lipophilic drugs by multidrug transporters was proposed (Zheleznova et al 1999). A drug-induced conformational change in the activator uncovers a buried charged residue and allows access to multiple hydrophobic residues in the substrate-binding pocket. An analogous mechanism of drug–protein interaction may be the basis of the 'promiscuity' of MDR1.

ABC domains

Drug transport by MDR1 requires energy from ATP hydrolysis. ATP hydrolysis is catalysed by the active sites localized in the ABC domains. The three-dimensional structures of several bacterial ABC units have been determined by X-ray crystallography in the past three years (HisP, Hung et al 1998; RbsA, Armstrong et al 1998; Rad50cd, Hopfner et al 2000; MalK, Diederich et al 2000). Comparison of these structures reveals an almost identical fold. This unique 'ABC fold' has an overall shape of an 'L', with two lobes or arms. The larger structure (lobe A or arm I) is composed of mostly β strands; lobe B (arm II) is mainly α helical. The nucleotide binds to a site that is formed by the β strands of arm I/lobe A and the adenine ring is involved in hydrophobic interactions with the protein. The nucleotide binding sites appear as shallow, more-or-less open grooves, forming rather atypical active sites, as compared to the structure of other ATPases. The conserved peptide motifs of the ABC domains are involved in creating the binding site: the glycine-rich loop of Walker A segment is in contact with the phosphate moiety (P loop), and the side-chains of the Walker B segment play a crucial role in the co-ordination of Mg^{2+}. On the basis of these structures, homology models of the human and other mammalian MDR1 ABC domains have been built and mutations have been designed. The analysis of these mutants led to the identification of the role of several conserved residues in catalysis (Urbatsch et al 2000a,b).

ATP hydrolytic cycle

Interaction with the drug substrate significantly enhances the basal ATPase activity of MDR1 ('drug-stimulated ATPase activity'; Sarkadi et al 1992, Ambudkar et al 1992) through molecular interaction between the TMDs and the ABCs. The transported drug-substrates increase the rate of ATP cleavage, without altering the K_m value (ATP) of the catalytic reaction. An elegant kinetic model of MDR1 ATP hydrolysis has recently been published (Krupka 1999), in which several unusual features (wide substrate-specificity, loose connection between ATP hydrolysis and drug transport) is discussed.

Assaying the drug-stimulated ATPase activity of MDR1 provides an experimental strategy to study drug–transporter interactions. The ATP hydrolytic cycle of MDR1 can be described by the following series of reactions (based on the model of Senior et al 1995, and Senior & Gatsby 1997).

$$MDR1 + MgATP \leftrightarrow MDR1 \cdot MgATP \leftrightarrow MDR1 \cdot MgADP \cdot P_i \leftrightarrow MDR1 \cdot MgADP$$
$$+ P_i \leftrightarrow MDR1 + MgADP + P_i$$

The transport and ATPase cycle of MDR1 is inhibited by vanadate, which stabilizes a transition state intermediate of the ATPase cycle, with an occluded nucleotide in the catalytic sites within the ABCs (Urbatsch et al 1995a,b):

$$MDR1 + MgATP \leftrightarrow MDR1 \cdot MgATP \leftrightarrow MDR1 \cdot MgADP \cdot P_i \leftrightarrow MDR1 \cdot MgADP$$
$$+ P_i \; (\leftrightarrow MDR1 + MgADP + P_i)$$
$$\updownarrow$$
$$\boxed{MDR1 \cdot MgADP \cdot V_i}$$

The MDR1·MgADP·V$_i$ complex most probably represents a high-energy transition state intermediate. This occluded ('trapped') nucleotide state can be visualized by covalent photoaffinity labelling, using $\alpha[^{32}P]$azido-ATP (which is an efficient energy donor substrate of the MDR1 transporter). Other anions, like BeF$_x$ and AlF$_4$ were also shown to inhibit the MDR1 ATPase catalytic cycle by trapping a nucleotide in the catalytic centre.

The individual steps of ATP hydrolysis can be studied by experiments with azidoATP. ATP binding, the first step of the interaction between the transporter and the catalytic substrate can be investigated under conditions that prohibit hydrolysis. Binding of MgATP and the drug substrates are independent processes (Cornwell et al 1987). MDR1 binds MgATP with a relatively low affinity (K_d is approx. 200–500 μM); the binding affinities of the two ABC domains are similar, and the protein can be saturated by two ATP molecules.

Bound ATP is rapidly hydrolysed by the wild-type MDR1 at 37 °C, in a process which involves the formation of a transition state complex. The complex — containing an occluded nucleotide in the catalytic site — can be stabilized by phosphate-mimicking anions like vanadate, AlF$_4$ or BeF$_x$ (Urbatsch et al 1995a,b, Sankaran et al 1997a,b). These anions occupy the place of the terminal phosphate and inhibit the MDR1 catalytic activity by stabilizing the occluded nucleotide complex. By following the transition state formation ('trapping activity') it is possible to gain insight into the initial phase of the catalytic cycle.

Similarly to the ATPase activity of MDR1, the rate of the vanadate- (Szabó et al 1998, Shepard et al 1998) as well as the AlF$_4$- or BeF$_x$-dependent (Szakács et al 2000) nucleotide occlusion is greatly accelerated by the transported drug substrates. This is consistent with a model where substrate recognition increases the rate of the transition state formation, the rate-limiting step of the catalytic cycle.

It has been shown recently, that the MDR1·MgADP·V$_i$ complex (i.e. the enzyme in the transition state) exhibits a dramatically reduced binding affinity for the transported drug substrate, as compared to the MDR1·MgATP complex (Sauna & Ambudkar 2000). This observation suggests that the hydrolytic step triggers conformational changes, which reduce drug binding to the binding site (and presumably makes drug binding to another site more favourable, from which the drug can then be released to the extracellular space). It was also demonstrated that hydrolysis of a second ATP molecule is required for conformational changes to reset the transporter to the high affinity drug-binding conformation. On the basis of the above results the stoichiometry of two ATP molecules/each transported drug substrate is suggested.

Intramolecular interactions regulating activity

Several lines of evidence indicate that both catalytic sites of MDR1 are active and the two ABC domains enter into the catalytic cycle alternatively (Hrycyna et al 1998a). The integrity of both of the catalytic domains is required for transport and ATPase activity. It was found that mutations in either ATP-binding sites prevent ATP hydrolysis and drug transport (Azzaria et al 1989, Müller et al 1996) as well as vanadate-dependent nucleotide occlusion (Szabó et al 1998, Urbatsch et al 1998). We have shown earlier that the replacement of a lysine residue with methionine in the catalytic Walker A motif in either ABC domains of the human MDR1 (K433M and K1076M) eliminated drug-stimulated ATPase activity, while these mutants could still bind ATP (Müller et al 1996). It was also demonstrated that several unilateral mutations, targeted to the evolutionarily conserved ABC-signature region of any of the ABC-domains, are accompanied with the loss of ATPase activity, while the ATP-binding activity was preserved in these mutants (Bakos et al 1997, Szakács et al 2001).

Interaction between the two halves of the MDR1 is crucial for the drug-stimulated ATPase and drug-transport activity of the transporter. This functional interaction was shown to be dependent on the flexibility of the region connecting the two halves of the MDR1 protein (Hrycyna et al 1998b). It was also demonstrated that the ABC domains expressed as individual polypeptides possessed very low ATPase activity (Sharma & Rose 1995, Wang et al 1999). The most plausible interpretation of the above findings is that the ATP sites within the MDR1 protein are very poor ATPases, unless they can interact with each other.

In our recent work we have studied the transition state formation in catalytically incompetent Walker A mutants of MDR1 (Szakács et al 2000). We have found that the inactivating mutations (K to M at positions 433 or 1076) targeted to either of the ABC domains, still allowed transition state complex formation when stabilized by AlF_4 or BeF_x. In these mutants the stimulatory effect of drugs on the transition state formation was also preserved. The finding that the ATPase-deficient mutants are engaged in the early steps of the catalytic cycle allowed us to explore the involvement of the mutated and 'wild-type' ATP sites in the transition state formation. We found that — regardless of the mutations — both catalytic sites trapped adenine nucleotides. The results of this study show that the unilateral mutations have the same effect on both sites: the N-terminal mutation results in an altered conformation, and this minute alteration of the mutated active centre is 'propagated' to the other (native) catalytic site. Furthermore, the C-terminal mutation has the same effect on the N-terminal site, suggesting a bidirectional cross-talk between the two catalytic centres. All these results are in favour of a model where catalysis at the two ABC units is intimately linked through extensive molecular interactions between the two ABC domains.

As mentioned above, interaction with the transported drugs enhances the catalytic ATPase activity of MDR1. Thus an allosteric control of the drugs' effects on the ATPase activity requires intramolecular interaction between the drug binding and the catalytic regions of the protein. The mechanism by which the transported drugs accelerate ATP hydrolysis is presently unknown. In order to study the role of a universally conserved glycine residue in the fourth position of the MDR1 signature region in each ABC domain (Gly534 and Gly1179 of the LSGG segments), we have generated MDR1 variants containing valine or aspartate at these positions. We found that these mutations abolished the ATPase activity of the protein but still allowed the formation of a transition state intermediate of the ATP hydrolytic cycle (Szakács et al 2001). In these mutants, in contrast to the wild-type MDR1, the transported drug substrates inhibited this partial reaction. Our results showed that mutations of the conserved glycine residue in the fourth position of the LSGG motifs of either ABC domains resulted in an error in the allosteric control of the ATPase activity upon drug binding.

The lack of a high-resolution structure limits the better understanding of the mechanism of these important intramolecular interactions (between the two ABC-domains and between the drug binding and the catalytic sites) that regulate MDR1 activity. At present, there are three different models for the arrangement of the ABC domains in the ABC–ABC dimers. The first model predicts the MDR1-ABCs to adopt the dimeric assembly that was found in the HisP crystal structure (Hung et al 1998), with the monomers arranged in a back-to-back position. The ATP-interacting sites (active sites) in this HisP dimer are in an exposed, peripheral location, practically excluding direct interaction between the two sites.

The other model, proposed on the basis of the crystallographic study of an alternative HisP dimer and on extensive sequence alignments (Jones & George 1999), suggests that the ABCs dimerize in a way that each ABC signature sequence interacts with the ATP molecule bound in the opposite monomer.

The same arrangement was seen in the crystal structure of the catalytic ABC ATPase domain of Rad50 of *Pyrococcus furiosus*, a core element of the DNA double-strand break repair complex (Hopfner et al 2000). The structure represents two functionally interacting ABC subunits with a 'head to tail' orientation. In the ATP-bound form, both subunits bind one MgATP molecule, and the two ATPs are buried in the dimer interface. In this dimeric structure the two ABC subunits complement each other's active sites: the Walker A segment (P loop) of one Rad50cd subunit and the ABC signature motif of the opposite Rad50cd subunit are involved in the formation of a single ATP-binding site. The ATP hydrolytic sites (catalytic sites) in this dimer are completely buried, resembling the nucleotide binding sites of other ATPases/GTPases. A recent report indicates that the distance between the Walker A motifs of the two ABC domains within MDR1 is 16–22 Å (Qu & Sharom 2001), and this result is in harmony with the Rad50cd-based model.

The crystal structure of MalK, the ABC-ATPase dimer of the maltose transporter of an archaeon *Thermococcus litoralis* shows an alternative dimer structure in which the two ABC subunits are oriented 'head to head' (Diederichs et al 2000), with significant deviation from the twofold symmetry. Residues of the Walker A region (P loop) interact with the α and β phosphate of the bound nucleotide at the inter-subunit interface. The ABC signature segments are located far from the active sites.

In the present paper we have paid special attention to the interdomain interactions regulating MDR1 activity. By using a combination of primary structural data and model-building strategies with mutagenesis we hope to soon be able to map the contact interfaces between the domains. These contacts should be considered as targets for drug design, and compounds perturbing these interactions may inhibit MDR1-mediated drug extrusion.

Acknowledgements

This work has been supported by research grants from OMFB, OTKA, and ETT, Hungary (D32847, T022072, T029921, F023655). G. Szakács is a recipient of a Soros Predoctoral Fellowship. É. Bakos is supported by an OTKA postdoctoral fellowship. B. Sarkadi is a recipient of a Howard Hughes International Scholarship. Artwork was prepared by G. Tusnády.

References

Ambudkar SV, Lelong IH, Zhang J, Cardarelli CO, Gottesman MM, Pastan I 1992 Partial purification and reconstitution of the human multidrug-resistance pump: characterization of the drug-stimulatable ATP hydrolysis. Proc Natl Acad Sci USA 89:8472–8476

Armstrong S, Tabemero L, Zhang H, Hermodsen M, Stauffacher C 1998 Powering the ABC transporters: the 2.5A of the ABC domain of RbsA. Pediatr Pulmonol 17:91–93

Azzaria M, Schurr E, Gros P 1989 Discrete mutations introduced in the predicted nucleotide-binding sites of the mdr1 gene abolish its ability to confer multidrug resistance. Mol Cell Biol 9:5289–5297

Bakos É, Klein I, Welker E et al 1997 Characterization of the human multidrug resistance protein containing mutations in the ATP-binding cassette signature region. Biochem J 323: 777–783

Chen CJ, Chin JE, Ueda K et al 1986 Internal duplication and homology with bacterial transport proteins in the mdr1 (P-glycoprotein) gene from multidrug-resistant human cells. Cell 47:381–389

Cordon-Cardo C, O'Brien JP, Casals D et al 1989 Multidrug-resistance gene (P-glycoprotein) is expressed by endothelial cells at blood-brain barrier sites. Proc Natl Acad Sci USA 86:695–698

Cornwell MM, Tsuruo T, Gottesman MM, Pastan I 1987 ATP-binding properties of P glycoprotein from multidrug-resistant KB cells. FASEB J 1:51–54

Diederichs K, Diez J, Greller G et al 2000 Crystal structure of MalK, the ATPase subunit of the trehalose/maltose ABC transporter of the archaeon *Thermococcus litoralis*. EMBO J 19: 5951–5961

Gros P, Croop J, Housman D 1986 Mammalian multidrug resistance gene: complete cDNA sequence indicates strong homology to bacterial transport proteins. Cell 47:371–380

Hopfner KP, Karcher A, Shin DS et al 2000 Structural biology of the Rad50 ATPase. ATP-driven conformational control in DNA double-strand break repair and the ABC-ATPase superfamily. Cell 101:789–800

Hrycyna CA, Ramachandra M, Ambudkar SV et al 1998a Mechanism of action of human P-glycoprotein ATPase activity: photochemical cleavage during a catalytic transition state using othovanadate reveals cross-talk between the two ATP sites. J Biol Chem 273: 16631–16634

Hrycyna CA, Airan LE, Germann UA, Ambudkar SV, Pastan I, Gottesman MM 1998b Structural flexibility of the linker region of human P-glycoprotein permits ATP hydrolysis and drug transport. Biochemistry 37:13660–13673

Hung LW, Wang IX, Nikaido K, Liu PQ, Ames GF, Kim SH 1998 Crystal structure of the ATP-binding subunit of an ABC transporter. Nature 396:703–707

Jones PM, George AM 1999 Subunit interactions in ABC transporters: towards a functional architecture. FEMS Microbiol Lett 179:187–202

Klein I, Sarkadi B, Váradi A 1999 An inventory of the human ABC proteins. Biochim Biophys Acta 1461:237–262

Krupka RM 1999 Uncoupled active transport mechanisms accounting for low selectivity in multidrug carriers: P-glycoprotein and SMR antiporters. J Membr Biol 127:129–143

Loo TW, Clarke DM 1999 The transmembrane domains of the human multidrug resistance P-glycoprotein are sufficient to mediate drug binding and trafficking to the cell surface. J Biol Chem 274:24759–24765

Müller M, Bakos É, Welker E et al 1996 Altered drug-stimulated ATPase activity in mutants of the human multidrug resistance protein. J Biol Chem 271:1877–1883

Qu Q, Sharom SJ 2001 FRET Analysis indicates that the two ATPase active sites of the P-glycoprotein multidrug transporter are closely associated. Biochemistry 40:1413–1422

Rao VV, Dahlheimer JL, Bardgett ME et al 1999 Choroid plexus epithelial expression of *MDR1* P glycoprotein and multidrug resistance-associated protein contribute to the blood-cerebrospinal-fluid drug-permeability barrier. Proc Natl Acad Sci USA 96:3900–3905

Rosenberg MF, Callaghan R, Ford RC, Higgins CF 1997 Structure of the multidrug resistance P-glycoprotein to 2.5 nm resolution determined by electron microscopy and image analysis. J Biol Chem 272:10685–10694

Sankaran B, Bhagat S, Senior AE 1997a Inhibition of P-glycoprotein ATPase activity by procedures involving trapping of nucleotide in catalytic sites. Arch Biochem Biophys 341:160–169

Sankaran B, Bhagat S, Senior AE 1997b Inhibition of P-glycoprotein ATPase activity by beryllium fluoride. Biochemistry 36:6847–6853

Sarkadi B, Price EM, Boucher RC, Germann UA, Scarborough GA 1992 Expression of the human multidrug resistance cDNA in insect cells generates a high activity drug-stimulated membrane ATPase. J Biol Chem 267:4854–4858

Sauna ZE, Ambudkar SV 2000 Evidence for a requirement for ATP hydrolysis at two distinct steps during a single turnover of the catalytic cycle of human P-glycoprotein. Proc Natl Acad Sci USA 97:2515–2520

Schinkel AH, Smit JJ, van Tellingen O et al 1994 Disruption of the mouse mdr1a P-glycoprotein gene leads to a deficiency in the blood-brain barrier and to increased sensitivity to drugs. Cell 77:491–502

Schinkel AH, Mayer U, Wagenaar E et al 1997 Normal viability and altered pharmacokinetics in mice lacking mdr1-type (drug-transporting) P-glycoproteins. Proc Natl Acad Sci USA 94:4028–4033

Senior AE, Al-Shawi MK, Urbatsch IL 1995 The catalytic cycle of P-glycoprotein. FEBS Lett 377:285–289

Senior AE, Gadsby DC 1997 ATP hydrolysis cycles and mechanism in P-glycoprotein and CFTR. Semin Cancer Biol 8:143–150

Sharma S, Rose DR 1995 Cloning, overexpression, purification, and characterization of the carboxyl-terminal nucleotide binding domain of P-glycoprotein. J Biol Chem 270:14085–14093

Shepard RL, Winter MA, Hsaio SC, Pearce HL, Beck WT, Dantzig AH 1998 Effect of modulators on the ATPase activity and vanadate nucleotide trapping of human P-glycoprotein. Biochem Pharmacol 56:719–727

Szabó K, Welker E, Bakos É et al 1998 Drug-stimulated nucleotide trapping in the human multidrug transporter MDR1: cooperation of the nucleotide binding domains. J Biol Chem 273:10132–10138

Szakács G, Özvegy CS, Bakos É, Sarkadi B, Váradi A 2000 Transition-state formation in ATPase-negative mutants of human MDR1 protein. Biochem Biophys Res Commun 276:1314–1319

Szakács G, Özvegy CS, Bakos É, Sarkadi B, Váradi A 2001 Role of the conserved Gly residue in the ABC-signature motif of human MDR1 in the drug-induced allosteric control of ATPase activity. Biochem J 356:71–75

Thiebaut F, Tsuruo T, Hamada H, Gottesman MM, Pastan I, Willingham MC 1987 Cellular localization of the multidrug-resistance gene product P-glycoprotein in normal human tissues. Proc Natl Acad Sci USA 84:7735–7738

Urbatsch IL, Gimi K, Wilke-Mounts S, Senior AE 2000a Conserved Walker A Ser residues in the catalytic sites of P-glycoprotein are critical for catalysis and involved primarily at the transition state step. J Biol Chem 275:25031–25038

Urbatsch IL, Gimi K, Wilke-Mounts S, Senior AE 2000b Investigation of the role of glutamine-471 and glutamine-1114 in the two catalytic sites of P-glycoprotein. Biochemistry 39:11921–11927

Urbatsch IL, Beaudet L, Carrier I, Gros P 1998 Mutations in either nucleotide-binding site of P-glycoprotein (mdr3) prevent vanadate trapping of nucleotide at both sites. Biochemistry 37:4592–4602

Urbatsch IL, Sankaran B, Weber J, Senior AE 1995a P-glycoprotein is stably inhibited by vanadate-induced trapping of nucleotide at a single catalytic site. J Biol Chem 270:19383–19390

Urbatsch IL, Sankaran B, Bhagat S, Senior AE 1995b Both P-glycoprotein nucleotide-binding
    sites are catalytically active. J Biol Chem 270:26956–26961
van Helvoort A, Smith A J, Sprong H et al 1996 MDR1 P-glycoprotein is a lipid translocase of
    broad specificity, while MDR3 P-glycoprotein specifically translocates phosphatidylcholine.
    Cell 87:507–517
Walker JE, Saraste M, Runswick M J, Gay N J 1982 Distantly related sequences in the alpha- and
    beta-subunits of ATP synthase, myoisn, kinases and other ATP-requiring enzymes and a
    common nucleotide binding fold. EMBO J 1:945–951
Wang C, Castro FA, Wilkes DM, Altenberg G A 1999 Expression and purification of the first
    nucleotide-binding domain and linker region of human multidrug resistance gene product:
    comparison of fusions to gluthation S-transferase, thioredoxin and maltose-binding protein.
    Biochem J 338:77–81
Zheleznova EE, Markham PN, Neyfakh AA, Brennan RG 1999 Structural basis of multidrug
    recognition by BmrR, a transcription activator of a multidrug transporter. Cell 96:353–336

DISCUSSION

Ling: Could your model of the transition states be used as a general model to test
anti-epileptic drugs (AEDs) to see whether they will interact with a molecule and
potentially be substrates?

Varadi: Yes, I think it could be a general model. One problem is that it is not a
cheap analytical technique, because the reagent is rather expensive. Drugs or
compounds interacting with a transporter can be studied, but you won't be able
to tell from a single labelling experiment whether it is a good drug or a good
inhibitor that is interacting with the drug binding site. You can get more-or-less
the same information about the drug from the ATPase activity. This measures the
whole cycle. If there is a drug that arrests the cycle at an 'inhibited' stage, it cannot
stimulate the ATPase activity because you are measuring many cycles. In the
transition state formation, what we observe is nothing more than the first
turnover. We cannot complete the first turnover, and we arrest the protein in the
transition state. Whatever happens before this state can be separated from all the
events that follow. I think there are drugs such as cyclosporin A that inhibit
ATPase but stimulate this nucleotide trapping reaction. The reason for this is
that the inhibition target of cyclosporin A comes into play after the transition
state formation.

Bates: My understanding is that the compounds that stimulate ATPase and are
inhibitors actually have a rapid diffusion back through the membrane, so that the
pump is continually in use and therefore unavailable for other substrates. This is
the theory for verapamil. Thus, the inhibitors that stimulate ATPase are very good
substrates.

Varadi: But you can measure other inhibitors that stimulate transition state
formation because they act on the primary drug binding site, if one supposes that

the information comes from there. But they leave the enzyme very slowly. Therefore the whole cycle slows down.

Bates: That is a description for non-competitive inhibition (Litman et al 1997). Some of the third-generation Pgp inhibitors are non-competitive — they have a very high affinity and they tend to inhibit the ATPase activity.

Varadi: But they can easily stimulate the transition state formation.

Ling: Perhaps I can phrase the question in another way. If you find a drug that does not affect the transition state assay, could you conclude that it is not a Pgp-interacting molecule?

Varadi: That is possible. If this drug just sits somewhere outside and blocks the off-site, and if we suppose this is accessible from the outside, then it will never interact with the pathway I described, yet it can still block Pgp. Theoretically this is a possibility. The other question is whether this so-called off-site, where the drug is released, is accessible from outside the cell. This is not clear. Most probably it is not.

Bates: There is a conformational change that occurs when the drug binding site in Pgp moves from the on-site to the off-site. I think you could design an experiment where you have the inhibitor on a bead, so that it sits on the outside of the cell. There are antibody experiments that show inhibition without the drug binding at the binding sites.

Scheper: There is an antibody that shows the conformational change after binding.

Bates: That is the UIC2 (Mechetner et al 1997). Furthermore MRK-16 may actually inhibit the conformational change when it inhibits Pgp activity (Vasudevan et al 1998).

Varadi: It would be a good idea to try these experiments, using inhibitory antibodies that inhibit the whole cycle.

Vezzani: Is there any mutation that provokes a gain-of-function in the Pgp pump?

Varadi: There was one naturally occurring mutation detected back in the late 1980s. There is also a similar situation in BCRP; this is a mutation in an intracellular loop. It triggers a change in the activity of the pump such that colchicine became a better substrate of MDR1.

Bates: I don't think that you would want to use ATPase activity as a definitive test of whether or not an AED is a substrate.

Ling: I didn't think that I would. There is still an issue about the different ways of asking the question as to whether a drug could potentially be a Pgp substrate.

Bates: The advantage of using it as a screen, of course, is that then you don't have to use the more cumbersome cytotoxicity assay, and you don't have to radiolabel every drug for drug accumulation assays. The ATPase assay could be a first-level screen for all 20 AED drugs.

Newman: When you look at ATPase activity, would the prediction be that a substrate should stimulate ATPase activity?

Varadi: Yes. But it is not only a 'yes' or 'no' answer; you could measure the K_m values.

Sander: Have all the AEDs been tested?

Löscher: There are very few studies on this.

Sills: We have preliminary data on eight AEDs, four established drugs (phenytoin, carbamazepine, phenobarbitone, sodium valproate) and also four newer drugs (gabapentin, lamotrigine, vigabatrin, topiramate). Of the eight, topiramate stands out as the most likely candidate. I wouldn't like to say any more than this, given the preliminary nature of the data, but the results are encouraging.

Pirmohamed: We have looked at carbamazepine in three different systems, and we can't find it acting as a substrate for Pgp.

Newman: We do see some potential for that in one system.

Kwan: I would like to comment from the clinical epileptologist's perspective. My impression reading through the literature about Pgp in oncology is that its mechanism of action is still unknown. From the epileptologist's point of view, we don't know the mechanisms of action of the AEDs. It would be nice if the structural chemists from the oncology side can help us to work out whether the AEDs are likely Pgp substrates based on their structures and properties. There are some 15 or 16 available AEDs and we don't want to screen them all in these different systems: it would take a very long time.

Bates: That is true, but in the time it would take to go through the structures, you could do the ATPase assay.

Ling: Perhaps it would help to have a historical perspective: how were the first AEDs discovered?

Sander: The first AED discovered was bromide, which was found because the French were using bromides in the army for some other reason (see Scott 1993). Locock then recognized this; he thought that epilepsy was a form of hysteria, so he used bromides to treat his female patients with epilepsy. He reported that it worked. A trial from the late 1940s showed that this is as effective as phenobarbitone, which was the second drug. This came out in 1912. The story goes that a registrar in psychiatry in Freiburg, Germany called Hauptman, used a new sleeping pill called luminal. Using the old doctor's trick of when you can't sleep put someone else to sleep, he went down to the ward where they had patients with epilepsy (his quarters were above the ward). About three months later he noticed that these patients were much better. This was the first modern AED. The next drug was phenytoin in 1936. This was supposed to be the first drug screened using the electroshock model. They wrote to all the pharmaceutical companies in the Boston area asking for any drugs that look like phenobarbitone. The first drug to arrive was phenytoin. They discovered it was effective in 1936, the work was published in early 1937 and the drug was on the market in late 1937. After phenytoin's discovery, everyone started screening drugs. They screened thousands of compounds in animal models for epilepsy. The next drug came from France, which was sodium valproate. This was followed by carbamazepine, which was developed as an antidepressant.

Löscher: Researchers optimized thousands of structures after finding phenytoin, because now they had a model of the disease. This model probably preselected a certain category of drugs.

Deisz: May I add that the cellular mechanisms of phenytoin and other first-generation AEDs are not fully understood. To the best of my knowledge, phenytoin has not been investigated in human epileptogenic tissue, for example. We demonstrated a prolongation and enhancement of GABAergic inhibition by phenytoin (Deisz & Lux 1977). Subsequently such an effect was also shown to occur at mammalian $GABA_A$ receptors if the right composition of subunits is present (Granger et al 1995). Considering that the stoichiometry of $GABA_A$ receptors changes in an animal model during the development of epilepsy (Brooks-Kayal et al 1998), a potentiation of $GABA_A$ receptor function may be switched on or off during the course of epilepsy in a given array of neurons.

References

Brooks-Kayal AR, Shumate MD, Jin H, Rikhter TY, Coulter DA 1998 Selective changes in single cell $GABA_A$ receptor expression in temporal lobe epilepsy. Nat Med 4:1166–1172

Deisz RA, Lux HD 1977 Diphenylhydantoin prolongs post-synaptic inhibition and iontophoretic GABA action in the crayfish stretch receptor. Neurosci Lett 5:199–203

Granger P, Biton B, Faure C et al 1995 Modulation of the γ-aminobutyric acid type A receptor by the antiepileptic drugs carbamazepine and phenytoin. Mol Pharmacol 47:1189–1196

Litman T, Zeuthen T, Skovsgaard T, Stein WD 1997 Competitive, non-competitive and cooperative interactions between substrates of P-glycoprotein as measured by its ATPase activity. Biochim Biophys Acta 1361:169–176

Mechetner EB, Schott B, Morse BS et al 1997 P-glycoprotein function involves conformational transitions detectable by differential immunoreactivity. Proc Natl Acad Sci USA 94:12908–12913

Scott DF 1993 History of epileptic therapy. Parthenon, New York

Vasudevan S, Tsuruo T, Rose DR 1998 Mode of binding of anti-P-glycoprotein antibody MRK-16 to its antigen. A crystallographic and molecular modeling study. J Biol Chem 273:25413–25419

Drug resistance caused by multidrug resistance-associated proteins

Jan Wijnholds

Department of Ophthalmogenetics, The Netherlands Ophthalmic Research Institute, Meibergdreef 47, 1105 BA, Amsterdam and Division of Molecular Biology, The Netherlands Cancer Institute, Plesmanlaan 121, 1066 CX, Amsterdam, The Netherlands

Abstract. Three types of drug efflux pumps, the multidrug resistance gene 1 (*MDR1* or *ABCB1*)-encoded P glycoprotein, the multidrug resistance-associated protein (MRP or ABCC1) and breast cancer resistance protein (BCRP or ABCG2) may play an important part in the intrinsic or acquired defence of cells against drugs. Recent studies have begun to show the broad tissue distribution and drug substrate specificity of the seven MRP family members (MRP1–7; or ABCC1–6 and ABCC10). MRPs are (multispecific) organic anion transporters, which can transport negatively charged anionic drugs and neutral drugs conjugated to glutathione, glucuronate or sulfate. MRP4 and MRP5 broaden the spectrum of drug resistance to nucleotide analogue drugs. Some MRPs can also transport neutral drugs if co-transported with glutathione. MRP1 and MRP5 are abundant in almost every organ and are prominently present in the brain. High levels of MRP1 are present in the epithelium of the choroid plexus. Using mutant mice lacking a functional *Mrp1* gene, we have previously shown the contribution of MRP1 to the blood–CSF (cerebrospinal fluid) drug permeability barrier. Recent studies indicate that the very low levels of MRP1 or MDR1 present in fibroblasts affect their sensitivity to a wide range of clinically important cytotoxic drugs. Even low concentrations of drug transporters may therefore protect cells against drugs.

2002 Mechanisms of drug resistance in epilepsy: lessons from oncology. Wiley, Chichester (Novartis Foundation Symposium 243) p 69–82

Drug efflux pumps are present in almost all tissues and cell types investigated. They are an important part of the defence of cells against cytotoxic and non-toxic drugs. Cole et al (1992) cloned the first multidrug resistance-associated protein gene, now called MRP1 or ABCC1. Currently, the MRP family consists of seven members called MRP1–7, or ABCC1–6 and ABCC10. The structural features of these plasma membrane transporters have been described in depth in reviews (Borst et al 2000, Hipfner et al 1999, Keppler et al 2000) and in bioinformatics papers on MRP3, MRP5 and MRP7 (Belinsky et al 1998, Hopper et al 2001). Some of these proteins are known by other names, as summarized in Table 1. The same table

TABLE 1   Abbreviations in use for members of the human multidrug resistance-associated protein (MRP) family and their main location in the body

Members	Other names	Main location in body	In polarized epithelia
MRP1	ABCC1 and MRP	Ubiquitous, high in choroid plexus	Basolateral
MRP2	ABCC2, cMOAT and cMRP	Liver, kidney and intestine	Apical
MRP3	ABCC3, MOAT-D and cMOAT-2	Liver, kidney, intestine, adrenal glands	Basolateral
MRP4	ABCC4 and MOAT-B	Prostate	?
MRP5	ABCC5, MOAT-C and pABC11	Ubiquitous, high in all brain segments	Basolateral
MRP6	ABCC6, MOAT-E and MLP-1	Liver and kidney	Unknown, but basolateral and apical for rat MRP6
MRP7	ABCC10	Low in all tissues tested	?

ABC, ATP-binding cassette; ABCC, C group of ABC transporters; MLP-1, MRP-like protein 1; MOAT, multispecific organic anion transporter; cMOAT, canalicular MOAT.

shows the main location of the MRP family members in the human body. The *in vivo* and *in vitro* functions of the MRPs are shown in Tables 2 and 3, respectively.

At least three of the MRP family members play a role in normal physiology and two members are associated with human disease. MRP2 is a canalicular multispecific organic anion transporter (cMOAT), and mutations lead to errors in biliary secretion resulting in the mild liver disease called Dubin–Johnson syndrome (Kartenbeck et al 1996, Paulusma et al 1997). MRP6 is an orphan transporter; its substrates are not well known (Kool et al 1999, Madon et al 2000). It is mainly expressed in the skin, liver and kidney, and mutations lead to a skin and eye disease called pseudoxanthoma elasticum (Bergen et al 2000, Le Saux et al 2000, Ringpfeil et al 2000). Mice without MRP1, the high affinity leukotriene C_4 transporter, have an altered response to inflammatory stimuli but are otherwise healthy and fertile (Wijnholds et al 1997, Robbiani et al 2000, Schultz et al 2001). The physiological roles of the other MRPs are not known.

MRP1, -2 and -3 have broad substrate specificities and can render cells resistant to anticancer drugs such as anthracyclins, epipodophyllotoxins and vinca alkaloids. Co-transport with glutathione is required for the transport of neutral drugs by MRP1 an MRP2 (Evers et al 2000, Loe et al 1998). MRP1, -2, and -3 can also transport organic anion substrates (e.g. methotrexate) or drugs conjugated to acidic ligands such as glutathione, glucuronate and sulfate (reviewed in Borst

TABLE 2 Demonstrated *in vivo* functions of human multidrug resistance proteins (MRPs)

MRP	In vivo function
MRP1	Transporter that mediates inflammation processes by the export of leukotriene C_4 from mast cells and macrophages. Drug permeability barrier activity at the blood–CSF and blood–testis barriers, due to its presence in choroid plexus and Sertoli cells, respectively. Protective drug efflux pump in epithelia (e.g. the urinary collecting duct, colon, and tongue and cheek), bone marrow and tumour cells.
MRP2	Transporter of organic anions (e.g. bilirubin glucuronides) from liver into bile. Transporter involved in the mild liver disease called Dubin–Johnson syndrome.
MRP3	?
MRP4	?
MRP5	?
MRP6	Transporter involved in the skin and eye disease pseudoxanthoma elasticum.
MRP7	?

TABLE 3 Demonstrated *in vitro* functions of human multidrug resistance proteins (MRPs)

MRP	In vitro function
MRP1	Transporter of glutathione-, glucuronide- and sulfate-conjugated substrates. Transporter of organic anions (e.g. methotrexate). Transporter of neutral multidrug resistance drugs and arsenite by co-transport with glutathione.
MRP2	Transporter of glutathione-, glucuronide- and sulfate-conjugated substrates. Transporter of organic anions (e.g. methotrexate). Transporter of neutral multidrug resistance drugs and cisplatin by co-transport with glutathione.
MRP3	Transporter of sulfate-, glucuronide- and glutathione-conjugated substrates. Transporter of organic anions (e.g. methotrexate) and glycocholate. Transporter of neutral multidrug resistance drugs (e.g. etoposide).
MRP4	Transporter of nucleotide (analogue) monophosphates.
MRP5	Transporter of organic anions (glutathione conjugates and fluorochromes). Transporter of nucleotide (analogue) monophosphates including cGMP.
MRP6	Transporter of anionic cyclic pentapeptides?
MRP7	?

et al 2000, Hipfner et al 1999, Keppler et al 2000). These transporters are able to transport conjugated drugs out of the cell. MRP5 has been shown to transport at least some glutathione conjugates such as dinitrophenyl glutathione (Wijnholds et al 2000a). For MRP4 and MRP7 this remains to be shown. MRP6 can transport an anionic pentapeptide but not the typical glutathione, glucuronide or sulfate conjugate substrates for MRP1, MRP2 and MRP3 (Madon et al 2000).

The drug resistance profiles for MRP4, -5, and -6 are not yet complete but seem to be less broad. However, MRP4 and -5 can mediate resistance to base and nucleotide analogues used as antiviral drugs and chemotherapeutics. These latter two transporters have been shown to be good transporters of a subclass of organic anions, that contains nucleotide monophosphates including guanosine $3',5'$-cyclic monophosphate or cGMP (Jedlitschky et al 2000, Schuetz et al 1999, Wijnholds et al 2000a). The substrate specificity of MRP7 is not known.

This paper will focus on the broadly expressed MRP family members, MRP1 and MRP5, that might have functions in the brain. The contribution of these transporters to drug resistance and to the protection of normal tissues will be discussed.

Protection of brain and testis tissues by MRP1

The contribution of the multidrug resistance gene 1 (*MDR1*)-encoded P glycoprotein to the protection of tissues (e.g. brain) has been clearly demonstrated. Analysis of mice lacking *Mdr1a* established an important role for MDR1a in the intestine, where it actively excretes drugs from the bloodstream into the intestinal lumen, and limits the entry of these MDR1 substrates from the intestinal lumen (for review see Schinkel 1999). The presence of MDR1 in the endothelium of the blood–brain capillaries protects the brain against the entry of substrate drugs, showing that MDR1 is an important contributor to the blood–brain barrier. In recent years, a significant contribution of MRP1 to the protection of several tissues, including the brain, could be demonstrated.

In order to characterize the normal physiological functions of MRP1, we generated mice that lack a functional *Mrp1* gene. These mice are healthy and fertile, have a normal lifespan and show no physiological, clinical or histological abnormalities under laboratory conditions. Therefore, inhibition of MRP1 in wild-type mice, and probably also in humans, would not lead to severe abnormalities. It cannot be excluded, however, that humans lacking MRP1 will show a phenotype due to, for example, a broad exposure to toxins in food and the use of drugs. As expected for a broad-specificity drug-efflux pump, *Mrp1* knockout mice show increased sensitivity to the anticancer drug etoposide (Lorico et al 1997, Wijnholds et al 1997). Analysis of these mice has demonstrated that a high level of MRP1 in the oropharyngeal mucosa protects against etoposide-induced oral mucositis caused by direct damage of the epithelium of the tongue and cheek. A high level of MRP1 in the epithelium of the urinary collecting ducts protects against etoposide-induced diabetes insipidus. High levels of MRP1 in the basal plasma membrane of the epithelium of the testicular tubules, the Sertoli cells, protects against the etoposide-induced abrogation of spermatogenesis. In fact, MRP1 is an important contributor to the blood–testis barrier (Wijnholds et al 1998), as MRP1 pumps the drugs back towards the blood. This latter finding prompted us to look at another blood–tissue barrier, the blood–CSF (cerebrospinal fluid) barrier since high levels of MRP1 were detected in the choroid plexus (Rao et al 1999, Wijnholds et al 2000b).

Whereas the blood–brain barrier is physically formed by the blood capillary endothelium in the brain, the blood–CSF barrier is formed by the epithelium of the choroid plexus. These epithelial cells are joined together by tight junctions, and drugs are forced to enter the epithelial cells to pass the barrier. The choroid plexus epithelium contains organic anion transporter proteins in the apical plasma membrane (e.g. OATP1), which may be responsible for the uptake of organic anions from the CSF into the choroid plexus (Angeletti et al 1997). *In vivo* transport studies suggested the existence of organic anion efflux pumps at the basolateral plasma membrane of the choroid plexus (Nishino et al 1999). MRP1 routes to the basolateral plasma membrane in all the epithelia analysed (Evers et al 1996, Wijnholds et al 1998), including the rat choroid plexus epithelium (Rao et al 1999). Therefore, MRP1 may be involved in the transport of organic anions from the choroid plexus epithelium towards the blood. Other experiments indicated the existence of a drug-permeability barrier for MRP1 substrates at the blood–CSF barrier. Murine MRP1 is localized in the basolateral membrane of the choroid plexus epithelium indicating that it may limit the entry of drugs into the CSF, whereas P glycoprotein is localized subapically indicating that it may transport drugs into the CSF (Rao et al 1999).

To explore the transport function of MRP1 in the choroid plexus we used mice that had wild-type levels of *Mrp1*, but lacked *Mdr1a* and *Mdr1b*, and mice that lacked *Mrp1* as well as *Mdr1a* and *Mdr1b*. These mice enabled us to determine the effect of MRP1 without the interference of MDR1. The mice were cannulated for CSF, and we were able to show that the lack of MRP1 protein caused etoposide levels to increase about 10-fold in the CSF after intravenous administration of the drug. These results indicate that MRP1 contributes significantly to the blood–CSF drug-permeability barrier (Wijnholds et al 2000b). The studies with the *Mrp1* knockout mice point toward the possibility of disrupting the blood–testis and blood–CSF barriers by the use of inhibitors of MRP1. Disruption of the blood–testis barrier could be useful for the development of male contraceptives, whereas disruption of the blood–CSF barrier could help to deliver drugs into the brain via the CSF. Since MRP1 and MDR1 share a broad spectrum of drug substrates, a combination of specific inhibitors for MRP1 and MDR1 may be useful in increasing the (anticancer or anti-epileptic) drug concentration in the brain.

Contribution to basal drug resistance by MRP1

Acquired drug resistance or innate insensitivity to drugs may be caused by one of many mechanisms (Borst 1991):

- activation of drugs may be reduced;
- inactivation of drugs may be increased;
- formation of drug target complexes may be decreased;
- tolerance of drugs may be increased;
- repair of drug damage may be increased;
- cellular uptake may be reduced;
- extrusion of the drug from the cell may be increased by plasma membrane efflux pumps; and
- the target cells or tissues may be hidden behind a blood–tissue drug permeability barrier.

MRPs contribute to the latter two resistance mechanisms. It is conceivable that in the absence of any drug efflux pump there will be a baseline drug resistance caused by the mechanisms described above.

Overproduction of high levels of MRP1 and MDR1 render cells resistant to many drugs, and high levels of these transporters in polarized epithelia increases the basolateral MRP1 and apical MDR1 cellular efflux activity, respectively. But do basal levels of these transporters significantly contribute to drug resistance in cells and tissues? Does the pump activity add drug resistance capacity above the baseline resistance? Initial proof that this is the case came from mouse cells lacking one of the functional drug resistance genes. Mouse embryonic stem cells and bone marrow-derived mast cells in which the *Mrp1* gene was inactivated showed an increased sensitivity to anthracyclins, vinca alkaloids, epipodophyllotoxins and sodium arsenite (Lorico et al 1996, Wijnholds et al 1997). A recent report showed that the contribution of the multidrug transporters MDR1 and MRP1 to basal drug resistance is extensive (Allen et al 2000). The drug sensitivities of wild-type mouse embryonic fibroblast cell lines were compared with cell lines in which the *Mdr1a* and *Mdr1b* genes encoding MDR1 were inactivated and with cell lines in which the *Mrp1* gene was inactivated in addition to *Mdr1a* and *Mdr1b*. Multiple independent cell lines of each genotype were examined. This permitted a clean dissection of the contribution of MRP1 and MDR1 to drug resistance at expression levels similar as those found in normal cells and tissues. Cell lines lacking MDR1 compared to wild-type cells were markedly more sensitive to anticancer drugs such as paclitaxel (16-fold), vincristine (threefold) and doxorubicin (fivefold). Cell lines lacking both MDR1 and MRP1 were markedly more sensitive than cell lines lacking only MDR1 to anticancer drugs like vincristine (over 10-fold), etoposide (sevenfold), and sodium arsenite (sevenfold). Most interestingly, cell lines lacking both MDR1 and MRP1 compared to the wild-type cell lines showed hypersensitivity to a broad array of drugs like paclitaxel (22-fold), vincristine (28-fold), doxorubicin (sevenfold), etoposide (sevenfold), and sodium arsenite (fourfold). These studies indicate that very low levels of MRP1 and MDR1 in cells and tissues may significantly affect their basal resistance to cytotoxic (or e.g. anti-epileptic) drugs if they are substrates for the pump. Similarly, drug transporters with other substrate specificities that are present at very low levels in cells or tissues may contribute to the basal drug resistance. The studies above indicate that an increased sensitization of (drug-resistant) target tissues to baseline levels could in principal be achieved once specific non-toxic inhibitors are available. For successful drug resistance reversal with pump inhibitors, it is important to determine for each substrate the relevant drug transporter activity in the target cell, not only its mere presence, and to determine whether this activity contributes significantly above the baseline drug resistance. Mice with gene disruptions in the relevant transporter genes will be helpful in these analyses.

Contribution to drug resistance by MRP5

MPR5 is ubiquitously expressed in almost all tissues with relatively high levels of gene transcripts in skeletal muscle and various segments of the brain (Kool et al 1997, McAleer et al 1999). MRP5 is an organic anion transporter of molecules such as glutathione conjugates (e.g. dinitrophenyl glutathione) and fluorochromes, and can be inhibited by typical inhibitors of organic anion transport (e.g. sulfinpyrazone, benzbromarone and probenecid) (Jedlitschky et al 2000, McAleer et al 1999, Wijnholds et al 2000a). MRP5 may be a low affinity glutathione conjugate pump or may prefer another group of glutathione conjugates than MRP1–3 since leukotriene C_4 is not transported by MRP5 (Jedlitschky et al 2000). We found no significant resistance to anthracyclins, vinca alkaloids or methotrexate, and only marginal resistance against epipodophyllotoxins. However, although the cells used for determining the drug resistance spectrum contained high levels of MRP5, only a small fraction of this was localized at the plasma membrane; the resistance spectrum may therefore not be complete. Interestingly, we found that cells overexpressing MRP5 confer resistance to anticancer base analogues such as thiopurines (e.g. 6-mercaptopurine and thioguanine) and antiviral drugs such as 9-(2-phosphonylmethoxyethyl) adenine (PMEA). MRP1–3 do not confer resistance to these drugs. Schuetz et al (1999) showed that MRP4 is functioning as a cellular efflux pump for PMEA and azidothymidine monophosphate. We showed that MRP5 functions as a cellular efflux pump for 6-thioinosine monophosphate and PMEA (Wijnholds et al 2000a). MRP5 is present in the basolateral membrane of polarized cells overproducing MRP5. In accordance with its location in the plasma membrane, MRP5 transports PMEA to the basal side of the cell monolayer (J. Wijnholds, L. van Deemter, J. Balzarini & P. Borst, unpublished results). Other recent experiments indicate that not only purine monophosphate but also pyrimidine monophosphate analogues are transported by MRP5. Cells containing MRP5 and incubated with the prodrug So324, a lipophilic 5′ monophosphate triester prodrug of 2′, 3′-didehydro-2′, 3′-dideoxythymidine (d4T or stavudine), extrude increased amounts of alaninyl-d4T monophosphate from the cell (J. Wijnholds, P. Wielinga, M. de Haas, J. Balzarini & P. Borst, unpublished results).

Interestingly, transport of antiviral drugs across the blood–brain barrier, from the brain towards the blood, and across the blood–CSF barrier, from the CSF towards the blood, has been reported for radiolabelled 2′, 3′-dideoxyinosine (Takasawa et al 1997). It is not known whether 2′, 3′-dideoxyinosine monophosphate or 2′, 3′-dideoxyadenosine monophosphate are transported across these barriers, but the transporter(s) do have organic anion transporter properties. It will be interesting to see if MRP5 (or MRP4) is involved in this transport. However, the presence of MRP5 (or MRP4) at the blood–CSF and blood–brain barriers needs to be shown. The use of mice lacking functional *Mrp5* and *Mrp4* will be useful to determine the putative role of these transporters at these drug permeability barriers.

In order to characterize the normal physiological functions of MRP5, we generated mice with a disruption of the *Mrp5* gene (J. Wijnholds, C. A. Neefjes-Mol, P. Krimpenfort, M. van der Valk & P. Borst, unpublished results 1999). Similarly to our *Mrp1* knockout mice, the *Mrp5* mutant mice are healthy and fertile, show a normal lifespan and no physiological, clinical or histological abnormalities under laboratory conditions. Jedlitschky et al (2000) showed that cyclic nucleotides are physiological substrates for MRP5. cGMP is a high affinity substrate, whereas cAMP is a low affinity substrate for MRP5. Transport mediated by MRP5 can be efficiently inhibited by compounds structurally related to cGMP, which are used as phosphodiesterase inhibitors, e.g. sildenafil, trequinsin and zaprinast (Jedlitschky et al 2000).

Increased intracellular levels of cGMP can be induced by nitric oxide. cGMP mediates as a second messenger physiological processes such as vasodilation and neurotransmission in the cardiovascular system and CNS (Garthwaite & Boulton 1995). The physiological importance of a cGMP efflux pump is not clear since intracellular levels of cGMP are lowered by phosphodiesterases (Bellamy & Garthwaite 2001), but cellular extrusion may be an alternative strategy to decrease cGMP levels. Therefore, it will be interesting to look for differences in response of the *Mrp5* mutant and wild-type mice exposed to continuously high levels of cGMP induced by phosphodiesterase inhibitors that do not inhibit MRP5. Obviously, mice can do without MRP5 and future studies will have to reveal the physiological role of this cGMP transporter.

Conclusions and prospects

The brain contains significant levels of MRP1 and MRP5. Whereas MRP5 is broadly expressed in the brain, MRP1 protein is mainly localized at the choroid plexus where it contributes to the blood–CSF barrier. MRP1 localized at the basolateral plasma membrane of the choroid plexus epithelial cells limits the passage of drugs from the blood towards the cerebrospinal fluid. It is conceivable that inhibitors of MRP1 would disrupt the drug permeability barrier, and would allow increased drug levels in the cerebrospinal fluid and brain. Obviously, this will only be the case for MRP1 substrates for which there is no other redundant transporter available or up-regulated. Our experiments indicated that in the mouse MRP1 plays a pivotal role at least for some drugs (e.g. etoposide) at the blood–CSF drug permeability barrier.

High amounts of MRP1 and/or MDR1 are believed to render tumours resistant to a broad array of (cytostatic) drugs. Recent experiments showed that low amounts of MRP1 and/or MDR1 in different cell types (e.g. mast cells, embryonic stem cells, fibroblasts) could make a considerable contribution to drug resistance. It is likely that other drug efflux pumps present at low levels contribute similarly, although maybe with a less broad substrate specificity. Inhibition of the low drug efflux pump activity may render cells more sensitive to drugs used in anticancer or epilepsy therapy.

The role of MRP5 in the brain is much less clear at the moment, but it is conceivable that MRP5 protects brain cells against nucleobase analogues and other anionic drugs. Although not shown yet, the protection may also be caused by the presence of MRP5 at the blood–brain and/or blood–CSF barriers. Such transport activities are known to reside at these barriers. MRP5 transports cGMP, but the physiological importance of this transport activity as well as its role in *in vivo* drug handling needs to be revealed. The viable *Mrp5* knockout mice will tell us this.

Acknowledgements

We thank Dr P. Borst (The Netherlands Cancer Institute, Amsterdam, The Netherlands) for critical advice on the manuscript. This work was supported in part by grants from the Dutch Cancer Society.

References

Allen JD, Brinkhuis RF, van Deemter L, Wijnholds J, Schinkel AH 2000 Extensive contribution of the multidrug transporters P-glycoprotein and Mrp1 to basal drug resistance. Cancer Res 60:5761–5766

Angeletti RH, Novikoff PM, Juvvadi SR, Fritschy JM, Meier PJ, Wolkoff AW 1997 The choroid plexus epithelium is the site of the organic anion transport protein in the brain. Proc Natl Acad Sci USA 94:283–286

Belinsky MG, Bain LJ, Balsara BB, Testa JR, Kruh GD 1998 Characterization of MOAT-C and MOAT-D, new members of the MRP/cMOAT subfamily of transporter proteins. J Natl Cancer Inst 90:1735–1741

Bellamy TC, Garthwaite J 2001 'cAMP-Specific' phosphodiesterase contributes to cGMP degradation in cerebellar cells exposed to nitric oxide. Mol Pharmacol 59:54–61

Bergen AA, Plomp AS, Schuurman EJ et al 2000 Mutations in ABCC6 cause pseudoxanthoma elasticum. Nat Genet 25:228–231

Borst P 1991 Genetic mechanisms of drug resistance. A review. Acta Oncol 30:87–105

Borst P, Evers R, Kool M, Wijnholds J 2000 A family of drug transporters: the multidrug resistance-associated proteins. J Natl Cancer Inst 92:1295–1302

Cole SP, Bhardwaj G, Gerlach JH et al 1992 Overexpression of a transporter gene in a multidrug-resistant human lung cancer cell line. Science 258:1650–1654

Evers R, Zaman GJ, van Deemter L et al 1996 Basolateral localization and export activity of the human multidrug resistance-associated protein in polarized pig kidney cells. J Clin Invest 97:1211–1218

Evers R, de Haas M, Sparidans R et al 2000 Vinblastine and sulfinpyrazone export by the multidrug resistance protein MRP2 is associated with glutathione export. Br J Cancer 83:375–383

Garthwaite J, Boulton CL 1995 Nitric oxide signaling in the central nervous system. Annu Rev Physiol 57:683–706

Hipfner DR, Deeley RG, Cole SP 1999 Structural, mechanistic and clinical aspects of MRP1. Biochim Biophys Acta 1461:359–376

Hopper E, Belinsky MG, Zeng H, Tosolini A, Testa JR, Kruh GD 2001 Analysis of the structure and expression pattern of MRP7 (ABCC10), a new member of the MRP subfamily. Cancer Lett 162:181–191

Jedlitschky G, Burchell B, Keppler D 2000 The multidrug resistance protein 5 functions as an ATP-dependent export pump for cyclic nucleotides. J Biol Chem 275: 30069–30074

Kartenbeck J, Leuschner U, Mayer R, Keppler D 1996 Absence of the canalicular isoform of the MRP gene-encoded conjugate export pump from the hepatocytes in Dubin–Johnson syndrome. Hepatology 23:1061–1066

Keppler D, Kamisako T, Leier I et al 2000 Localization, substrate specificity, and drug resistance conferred by conjugate export pumps of the MRP family. Adv Enzyme Regul 40:339–349

Kool M, de Haas M, Scheffer GL et al 1997 Analysis of expression of cMOAT (MRP2), MRP3, MRP4, and MRP5, homologues of the multidrug resistance-associated protein gene (MRP1), in human cancer cell lines. Cancer Res 57:3537–3547

Kool M, van der Linden M, de Haas M, Baas F, Borst P 1999 Expression of human *MRP6*, a homologue of the multidrug resistance protein gene *MRP1*, in tissues and cancer cells. Cancer Res 59:175–182

Le Saux O, Urban Z, Tschuch C et al 2000 Mutations in a gene encoding an ABC transporter cause pseudoxanthoma elasticum. Nat Genet 25:223–227

Leier I, Jedlitschky G, Buchholz U, Cole SP, Deeley RG, Keppler D 1994 The MRP gene encodes an ATP-dependent export pump for leukotriene C4 and structurally related conjugates. J Biol Chem 269:27807–27810

Loe DW, Almquist KC, Deeley RG, Cole SP 1996 Multidrug resistance protein (MRP)-mediated transport of leukotriene C4 and chemotherapeutic agents in membrane vesicles. J Biol Chem 271:9675–9682

Loe DW, Deeley RG, Cole SP 1998 Characterization of vincristine transport by the M(r) 190,000 multidrug resistance protein (MRP): evidence for cotransport with reduced glutathione. Cancer Res 58:5130–5136

Lorico A, Rappa G, Flavell RA, Sartorelli AC 1996 Double knockout of the MRP gene leads to increased drug sensitivity in vitro. Cancer Res 56:5351–5355

Lorico A, Rappa G, Finch RA, Yang D, Flavell RA, Sartorelli AC 1997 Disruption of the murine MRP (multidrug resistance protein) gene leads to increased sensitivity to etoposide (VP-16) and increased levels of glutathione. Cancer Res 57:5238–5242

Madon J, Hagenbuch B, Landmann L, Meier PJ, Stieger B 2000 Transport function and hepatocellular localization of mrp6 in rat liver. Mol Pharmacol 57:634–641

McAleer MA, Breen MA, White NL, Matthews N 1999 pABC11 (also known as MOAT-C and MRP5), a member of the ABC family of proteins, has anion transporter activity but does not confer multidrug resistance when overexpressed in human embryonic kidney 293 cells. J Biol Chem 274:23541–23548

Nishino J, Suzuki H, Sugiyama D et al 1999 Transepithelial transport of organic anions across the choroid plexus: possible involvement of organic anion transporter and multidrug resistance-associated protein. J Pharmacol Exp Ther 290:289–294

Paulusma CC, Kool M, Bosma PJ et al 1997 A mutation in the human canalicular multispecific organic anion transporter gene causes the Dubin–Johnson syndrome. Hepatology 25:1539–1542

Rao VV, Dahlheimer JL, Bardgett ME et al 1999 Choroid plexus epithelial expression of *MDR1* P glycoprotein and multidrug resistance-associated protein contribute to the blood–cerebrospinal-fluid drug-permeability barrier. Proc Natl Acad Sci USA 96:3900–3905

Ringpfeil F, Lebwohl MG, Christiano AM, Uitto J 2000 Pseudoxanthoma elasticum: mutations in the *MRP6* gene encoding a transmembrane ATP-binding cassette (ABC) transporter. Proc Natl Acad Sci USA 97:6001–6006

Robbiani DF, Finch RA, Jäger D, Muller WA, Sartorelli AC, Randolph GJ 2000 The leukotriene C4 transporter MRP1 regulates CCL19 (MIP-3β, ELC)-dependent mobilization of dendritic cells to lymph nodes. Cell 103:757–768

Schinkel AH 1999 P-Glycoprotein, a gatekeeper in the blood–brain barrier. Adv Drug Deliv Rev 36:179–194

Schuetz JD, Connelly MC, Sun D et al 1999 MRP4: A previously unidentified factor in resistance to nucleoside-based antiviral drugs. Nat Med 5:1048–1051

Schultz MJ, Wijnholds J, Peppelenbosch MP et al 2001 Mice lacking the multidrug resistance protein 1 are resistant to Streptococcus pneumoniae-induced pneumonia. J Immunol 166:4059–4064

Takasawa K, Terasaki T, Suzuki H, Sugiyama Y 1997 *In vivo* evidence for carrier-mediated efflux transport of 3′-azido-3′-deoxythymidine and 2′,3′-dideoxyinosine across the blood-brain barrier via a probenecid-sensitive transport system. J Pharmacol Exp Ther 281:369–375

Wijnholds J, Evers R, van Leusden MR et al 1997 Increased sensitivity to anticancer drugs and decreased inflammatory response in mice lacking the multidrug resistance-associated protein. Nat Med 3:1275–1279

Wijnholds J, Scheffer GL, van der Valk M et al 1998 Multidrug resistance protein 1 protects the oropharyngeal mucosal layer and the testicular tubules against drug-induced damage. J Exp Med 188:797–808

Wijnholds J, Mol CA, van Deemter L et al 2000a Multidrug-resistance protein 5 is a multispecific organic anion transporter able to transport nucleotide analogs. Proc Natl Acad Sci USA 97:7476–7481

Wijnholds J, de Lange EC, Scheffer GL et al 2000b Multidrug resistance protein 1 protects the choroid plexus epithelium and contributes to the blood–cerebrospinal fluid barrier. J Clin Invest 105:279–285

DISCUSSION

Pirmohamed: Is your triple knockout physiologically normal?

Wijnholds: Yes. The mice are healthy and fertile, show a normal lifespan and no other abnormalities when kept in our animal facility at the Netherlands Cancer Institute. If we compare the *Mrp1* knockout mouse with the normal mouse, in ear inflammation tests *Mrp1* has a function as a leukotriene C_4 exporter. In experiments in which we treated ears of the mice with arachadonic acids, which are precursors for leukotriene C_4, we found a reduced swelling effect on the ears of the *Mrp1* knockout mouse. We also injected some dye, and the wild-type mice had strongly blue ears because of oedema and vasodilation caused by the leukotriene C_4, whereas the MRP1 knockout mice have much less blue ears.

Pirmohamed: MRP5 is a nucleoside analogue transporter. These are used in leukaemia and HIV. Is MRP5 highly expressed in different white blood cells? Can you use these white cells as a surrogate for the blood–brain barrier?

Wijnholds: We know that MRP5 is present in blood cells, but we haven't yet looked at which ones express it. It is interesting that some white cells are the homing sites for HIV.

Pirmohamed: If you could show a correlation between the white cell and blood–brain barrier, you could use a white cell as a surrogate for the blood–brain barrier in humans to look at transport of drugs. Clearly, one can't get to the blood–brain barrier in humans.

Wijnholds: I don't think this would work. If it is a genetic effect you would expect it also to occur in the white blood cells, but since there is probably not a genetic effect in epilepsy you would not see any effects in white blood cells. Also, there is not necessarily a correlation between the levels of MRPs in white blood cells and the blood–brain barrier.

Ling: Your triple knockout experiments demonstrate that even a small number of molecules in a cell that doesn't normally have this molecule, could make a big difference in terms of its ability to control the amount of drug that goes in or comes out of the cell.

Wijnholds: This may even happen with low levels not detectable by normal techniques.

Ling: This raises an interesting question. If MRP1, for example, is normally present at a high level in the brain, what difference would a 10% increase in expression make in terms of causing additional drug resistance?

Wijnholds: I think it would make a difference. It may not make much difference to the cytotoxicity, but if the drug has an effect on a biochemical process in the cell, this effect may be more than just the 10% increase in protein.

Ling: Do you think, for example, that in drug therapy for epilepsy, a small increase in transporter level overall could make a big difference?

Wijnholds: That could be the case, yes.

Abbott: With regard to CSF flow through brain: the choroid plexuses secrete CSF into the ventricles, from where it flows through foramina into the subarachnoid space and back into the venous circulation via arachnoid granulations. While the CSF and brain interstitial fluid (ISF) are in diffusional exchange across the ependymal wall and pial surface, there is very limited penetration of CSF into the brain, and drugs in the CSF will not spread widely into the brain. One reason is that the brain capillaries appear to be secreting ISF, which drains partly into neck lymphatics and partly into the CSF, opposing bulk flow from the CSF (Begley et al 2000). This means that drugs in CSF will move into the brain parenchyma mainly by diffusion. Diffusion is an inefficient mechanism for movement over long distances because the concentration falls off as the square of the distance, hence the effective penetration distance will be short (millimetres rather than centimetres). It is wrong to think of the CSF as percolating through the brain, and therefore raising drug concentration in CSF will not necessarily result in greater drug delivery to the brain. I agree that efflux transporters on the choroid plexuses help protect the neurons close to the ventricular surface, but blocking these transporters is not a way to deliver drugs to the bulk of the CNS; drug access is predominantly determined by the brain capillaries.

Wijnholds: The brain capillaries are probably the primary sites for getting things into the brain. But as you say, if compounds enter the CSF they will penetrate a few micrometres into the brain. How much they penetrate depends on the properties of the drug. It depends what is going on with the fluid flow, too.

Abbott: Human brain CSF has a turnover time of $\sim 4\,$h, or 0.4% per min (Davson & Segal 1996). Even drugs present in high concentrations will be subject to dilution and drainage of CSF. Diffusion from CSF will not be an efficient mechanism for delivery to most of the CNS, especially in the large human brain, and even for very lipophilic drugs.

Löscher: There are some arguments against this. In pharmacology, if we test drugs that do not penetrate into the brain after systemic injection, we apply them intracerebroventricularly (ICV) into the CSF. Normally, we then see functional alterations mediated by the drug. The second argument is a clinical one. After systemic administration, drugs such as penicillin do not penetrate the blood–brain barrier if you treat patients with brain infections. However, if you inject penicillin directly into the CSF it has antibacterial effects plus the neurotoxic side effects that are not seen with systemic injection. Certainly, there are functional alterations after such intrathecal drug administration.

Abbott: In the case of penicillin, most of the bacterial infection will be in the meninges, in surfaces bathed by CSF. With regard to side-effects, there may be as much as a 10^5-fold difference in CSF drug concentration following ICV injection compared to IV, which could explain the different effects, particularly in neurons close to the CSF.

Löscher: Do you obtain anticonvulsant effects with anticonvulsant drugs by injecting these drugs into the CSF?

Abbott: Again, I think this relies on the concentration effects.

Löscher: Very often the concentrations needed are low if the drug is given ICV. We are not talking about high concentrations.

Abbott: How is the epilepsy induced in this animal model?

Löscher: Whatever way you want. Brian Meldrum has done a lot of this work.

Meldrum: It works best in DBA2 mice. In this case you give a relatively low concentration of drug, but you flood the CSF.

Abbott: That may be different. Flooding the CSF or inducing high volume (convective) flow using pressure is a successful method to enhance drug penetration (Morrison et al 1994). In cases of chemically induced epilepsy using topical application on the brain surface, anticonvulsants applied to the same site will also be effective.

References

Begley DJ, Khan EU, Rollinson C, Abbott NJ, Regina A, Roux F 2000 The role of brain extracellular fluid production and efflux mechanisms in drug transport to the brain. In: Begley DJ, Bradbury MW, Kreuter J (eds) The blood–brain barrier and drug delivery to the CNS. Marcel Dekker, New York, p 93–108

Davson H, Segal MB 1996 Physiology of the CSF and blood–brain barriers. CRC Press, Boca Raton

Morrison PF, Laske DW, Bobo H, Oldfield EH, Dedrick RL 1994 High-flow microinfusion: tissue penetration and pharmacodynamics. Am J Physiol 266:R292–R305

Reversal of multidrug resistance: lessons from clinical oncology

Susan E. Bates, Clara Chen, Robert Robey, Min Kang, William D. Figg and Tito Fojo

Molecular Therapeutics Section, Medicine Branch, National Cancer Institute, Bethesda, MD 20892, USA

Abstract. Modulation of P glycoprotein (Pgp) in clinical oncology has had limited success. Contributing factors have included the limitation in our understanding of the tumours in which Pgp overexpression is mechanistically important in clinical drug resistance; the failure to prove that concentrations of modulators achieved in patients were sufficient to inhibit Pgp; and the inability to conclusively prove that Pgp modulation was occurring in tumours in patients. New approaches are needed to determine the clinical settings in which Pgp overexpression plays a major role in resistance. Clinical trials with third generation modulators are ongoing, including trials with the compounds LY335979, R101933 and XR9576. Using the Pgp substrate Tc-99m Sestamibi as an imaging agent, increased uptake has been seen in normal liver and kidney after administration of PSC 833, VX710 and XR9576. These studies confirm that the concentrations of modulator achieved in patients are able to increase uptake of a Pgp substrate. Furthermore, CD56$^+$ cells obtained from patients treated with PSC 833 demonstrate enhanced rhodamine retention in an *ex vivo* assay after administration of the antagonist. Finally, a subset of patients treated with Pgp antagonists show enhanced Sestamibi retention in imaged tumours. These results suggest that Pgp modulators can increase drug accumulation in Pgp-expressing tumours and normal tissues in patients. Using third generation Pgp antagonists and properly designed clinical trials, it should be possible to determine the contribution of modulators to the reversal of clinical drug resistance.

2002 Mechanisms of drug resistance in epilepsy: lessons from oncology. Wiley, Chichester (Novartis Foundation Symposium 243) p 83–102

The history of multidrug resistance begins with the 1973 discovery by Keld Dano of the active outward transport of daunomycin in drug-resistant cells that had been selected in daunomycin, but were cross-resistant to doxorubicin and the vinca alkaloids (Dano 1973). A series of studies then described the multidrug resistance (MDR) phenotype in which cells selected for drug resistance in a single anticancer agent developed resistance to a variety of structurally unrelated compounds. Victor Ling, with other investigators, correlated overexpression of a 170 kDa protein termed P glycoprotein (Pgp) with reduced drug accumulation and

TABLE 1   Pgp substrates and antagonists

| | *Pgp antagonists* | | |
Pgp substrates	*First generation*	*Second generation*	*Third generation*
Paclitaxel	Verapamil	Dexverapamil	VX 710
Docetaxel	Quinidine	Dexniguldipine	S9788
Vinblastine	Quinine	PSC 833	GF120918
Vincristine	Amiodarone		LY335979
Vinorelbine	Cyclosporin A		R101933
Adriamycin			XR9576
Daunorubicin			
Etoposide			
Teniposide			
Actinomycin D			
Homoharringtonine			

multidrug resistance in a series of mammalian cell lines (Kartner et al 1983). The gene encoding Pgp was cloned and named the *MDR1* gene; expression of this gene was found in a variety of cancers. In some tumours expression was found at the time of diagnosis (kidney, colon and adrenocortical); while in others, expression was found after relapse and treatment failure (breast cancer, lymphoma and leukaemia) (Sandor et al 1998). The potential relevance of this for clinical oncology received a boost in 1981 when Tsuruo observed that verapamil was able to overcome this MDR phenotype (Tsuruo et al 1981). Subsequently, it was recognized that several compounds already in use in the clinic were able to inhibit Pgp in the laboratory. In addition to verapamil, these 'first generation' compounds included quinidine, amiodarone, nicardapine, nifedipine, quinine, tamoxifen and cyclosporin (Table 1) (Ferry et al 1996).

Home-run trials

Subsequently, clinical trials were initiated that were aimed at inhibiting Pgp-mediated drug efflux, and thereby reversing clinical drug resistance. These first-generation trials incorporated a Pgp antagonist in combination with any of several different antineoplastic regimens in an array of different cancers (extensively reviewed by Tew et al 1993, Fisher & Sikic 1995). These trials were frequently designed as 'home-run' trials, in which a favourite antagonist was combined with a favourite antineoplastic agent, and the combination was used to treat a particular population of patients (Bates et al 1996). This type of trial had several major shortcomings: resistance to the antineoplastic drug in the combination was not clearly established; the role of Pgp as a mediator of resistance was not established in the tumours; lack of potency of the modulator at achievable serum concentrations; and lack of confirmation of efficacy of the modulator. These trials failed to prove convincingly the importance of Pgp inhibition in oncology. It has been assumed that lack of potency of the modulator was at least a contributing factor, although perhaps not the sole explanation. Two early modulator trials with quinine attempted to confirm inhibition of Pgp-mediated efflux by using an *ex vivo* biological assay. Serum from patients receiving quinine was added *in vitro* to multidrug resistant cells expressing high levels of Pgp. Drug accumulation studies were then performed — with doxorubicin in one study, and mitoxantrone in the other (Solary et al 1991, 1996). In both cases, increased drug accumulation ranging from 20–120% was observed. While this type of biological assay does not prove Pgp inhibition in tumours, it does confirm the presence of serum concentrations of Pgp antagonists sufficient to increase drug accumulation.

Other types of trial designs were also performed with the first-generation agents — both a crossover design and a randomized trial design. In the crossover design, the patient serves as his own control, and the modulator is not added until resistance is confirmed with a specific drug regimen. This design avoids the first weakness of the home-run design, where resistance to the antineoplastic drug has not been confirmed. However, the crossover design may induce resistance mechanisms other than Pgp, confounding the results of Pgp antagonism. At least five trials with first generation agents were conducted using a randomized design. Only one of these suggested efficacy for the Pgp antagonist; a trial in non-small cell lung cancer, where Pgp expression is not thought to be a major mechanism of resistance (Sandor et al 1998).

Pharmacokinetic interaction

Over the course of these trials, a new complication inherent in studies employing Pgp antagonists was recognized. When cyclosporin was used as the antagonist, the dose of the anticancer agent had to be reduced in order to avoid excess toxicity. Pharmacokinetic studies demonstrated that anticancer drug clearance was reduced, resulting in a prolonged terminal half-life, and an increased area under the concentration curve (AUC). If the dose of the anticancer agent was reduced, then the observed toxicity could be equalized to that observed for the anticancer agent in the absence of cyclosporin. Figure 1 represents a model of the AUC curves for anticancer agents with and without the addition of a Pgp antagonist. It was hoped that the AUCs would be more or less comparable, and efficacy would be

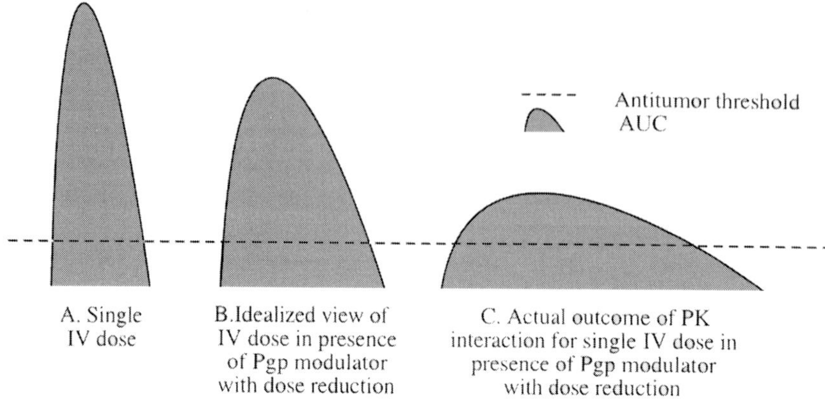

FIG. 1.   Model of AUC curves for anticancer agents.

improved (panels A and B). The cyclosporin analogue and more potent Pgp antagonist PSC 833 also elicited this interaction. Although the mechanism of the interaction has not been fully elucidated, the reduced clearance appears to be a product of both antagonism of Pgp-mediated drug excretion and inhibition of P450-mediated metabolism, possibly through the 3A4 isoenzyme. As observed in panel C, the long terminal half-life for some drugs may result in an AUC that is comparable to the AUC obtained in the absence of the antagonist, if both are calculated to infinity. However, if dose intensity or duration of time above a threshold is important, then a reduction in C_{max} (maximum concentration), C_{ss} (steady-state concentration), or time above the threshold could be detrimental to anticancer efficacy. Such a concern was dramatically echoed in xenograft studies performed by Krishna & Mayer (1997) (Table 2). In this study, animals were

TABLE 2   Doxorubicin pharmacokinetics with PSC 833 in mouse model system

Group	Plasma C_{max}	Plasma AUC^{a}	Tumour C_{max}	Tumour AUC	Liver C_{max}	Liver AUC	Heart C_{max}	Heart AUC
Dox 7.5 mg/kg	2.7	1.3	3.9	73.8	59.5	874.9	35.1	820.4
Dox 7.5 mg/kg + PSC	4.2	13.7	3.9	115.6	72.2	992.3	38.4	1229.4
Dox 2.0 mg/kg + PSC	1.6	0.3	2.9	39.1	24.8	602.9	27.9	790.6

[a]AUC was calculated using trapesoidal rule $(0-t_{last})$.
Dox, doxorubicin.
Adapted from Krishna & Mayer (1997).

TABLE 3 Pharmacokinetic interaction: C_{max} and AUC parameters measured at maximum tolerated dose (MTD) in clinical trials with Pgp antagonists

Antagonist	*Drug*	*Dose*[a]	*C_{max} at MTD without antagonist*	*C_{max} at MTD with antagonist*	*Ratio AUC+/ AUC− antagonist*	*Reference*
PSC 833	Etoposide	none	12.0 μg/ml	14.5 μg/ml	1.86 (0–24 h)	Boote et al 1996
PSC 833	Doxorubicin	25%	9.5 ng/ml	11.1 ng/ml	1.27 (0–96 h)	Sonneveld et al 1996
PSC 833	Dexamethasone	none	88 μg/ml	91 μg/ml	1.24 (0–tz)	Kovarik et al 1998
PSC 833	Doxorubicin[b]	30%	11.7 nM	11.3 nM	1.54 (0−∞) 1.19 (0–48 h)	Giaccone et al 1997
PSC 833	Paclitaxel 3 h infusion	30%	5.5 μM[c]	3.9 μM[c]	0.43–0.76 (0−∞)	Fracasso et al 2000
PSC 833	Paclitaxel 96 h infusion	50%	0.074 μg/ml	0.079 μg/ml	0.93 (0–96 h)	Chico et al 2001
VX710	Paclitaxel 3 h infusion	50%	2.17[c] μg/ml 3.65[d] μg/ml	1.56[c] μg/ml 2.15[d] μg/ml	1.15[c] (0−∞) 1.00[d] (0−∞)	Rowinsky et al 1998
GF120918	Doxorubicin	none	3.11 μg/ml	3.9 μg/ml	1.51 (0−∞)	Sparreboom et al 1999
R101933	Docetaxel	none	2.47 μg/ml	2.95 μg/ml	1.10 (0−∞)	van Zuylen et al 2000

[a]Dose reduction compared to MTD in the absence of antagonist.
[b]Values normalized to doxorubicin dose of 50 mg/m^2.
[c]Value for C_{max} and for AUC from historical controls treated with 135 mg/m^2 in a 3 h infusion, and from patients treated with 60 mg/m^2 paclitaxel in combination with VX710.
[d]Value for C_{max} and for AUC from historical controls treated with 175 mg/m^2 in a 3 h infusion, and from patients treated with 80 mg/m^2 paclitaxel in combination with VX710.
[e]Estimated from Fig. 1.

treated with PSC 833 and doxorubicin. The maximum tolerated dose (MTD) for doxorubicin was 7.5 mg/kg and 2.0 mg/kg in the absence and presence of PSC 833, respectively. While C_{max} and AUC were increased following the addition of PSC 833, without dose reduction, both were actually decreased in the animals treated at the MTD for the combination with PSC 833.

Clinical trials with Pgp antagonists in patients have been more difficult to interpret, and many trials have been published without complete pharmacokinetic (PK) data. Inspection of Table 3 suggests that there is a reduction in either C_{max} or AUC for paclitaxel with dose reduction following the addition of PSC 833 or VX710. No reduction was observed for the mean C_{max} and AUC resulting from the 96 h paclitaxel infusion in combination with PSC 833. However, as noted below, there was significant interpatient variability in this trial and several patients were clearly under-dosed at the established MTD (Chico et al 2001). The two third generation compounds listed in Table 3, R101933 and GF120918, required no associated dose reduction, and as a result, both C_{max} and AUCs were increased with the addition of the modulator. These studies confirm the importance of identifying a potent, non-toxic inhibitor, which provokes no significant PK interaction with the anticancer agent.

Knockout mouse studies — contribution of Pgp to pharmacokinetic interaction and blood–brain barrier

Based on the observation that some of the newer Pgp antagonists have a nominal PK, it is suspected that a large component of the interaction for cyclosporin, PSC 833 and VX710 is inhibition of P450. However, studies with knockout mice in which the mouse *Mdr1* gene orthologue has been deleted have confirmed that *MDR1* plays a measurable role in drug excretion. Depending upon the compound tested, plasma, liver, kidney and lung levels are increased approximately twofold in the mice lacking *Mdr1* (Table 4). Thus it appears that Pgp alone can account at least a portion of the PK interaction. Interestingly, CNS accumulation of vinblastine, digoxin and cyclosporin A are increased 22-, 27-, and 17-fold over that observed in the wild-type mice, respectively. The most remarkable increase in uptake, for ivermectin, was a finding sparked by the observation of ivermectin toxicity in mice following routine spraying of cages to eliminate a mite infestation (Schinkel et al 1994). This finding has suggested that Pgp contributes significantly to the blood–brain barrier in blocking the entry of antineoplastic agents and other compounds into the CNS. Humans may have additional mechanisms for protecting the CNS, since no evidence of CNS toxicity has emerged from the clinical trials with Pgp antagonists (other than ataxia as dose limiting toxicity for PSC 833). Interestingly, when the knockout mice are exposed to PSC 833, there is a further increase in vinblastine or digoxin accumulation in brain tissue (Mayer et al 1997). These results suggest that Pgp plays an important role in the blood–brain barrier; and that PSC 833 may be inhibiting a second transporter in the CNS or altering uptake in some other way.

Surrogate studies

With these difficulties in mind, we combined PK monitoring with surrogate assays designed to confirm Pgp antagonism in our Phase I trials. In our recently reported

TABLE 4A **Ratio of drug level 4 h post dose between *Mdr*-deficient (*Mdr1a*(−/−)) and wild-type mice**

Drug	Plasma	Liver	Kidney	Lung	Brain	Reference
Digoxin	1.9	2.0	1.9	2.2	35.3	(Schinkel et al 1995)
Vinblastine	1.7	2.4	2.3	2.1	22.4	(van Asperen et al 1996)
Doxorubicin	0.9	4.5	1.0	1.0	2.8	(van Asperen et al 1999)
Dexamethasone	1.0	1.1	1.2	0.8	2.5	(Schinkel et al 1995)
Cyclosporin A	1.4	1.2	1.0	1.2	17.0	(Schinkel et al 1995)
Loperamide	2.0	3.1	1.5	1.7	13.5	(Schinkel et al 1996)
Ivermectin	3.3	3.8	3.0	4.0	87	(Schinkel et al 1994)

TABLE 4B **Ratio of drug level 4 h post dose in the presence of antagonist to drug level 4 h post dose in absence of antagonist**

Compound		Wild-type		$Mdr1^{-/-}$ [c]				Reference
		Plasma	Brain	Plasma −PSC	Plasma +PSC	Brain −PSC	Brain +PSC	
Digoxin	PSC 833	2.4[a]	19	2.4	3.0	68.3	37.7	(Mayer et al 1997)
Colchicine	PSC 833	2.5[b]	>10					(Desrayaud et al 1997)

[a]4 h post injection.
[b]Ratio of $AUC_{0-6\,h}$.
[c]Ratio of indicated source from $Mdr1a/1b(-/-)$ mouse divided by wild-type.

trial, PSC 833 was combined with paclitaxel in a conventional dose-escalation schema (Chico et al 2001). CD56[+] circulating mononuclear cells were obtained from patients before and after treatment with the antagonist PSC 833 (Robey et al 1999). Rhodamine efflux was readily demonstrated in these CD56[+] cells in the absence of administered PSC 833, but was markedly inhibited in these cells beginning 2 h after administration of PSC 833. Figure 2 shows the time course in CD56[+] cells obtained from a patient administered oral PSC 833. Efflux of rhodamine (dashed line) results in reduced fluorescence relative to that observed when exogenous PSC 833 has been added (dotted line). However, the PSC 833, which the patient ingested, inhibits rhodamine efflux from CD56[+] cells maximally at the 120 min time point. These studies confirmed inhibition of Pgp by PSC 833 in all patients. Similar results have been obtained with other potent Pgp inhibitors, including GF120918 (Witherspoon et al 1996).

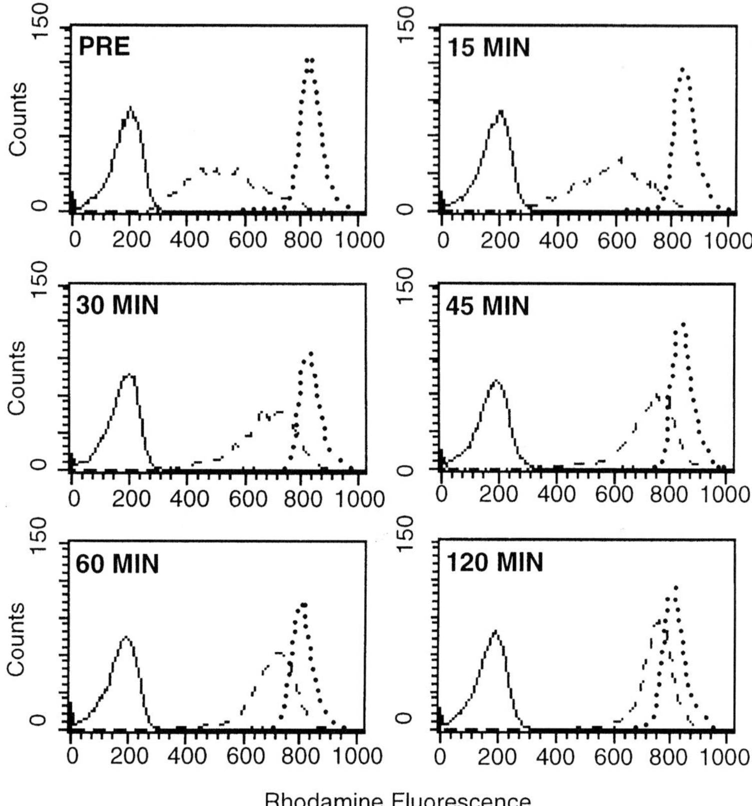

Rhodamine Fluorescence

FIG. 2.   Inhibition of rhodamine efflux from CD56[+] cells after administration of PSC 833. Whole blood was obtained at 0, 15, 30, 45, 60, and 120 min after a single oral dose of PSC 833. Rhodamine 123 was added and the blood was allowed to incubate for 30 min after which the mononuclear cells were separated and incubated for 60 min in rhodamine-free media and stained with CD56 antibody (dashed line); or rhodamine and PSC 833 were both added for the 30 min incubation period, the mononuclear cells were separated and the cells were incubated for 60 min in media with PSC 833 and stained with CD56 antibody (dotted line). Cell autofluorescence is shown as a solid line. Note some reversal of Pgp-mediated rhodamine efflux in the CD56[+] cells is seen after 30 min and reversal is near complete at 120 min.

Imaging studies

Another important lesson learned from clinical trials with Pgp antagonists has been the need for imaging studies. No anticancer agents were developed with confirmation of drug distribution into solid tumours; penetration was assumed from the success of the agents. As the first generation of Pgp antagonist trials failed to provide a role for Pgp antagonists in the clinic, the questions emerged:

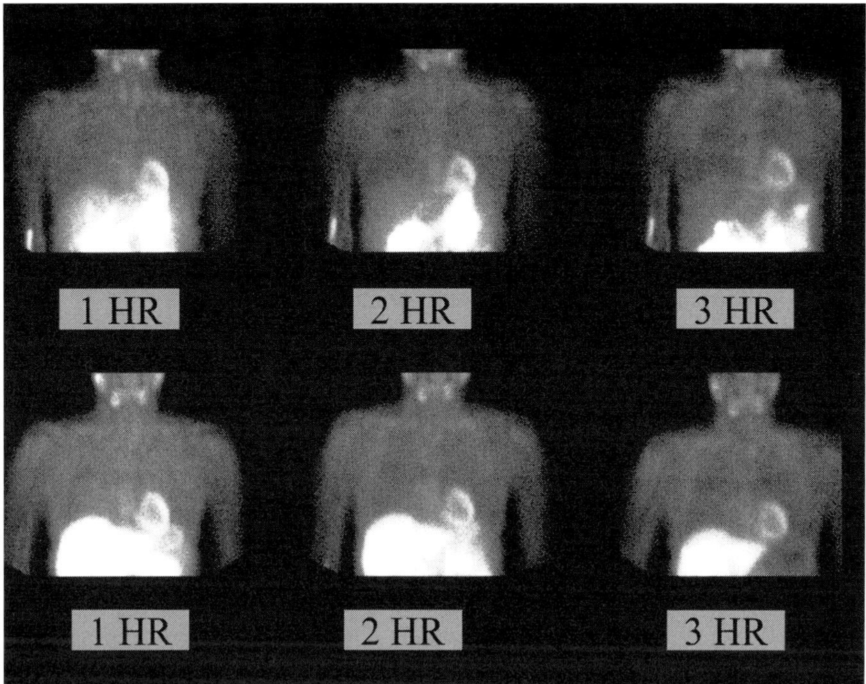

FIG. 3.   Sestamibi retention before and after PSC 833 administration. While intense uptake of Sestamibi is seen in the GI tract prior to PSC 833 administration as shown in the top series of images taken 1, 2 and 3 hours after Sestamibi injection, this is replaced by intense uptake in the liver following PSC 833 administration as shown in the bottom series of images.

were the antagonists reaching the intended target? Was it a failure of Pgp inhibition or a failure of drug action despite Pgp inhibition? The observation by Piwnica-Worms et al (1993) that Sestamibi, an imaging agent in clinical use as Cardiolyte®, was a substrate for Pgp, gave an opportunity to answer that question. Subsequently, studies demonstrated that increased Sestamibi retention could be demonstrated in patients following administration of several Pgp antagonists, including PSC 833 (Bakker et al 1999, Roepe et al 1993). A small fraction of patients imaged had demonstrable increases in Sestamibi retention in tumours. One striking finding in all patients was the increased Sestamibi retention in the liver following administration of the antagonist (Fig. 3) (Luker et al 1997). While not confirming that PSC 833 would be able to modulate retention in most tumours, the demonstration liver retention confirmed that PSC 833 was able to reach Pgp, and inhibit its activity in normal cells other than those circulating in the bloodstream. Similar uptake in the liver has been reported with Sestamibi in patients treated with VX710 and XR9576 (Abraham et al 2001, Peck et al 1996).

These studies also confirmed increased uptake in tumours in a subset of patients, suggesting that these third generation Pgp antagonists are able to penetrate tumours and reverse Pgp in cancer cells.

Interpatient variability

As noted above, studies reporting PK from trials in which a reduced anticancer drug dose was required, suggested that there was the risk of reduced drug exposure. Since dose reductions are determined by defining maximal tolerated dose in conventional Phase I dose escalation schedules, there is no opportunity to individualize dosing. The well-known interindividual variation in P450 activity may result in interindividual variation in the pharmacokinetic interaction observed when a Pgp antagonist is combined with an anticancer drug (Thummel et al 1994). In our recently reported Phase I study of paclitaxel (Taxol) in combination with PSC 833, the maximum tolerated dose of paclitaxel was $17.5\,\mathrm{mg/m^2}$ when administered over 96 h in combination with PSC 833 (Chico et al 2001). This dose was half that administered over 96 h without PSC 833 (Wilson et al 1994). However, in some patients, the reduced dose of paclitaxel administered with PSC 833 appeared to be insufficient, in that little bone marrow toxicity was observed. In other patients there was increased toxicity. These clinical observations were correlated with paclitaxel levels obtained from pharmacokinetic analysis. Thus, two problems appear to be inherent in the necessity to reduce doses in combination with Pgp antagonists. First, there is a reduction in C_{max}, and potentially of C_{ss}. Although the precise contribution of achieving C_{max} is unknown in cancer therapy, years of experience with conventional anticancer agents certainly suggest that treating at the MTD in any given schedule is important. Second, the significant intrapatient variability in the pharmacokinetic interaction results in some patients being overtreated and others undertreated at prescribed doses. While this has been ascribed to differences in P450, which vary widely among individuals, recent evidence regarding interindividual variation in Pgp-mediated efflux as a function of DNA polymorphism suggests that Pgp itself could also be a contributing factor (Hoffmeyer et al 2000).

Second- and third-generation agents

As noted above, Table 1 lists a number of compounds in preclinical or clinical development as potent Pgp antagonists. Ferry divides these compounds as second-generation agents — those closely related to first-generation agents, but with reduced toxicity; and third-generation agents — those highly potent with activity in the nanomolar range (Ferry et al 1996). These compounds hold the promise of being highly potent, non-toxic inhibitors of Pgp. Several are reported to have nominal effects on the pharmacokinetics of the anticancer agent. As described above, based on the mouse knockout work, a twofold increase in plasma concentrations of an anticancer agent could be expected from Pgp inhibition alone. Lack of a P450 interaction may allow a more predictable PK interaction, helping solve the problem of interpatient variability.

Realistic expectations

Finally, if trials with Pgp antagonists in oncology fail to confirm the role of Pgp as a major mediator of drug resistance, the ability of an antagonist to mediate intracellular concentrations of drug may still be important. In this view, Pgp would not be the principal mediator of resistance, but would be one component in a multifactorial process. Inhibition of Pgp would allow increased drug accumulation, but might not sensitize cells if downstream mediators of apoptosis, for example, were absent. Much of the early work with Pgp antagonists was performed using cell line models with very high levels of Pgp. These cell lines could be sensitized several hundred fold with the addition of antagonists. Use of these models led directly to the impression that similar degrees of sensitization could be expected in patients. That this impression would be mistaken can be surmised by comparison of *MDR1* levels in actual tumour samples with levels obtained from cell lines (Table 5). Using a PCR-based quantitative assay, selected cell lines in which preclinical studies were performed confirmed levels of *MDR1* expression in the range of 400- to 1000-fold over baseline levels in 'sensitive cells'. Yet, when patient samples were

TABLE 5   Expression of *MDR1* in selected cell lines and cancer samples assayed by quantitative PCR method[a]

KB 3–1	0.04	Breast cancer samples
KB 8–5	108	3.4, range <0.1–6.7
KB 8–5–11	410	Renal cell carcinoma metastases
KBV–1	5654	12.1, range <0.1–154
		Non-Hodgkin's lymphoma at diagnosis
8226/S	0.0	1.0, range <0.1–7.2
8226/dox6	401	pre EPOCH
8226/dox40	1823	2.2, range <0.1–10.6
		post EPOCH
SW620	10	8.0, range 0.2–162
SW620 Ad20	1600	

[a]Values are calculated based on the SW620 cell line having the arbitrary value of 10. From Kang et al (1995).

analysed for *MDR1* expression, it was observed that levels typically ranged up to 10-fold above the levels observed in the 'sensitive cells'. This type of expression could be expected to alter intracellular drug concentrations, but not to confer the tremendous degree of resistance observed in the *in vitro* selected models, or in the tumours of previously heavily pretreated cancer patients. Thus, overly high expectations led to the original home-run designs in the clinical trials, and ultimately to disappointment in the results obtained. More realistic expectations will lead to better trial design, and potentially, proof of concept for Pgp inhibition.

Conclusions

Systematic confirmation of increased drug uptake in tumours in patients will allow interpretation of negative results from a clinical trial: although the combination did not achieve clinical benefit, increased drug uptake could be observed. Since major efforts have been directed at increasing dose intensity over the past decade (bone marrow transplant studies; GCSF support for increased drug doses), a Pgp antagonist able to increase drug exposure could be seen in the light of those manoeuvres — rather than as the drug resistance reversal agent originally envisioned. This increase in drug exposure would be expected to be most beneficial in upfront treatment — at a time when cells are most sensitive to treatment — as a prevention tool.

References

Abraham J, Edgerley M, Wilson R et al 2001 A phase I study of the novel P-glycoprotein (Pgp) antagonist, XR9576 in combination with vinorelbine. Proc Am Soc Clin Oncol Annu Meet 37

Bakker M, van der Graaf WT, Piers DA et al 1999 99mTc-Sestamibi scanning with SDZ PSC 833 as a functional detection method for resistance modulation in patients with solid tumours. Anticancer Res 19:2349–2353

Bates SE, Wilson WH, Fojo AT et al 1996 Clinical reversal of multidrug resistance. Stem Cells 14:56–63

Boote DJ, Dennis IF, Twentyman PR et al 1996 Phase I study of etoposide with SDZ PSC 833 as a modulator of multidrug resistance in patients with cancer. J Clin Oncol 14:610–618

Chico I, Kang MH, Bergan R et al 2001 Phase I study of infusional paclitaxel in combination with the P-glycoprotein antagonist PSC 833. J Clin Oncol 19:832–842

Dano K 1973 Active outward transport of daunomycin in resistant Ehrlich ascites tumor cells. Biochim Biophys Acta 323:466–483

Desrayaud S, Guntz P, Scherrmann JM, Lemiare M 1997 Effect of the P-glycoprotein inhibitor, SDZ PSC 833, on the blood and brain pharmaconkinetics of colchicine. Life Sci 61:153–163

Ferry DR, Traunecker H, Kerr DJ 1996 Clinical trials of P-glycoprotein reversal in solid tumours. Eur J Cancer 32A:1070–1081

Fisher GA, Sikic BI 1995 Clinical studies with modulators of multidrug resistance. Hematol Oncol Clin North Am 9:363–382

Fracasso PM, Westerveldt P, Fears CA et al 2000 Phase I study of paclitaxel in combination with a multidrug resistance modulator, PSC 833 (Valspodar), in refractory malignancies. J Clin Oncol 18:1124–1134

Giaccone G, Linn SC, Welink J et al 1997 A dose-finding and pharmacokinetic study of reversal of multidrug resistance with SDZ PSC 833 in combination with doxorubicin in patients with solid tumors. Clin Cancer Res 3:2005–2015

Hoffmeyer S, Burk O, von Richter O et al 2000 Functional polymorphisms of the human multidrug-resistance gene: multiple sequence variations and correlation of one allele with P-glycoprotein expression and activity in vivo. Proc Natl Acad Sci USA 97:3473–3478

Kang YK, Zhan Z, Regis J et al 1995 Expression of MDR-1 in refractory lymphoma: quantitation by polymerase chain reaction and validation of the assay. Blood 86:1515–1524

Kartner N, Riordan JR, Ling V 1983 Cell surface P-glycoprotein associated with multidrug resistance in mammalian cell lines. Science 221:1285–1288

Kovarik JM, Purba HS, Pongowski M, Gerbeau C, Humbert H, Mueller EA 1998 Pharmacokinetics of dexamethasone and valspodar, a P-glycoprotein (MDR1) modulator: implications for coadministration. Pharmacotherapy 18:1230–1236

Krishna R, Mayer LD 1997 Liposomal doxorubicin circumvents PSC 833-free drug interactions, resulting in effective therapy of multidrug-resistant solid tumors. Cancer Res 57:5246–5253

Luker GD, Facasso PM, Dobkin J, Piwnica-Worms D 1997 Modulation of the multidrug resistance P-glycoprotein: detection with technetium-99m-sestamibi in vivo. J Nucl Med 38:369–372

Mayer U, Wagenaar E, Dorobek B, Beijnen JH, Borst P, Schinkel AH 1997 Full blockage of intestinal P-glycoprotein and extensive inhibition of blood–brain barrier P-glycoprotein by oral treatment of mice with PSC 833. J Clin Invest 100:2430–2436

Peck RA, Marshall J, Ziessman H et al 1996 A Phase I trial of doxorubicin and VX-710. Proc Am Assoc Cancer Res 87

Piwnica-Worms D, Chiu ML, Budding M, Kronauge JF, Kramer RA, Croop JM 1993 Functional imaging of multidrug-resistant P-glycoprotein with an organotechnetium complex. Cancer Res 53:977–984

Robey R, Bakke S, Stein W et al 1999 Efflux of rhodamine from CD56[+] cells as a surrogate marker for reversal of P-glycoprotein-mediated drug efflux by PSC 833. Blood 93:306–314

Roepe PD, Wei LY, Cruz J, Carlson D 1993 Lower electrical membrane potential and altered pH_i homeostasis in multidrug-resistant (MDR) cells: further characterization of a series of MDR cell lines expressing different levels of P-glycoprotein. Biochemistry 32:11042–11056

Rowinsky EK, Smith L, Wang YM et al 1998 Phase I and pharmacokinetic study of paclitaxel in combination with biricodar, a novel agent that reverses multidrug resistance conferred by overexpression of both MDR1 and MRP. J Clin Oncol 16:2964–2976

Sandor V, Fojo T, Bates SE 1998 Future perspectives for the development of P-glycoprotein modulators. Drug Resist Updates 1:190–200

Schinkel AH, Smit JJ, van Tellingen O et al 1994 Disruption of mouse *Mdr1a* P-glycoprotein gene leads to a deficiency in the blood–brain barrier and to increased sensitivity to drugs. Cell 77:491–502

Schinkel AH, Wagenaar E, van Deemter L, Mol CA, Borst P 1995 Absence of the *Mdr1a* P-glycoprotein in mice affects tissue distribution and pharmacokinetics of dexamethasone, digoxin, and cyclosporin A. J Clin Invest 96:1698–1705

Schinkel AH, Wagenaar E, Mol CA, van Deemter L 1996 P-glycoprotein in the blood–brain barrier of mice influences the brain penetration and pharmacological activity of many drugs. J Clin Invest 97:2517–2524

Schinkel AH, Mayer U, Wagenaar E et al 1997 Normal viability and altered pharmacokinetics in mice lacking Mdr1-type (drug-transporting) P-glycoproteins. Proc Natl Acad Sci USA 94:4028–4033

Solary E, Velay I, Chauffert B et al 1991 Sufficient levels of quinine in the serum circumvent the multidrug resistance of the human leukemic cell line K562/ADM. Cancer 68:1714–1719

Solary E, Witz B, Caillot D et al 1996 Combination of quinine as a potential reversing agent with
mitoxantrone and cytarabine for the treatment of acute leukemias: a randomized multicenter
study. Blood 88:1198–1205

Sonneveld P, Marie JP, Huisman C et al 1996 Reversal of multidrug resistance by SDZ PSC 833,
combined with VAD (vincristine, doxorubicin, dexamethasone) in refractory multiple
myeloma. A phase I study. Leukemia 10:1741–1750

Sparreboom A, Planting AS, Jewell RC et al 1999 Clinical pharmacokinetics of doxorubicin in
combination with GF120918, a potent inhibitor of MDR1 P-glycoprotein. Anticancer Drugs
10:719–728

Tew KD, Houghton PJ, Houghton JA 1993 Preclinical and clinical modulation of anticancer
drugs. CRC Press, Boca Raton

Thummel KE, Shen DD, Podoll TD et al 1994 Use of midazolam as a human cytochrome P450
3A probe: II. Characterization of inter- and intraindividual hepatic CYP3A variability after
liver transplantation. J Pharmacol Exp Ther 271:557–566

Tsuruo T, Iida H, Tsukagoshi S, Sakurai Y 1981 Overcoming of vincristine resistance in P388
leukemia *in vivo* and *in vitro* through enhancing cytotoxicity of vincristine and vinblastine by
verapamil. Cancer Res 41:1967–1972

van Asperen J, Schinkel AH, Beijnen JH, Nooijen WJ, Borst P, van Tellingen O 1996 Altered
pharmacokinetics of vinblastine in Mdr1 a P-glycoprotein-deficient mice. J Natl Cancer Inst
88:994–999

van Asperen J, van Tellingen O, Tijssen F, Schinkel AH, Beijnen JH 1999 Increased
accumulation of doxorubicin and doxorubicinol in cardiac tissue of mice lacking *Mdr1a*
P-glycoprotein. Br J Cancer 79:108–113

van Zuylen L, Sparreboom A, van der Gaast A et al 2000 The orally administered P-glycoprotein
inhibitor R101933 does not alter the plasma pharmacokinetics of docetaxel. Clin Cancer Res
6:1365–1371

Wilson WH, Berg SL, Bryant G et al 1994 Paclitaxel in doxorubicin-refractory or mitoxantrone
refractory breast cancer: a phase 1/11 trial of 96-hour infusion. J Clin Oncol 12:1621–1629

Witherspoon SM, Emerson DL, Kerr BM, Lloyd TL, Dalton WS, Wissel PS 1996 Flow
cytometric assay of modulation of P-glycoprotein function in whole blood by the multidrug
resistance inhibitor GG918. Clin Cancer Res 2:7–12

DISCUSSION

Hendrikse: What about the pharmacokinetics in the brains of these patients after
modulation with PSC 833: did you see any modulating effects?

Bates: There was no evidence of Sestamibi uptake in the brain. Sestamibi is also a
substrate for MRP, so it is possible that there is redundancy in the blood–brain
barrier that is keeping MRP out. But with and without XR9756, we still don't
see Sestamibi uptake in the brain. To me this suggests that there is redundancy of
transporters.

Sisodiya: Does that reflect the time resolution of SPECT (single photon emission
computed tomography) versus PET (positron emission tomography)? The time
resolution of SPECT is poor. If there is a lot of activity in the brain, it may
happen too quickly to be picked up.

Bates: If it is solely due to Pgp then that should be overcome. The bottom line is
that there is a redundancy in the transporters that we haven't yet figured out. With

all of these Pgp antagonists, surely we should have seen more CNS toxicity. One of the things that Dr Oza points out in his paper (Oza 2002, this volume) from the toxicity studies is that although at the dose where dose-limiting toxicity (DLT) occurs you may have toxicity due to the reversing agent, at the maximum tolerated dose patients don't have CNS toxicity with the anticancer agent. You would think that Adriamycin in the brain would cause toxicity, but it doesn't.

Ling: One question that has always puzzled me is why Sestamibi doesn't go into the brain. Is it because the Pgp in the blood–brain barrier is packed together in the membrane in such a way that it is less susceptible to modulation? Or do you think that the Pgp is modulated, but there are other mechanisms that keep Sestamibi out?

Bates: I suspect that redundancy is the answer, where multiple overlapping transporters comprise the blood–brain barrier in humans. Perhaps humans have a more complex blood–brain barrier than mice. Data from knockout mice in which the orthologue for Pgp has been deleted show a 22-fold increase in vinblastine accumulation in the brain, while ivermectin is increased 87-fold (Schinkel et al 1994). This result suggests that Pgp modulation would also increase vinblastine accumulation, an idea confirmed in animal models for several compounds. Redundancy could explain why there is more impact for some compounds than for others. If you note the opiate example mentioned elsewhere by Dr Wood: with the Xenova compound (XR 9576) people get sleepy when treated with Imodium (loperamide). This would suggest that it is possible to overcome brain Pgp for some compounds that don't have other pumps.

Newman: It's also possible that Sestamibi doesn't get across the blood–brain barrier because of its structure. Then it wouldn't be necessary to pump it out.

Hendrikse: Under physiological conditions Sestamibi is normally positively charged. It could be that the positive charge prevents it from being transported across the blood–brain barrier.

Abbott: If it is a large, positively charged molecule that is not hydrophobic, it is unlikely to cross the blood–brain barrier.

Schmutz: Playing the role of devil's advocate, in this meeting we have been looking at the lessons from drug resistance in oncology, mainly concentrating on Pgp. After all the unimpressive clinical trials, the relevance of Pgp may have been overestimated. There may be other mechanisms involved. Isn't there something else that is at least as important as drug-resistance-associated proteins for drug resistance in cancer therapy? Is Pgp still in the forefront?

Bates: The problem is the time lag between work in the lab and getting it to the clinic. The impact of inhibiting the 10 or so Pgp-related transporter proteins isn't yet being tested in the clinic; we don't have inhibitors for them and we don't know where they are expressed. The need to define uptake proteins as mentioned earlier is totally new. This is a real paradigm shift, to think that a tissue needs an uptake pump. This is nowhere near ready for the clinic. The issues of survival and apoptosis are also being worked on: there are compounds that are thought to directly induce apoptosis that are in preclinical development.

Ling: There's a huge jump from demonstrating a mechanism that is potentially capable of causing drug resistance in the lab, to saying that the same mechanism correlates with clinical drug resistance.

Deisz: I would like to underscore Dr Ling's comment about the limitations of laboratory conditions and extrapolation from one species to another. In a mouse model, it has been reported that cell death induced by TRAIL (tumour necrosis factor-related apoptosis-inducing ligand) is confined to tumour cells (Walczak et al 1999). Recently, we investigated the effects of TRAIL on slices from epilepsy surgery. We provided evidence that TRAIL induces apoptosis in all CNS cells: oligodendrocytes, astrocytes and neurons (Nitsch et al 2000). The limitations of the mouse model are quite obvious in this case.

Ruetz: Pgp is a part of a long series of events. One issue that is commonly forgotten is that tumour cells are actually quite sick. Normally, tumour cells have a hard time surviving. In a growing tumour, more cells are dying than in the normal tissue. Pgp could be involved in prevention of apoptosis. It is becoming clear that Pgp might be important to help cells get over the barrier to the next level where they can be resistant. Neurons in the brain do not recover from an acid load, whereas most other cells do. It might be that Pgp is expressed in these cells in the epileptic situation because they are getting sick or damaged. The elevated expression of Pgp may be an attempt by the cell to prevent apoptosis or death. In the tumour the same thing is going on: there is a comparable situation in both epilepsy and cancer.

Abbott: Suppose it turns out that the Pgp-expressing cancer cells are indeed the sick cells, the ones trying to overcome the stress; we may be able to kill them using cytotoxic agents plus Pgp inhibitors, but maybe they would have died anyway. Proliferating cancer cells could be less vulnerable to treatment if they express less Pgp. In cultured brain endothelial cells, which show Pgp expression when fully differentiated, we noticed less expression in actively proliferating cells. So in a tumour, maybe one can kill the dying cells, but still not achieve tumour regression. It may be that the problem has been our focus on the cells we can treat rather than the ones causing the pathology.

Newman: We don't have formal proof of this, but one of the major assumptions that we have made over the years is that the cells that we can't kill are the cells that are expressing Pgp. These cells express Pgp at higher levels after a Pgp substrate chemotherapeutic agent is used. For Pgp, the correlations that have been seen in the clinic with respect to outcome relative to Pgp expression suggest that we do need to hit Pgp. Stefan Ruetz has made an important point: the Pgp comes up early, but so do many other mechanisms. One of the major lessons that we have learned in oncology is that in order to make a difference with a Pgp inhibitor we have to hit the tumours right at the beginning, at first diagnosis. At this stage there may be a small amount of Pgp in the tumours, but not a huge amount, and additional resistance mechanisms haven't kicked in yet. If we can go in at that point, there is some hope.

Bates: I agree. In this field we have learned a lot of things the hard way. We need to show that Pgp is a modulator of intracellular drug concentration and that we are changing the drug concentrations in our clinical trials. If we can double or even triple the intracellular concentration of the anticancer agent, this offers more dose intensity than some transplant regimens have offered. In oncology we need to use the drug in the 'up-front' setting, before other resistance mechanisms become established. Lower anticancer drug concentrations actually facilitate over-expression of resistance mechanisms.

Newman: We should add that because of the PK interactions observed with so many of the first and second-generation Pgp inhibitors, most Pgp modulator trials to date have been carried out with highly resistant, refractory patients who have already undergone chemotherapy. We think this is an explanation for some of the failures.

Sander: Are you saying that you should do trials with this right at the beginning instead of chemotherapy, and that this has not been done?

Bates: For ethical reasons, most modulator trials have been conducted in the relapsed setting, where no curative potential exists. Once non-toxic inhibitors are developed that don't interfere with pharmacokinetics and are confirmed to increase accumulation of anticancer drugs in some tumours, then clinicians will feel confident in moving some of these inhibitors to an up-front setting. Then this question can be directly addressed.

Wood: There is a different strategy that hasn't been discussed at all: we have taken the approach that we should inhibit Pgp when a drug is a Pgp substrate. But if you take lessons from the drug metabolism area, what industry did was having identified that things were substrates, it then factored out that. So rather than inhibiting 2D6, people developed drugs that were not 2D6 substrates. The other, much more attractive approach is to develop drugs that are not Pgp substrates. This would allow us to get around the whole problem of Pgp versus MRP and so on. It is probably not all that difficult to do: it would be possible to screen thousands of compounds using high throughput screening.

Scheper: My worry is that there will not be any drugs that are not subject to one or more of these pumps.

Bates: We have two new anticancer agents that aren't good Pgp substrates, but are excellent substrates for BCRP. If the epilepsy community finds that the only transporter that gets overexpressed in epilepsy is Pgp, then a strategy to develop non-Pgp substrates would be better. But for cancer, the tissue is too pleiotropic and the force of selection is too great: there could be overexpression of a whole group of these transporters.

Newman: Alastair Wood is right in principle. A huge amount of effort has gone into trying to discover and develop chemotherapeutic agents related to the good ones that are currently available, but which are not Pgp substrates. The lack of progress in the area certainly isn't from a lack of effort. What has happened is that the companies have found out that it was a lot tougher than they thought it might be. After more than a decade of searching we only now have agents that are in the earliest stages of clinical development.

Ling: It seems to me that what we are saying is that it is important to define clearly what transporters there are for neurology. It doesn't mean that there will not be other mechanisms of resistance, but at least this is one mechanism that we know. The second question is whether we would prefer to try to avoid a transporter and compromise by having a less effective anti-epileptic drug (AED), or would we prefer the best AED possible and then try to modulate the way of getting the drug to the target.

Löscher: Of course, industry is doing this already in the development of neuroactive compounds, not only in terms of AEDs. This is also an issue for other diseases of the brain in which there is pharmacoresistance. The second strategy you mentioned — to look for lead compounds, and then only after you have them to change the structure so that they are no longer substrates of Pgp — is one that is being used.

Andermann: Can you predict whether what you get by modulation of Pgp will be an increase in effectiveness of AEDs, rather than an increase in side effects? Theoretically, you might also get an increase in side effects. One of the interesting issues is that people who have drug interactions may have relatively low serum levels of drugs, yet they may have quite considerable side effects. The side effects don't seem to be necessarily related to the serum level.

Löscher: There is an interesting point that has not been discussed at this meeting: some of these drug transporters are not equally distributed across the brain. Thinking about your question in a speculative way, in temporal lobe epilepsy and other focal epilepsies, the target for the anticonvulsant effect of an AED may be different from the targets for side effects. If drug transporters are involved here, their distribution across different brain regions could be very important. Not much is known about this. It has been reported that the MRPs are not evenly distributed.

Meldrum: This is an important general issue that challenges the concept behind this meeting. We give AEDs to patients. Those who aren't drug resistant stop having generalized seizures, but those who are continue to have seizures. But with regard to side effects, by definition the situation is reversed: those who are drug resistant show large side effects, and this stops us giving them higher doses. We know that the compound is getting into the brain and acting there, so resistance to AEDs can't be a generalized effect on transport; it can't be a Pgp effect that applies to the whole brain. The only hypothesis that supports this meeting has to be that there is a focal concentration of Pgp that is preventing the drug getting to that focus. But this doesn't make sense in the clinical context in that AEDs can exacerbate the focal discharge. An increase in interictal discharges is often observed in patients successfully treated with carbamazepine (Wilkus et al 1978, Rodin et al 1974).

Sisodiya: We have been looking at the cerebellum in some post-mortem cases. Whereas we see overexpression of drug-resistance proteins in the lesion we don't see overexpression in the cerebellum. In drug-resistant patients, even when we increase the dose, it is still not getting into the focus of the epilepsy, although it may get into other areas, such as the cerebellum. This may cause side-effects, even though the drug is not working.

Meldrum: The carbamazepine effect, for example, blocks the generalized seizures but may increase the interictal discharges in successfully treated patients. The evidence is that the focus is not the site of treatment. The site of treatment has to be the brain as a whole, or the interface between the focus and the brain — it can't be the focus.

Sills: How do you know that the increase in interictal spikes in these carbamazepine-treated patients is directly related to the drug and not the abolition of the generalized seizure itself?

Meldrum: That is one hypothesis: that what we are seeing in these spikes is an abortive form of what would have been a generalized seizure. The spikes are still occurring in the focus, and therefore you can't see the mechanism of action of the drug as being essentially on the focus, either. In the case of barbiturates, focal discharges are commonly abolished, but this is not the case for carbamazepine.

Pirmohamed: I wonder whether we are jumping too far by proposing the development of AEDs that are poor substrates for Pgp and MRP. We have established that there is increased expression of certain transporters in some parts of the brain, but surely the most crucial issue is that of the 15 AEDs available, the research has to identify that these are substrates for all the different transporters. If they are not, then we may be wasting our time.

Ling: The ABC transporter people will say that they would be astounded if there weren't some transporter that could affect any of the AEDs currently available or that will be invented in the future. Also, we don't know in either the normal or diseased brain which transporters are the ones actually expressed at a clinically relevant level. There are a lot of questions that are still unanswered.

References

Nitsch R, Bechmann I, Deisz RA et al 2000 Human brain-cell death induced by tumour-necrosis-factor-related apoptosis-inducing ligand (TRAIL). Lancet 356:827–828

Oza AM 2002 Clinical development of P glycoprotein modulators in oncology. In: Mechanisms of drug resistance in epilepsy: lessons from oncology. Wiley, Chichester (Novartis Found Symp 243) p 103–118

Rodin EA, Rim CS, Rennick PM 1974 The effects of carbamazepine on patients with psychomotor epilepsy: results of a double-blind study. Epilepsia 15:547–561

Schinkel AH, Smit JJ, van Tellingen O et al 1994 Disruption of the mouse mdr1a P-glycoprotein gene leads to a deficiency in the blood-brain barrier and to increased sensitivity to drugs. Cell 77:491–502

Walczak H, Miller RE, Ariail K et al 1999 Tumoricidal activity of tumor necrosis factor-related apoptosis-indcing ligand in vivo. Nat Med 5:157–163

Wilkus RJ, Dodrill CB, Troupin AS 1978 Carbamazepine and the electroencephalogram of epileptics: a double blind study in comparison to phenytoin. Epilepsia 19:283–291

Clinical development of P glycoprotein modulators in oncology

Amit M. Oza

Princess Margaret Hospital, 610 University Avenue, Toronto, Ontario, Canada M5G 2M9

Abstract. The last two decades have witnessed dramatic advances into the mechanisms of drug resistance in cancer. The identification of P glycoprotein (Pgp) as a specific mechanism led to the initial hope and expectation that it would be possible to modulate this and increase sensitivity to drug therapy. Clinical trials using first- and second-generation Pgp modulators did establish proof of principle that in some settings, clinical drug resistance could be overcome with the addition of a Pgp modulator — for example, clinical resistance to paclitaxel, a Pgp substrate, in women with ovarian cancer was shown to be overcome in approximately 20% with the addition of PSC 833, a highly effective Pgp modulator. However, evolutionary and adaptive redundancy in resistance mechanisms have tempered clinical results, even with very effective second- and third-generation modulators. The lessons from oncology establish sound methodology for the evaluation of Pgp modulators for safety, tolerability and efficacy in Phase I, II and III clinical trials. This review will focus on some of the early-phase clinical trials with earlier and newer Pgp modulators, either as single agents or in combination with chemotherapy.

2002 Mechanisms of drug resistance in epilepsy: lessons from oncology. Wiley, Chichester (Novartis Foundation Symposium 243) p103–118

Systemic chemotherapy has been used in the treatment of cancer for four decades, with gradual improvement in the efficacy of therapy. A wide variety of anticancer agents are in current clinical use with increasing specificity of action. Recent anticancer agents are specifically targeting aberrant cellular processes in the cancer cell with the hope and expectation of improving activity and reducing non-specific toxicity. Over the past 10–20 years, it has become apparent that during the course of evolution, our bodies have developed many different protective ways of overcoming and adapting to pharmacological assaults. Whilst these adaptive and protective mechanisms are extremely important, the same mechanisms are also present in malignant cells and therefore potentially reduce the efficacy of anticancer drug therapy. Although this review will primarily focus on P glycoprotein (Pgp), and lessons learnt over the past decade or two when there was a major drive to modulate Pgp-based drug resistance to improve results, it is important to realize that there is a tremendous amount of protective evolutionary redundancy in resistance mechanisms in malignant and non-malignant tissues. This is one of the prime reasons for the limited clinical impact of Pgp modulation. From a simplistic point of view, the goal of using Pgp modulators in oncology is to increase anticancer drug concentration in cancer cells by reducing efflux and clearance. As anticancer drugs are generally administered in a cyclical fashion, the Pgp modulators were also administered in temporal relation to cyclical therapy. For non-malignant indications however, such as anticonvulsant therapy, drugs have to be administered continuously and therefore the challenges of Pgp modulation are quite distinct.

Pgp in cancer

Drug resistance, either intrinsic or acquired, is a frequently encountered problem in the failure of antineoplastic agents. Pgp, an efflux pump that extrudes hydrophobic cytotoxic drugs from cancer cells, plays a key role in multidrug resistance (MDR) and may contribute to clinical drug resistance. Pgp is a 170 kDa cell-surface glycoprotein, encoded for by the *MDR1* gene (Riordan & Ling 1985). The presence of MDR has been correlated with poor outcome in acute myeloid leukaemia, non-Hodgkin's lymphoma, acute lymphoblastic leukaemia and multiple myeloma (Arceci 1993, Fojo et al 1987, Goldstein et al 1989, Ro et al 1990, Pastan & Gottesman 1987, Epstein et al 1989, Herweijer et al 1990, Campos et al 1992). Many chemotherapeutic agents were also confirmed to be excellent substrates for the Pgp pump (Pastan & Gottesman 1987, Dorr et al 1987, Ford & Hait 1990, Epstein et al 1989, Herweijer et al 1990, Campos et al 1992). Many studies analysed the expression of Pgp in normal and malignant tissues and found that several tumours that showed high levels of expression of Pgp also seemed to show considerable clinical resistance to Pgp substrates — for example, colon cancer has very high levels of Pgp and is very resistant to doxorubicin, a Pgp substrate. It is also important to note that epithelial surfaces such as the biliary tract and gall bladder show high levels of Pgp and show chemoresistance to most drugs. Intrinsically resistant malignancies that are associated with high levels of Pgp are colon cancer, renal cell cancer, non-small-cell lung cancer, gliomas, meningiomas and primitive neuroectodermal tumours.

Many different resistance modulators have been identified to date, illustrated in Fig. 1. It is also now apparent that the mechanisms of resistance also differ with the different chemotherapeutic agents, and there may be several different mechanisms that are active simultaneously. Examples of the different resistance mechanisms which are in part responsible for clinical drug resistance are provided in Table 1. In addition to multiple mechanisms of drug resistance, it is also apparent that treatment will also induce resistance. Several studies have compared the level of

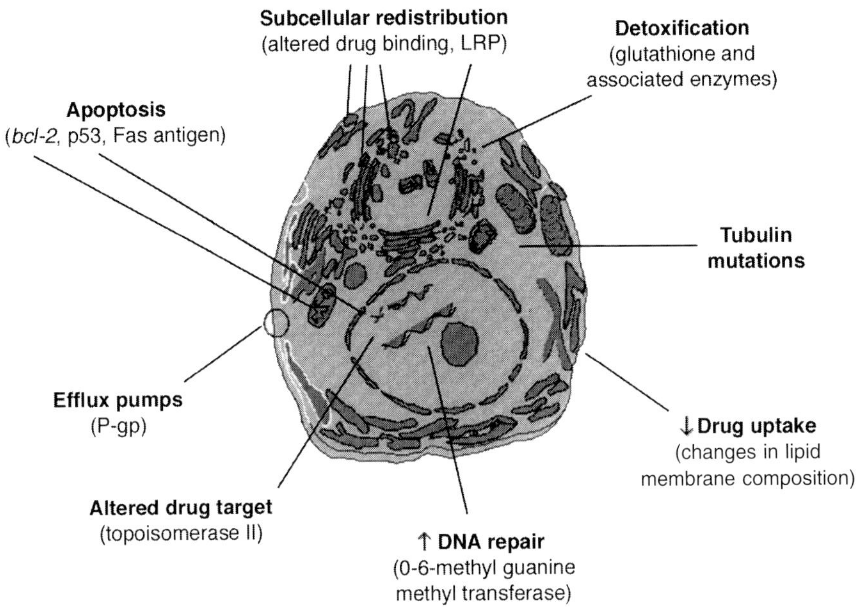

FIG. 1.   Potential mechanisms of drug resistance. Modified from Dalton et al (1993).

TABLE 1   Mechanisms of resistance to different chemotheraputic drugs

Drug	Mechanism of resistance
Doxorubicin, Daunorubicin, Idarubicin	Pgp, MRP, LRP, topoisomerase II
Mitoxantrone	Pgp, topoisomerase II
Vincristine	Pgp, tubulins
Melphalan	GSH/GST, LRP
Etoposide	Pgp, MRP, topoisomerase II
Paclitaxel	Pgp, tubulin mutations

Pgp expression at diagnosis and at relapse, with a fairly consistent trend showing increase in amount of Pgp with recurrence (Table 2).

Evidence to support the hypothesis that clinical resistance is dependent on Pgp expression in some malignancies was provided by the demonstration that Pgp expression could inversely correlate with response to therapy. This was elegantly demonstrated by Willman (1997), who evaluated 211 elderly patients with acute myeloid leukaemia and assessed both overall Pgp expression and functional

TABLE 2 Acquired drug resistance

| | Pgp level (%) | |
Disease	At diagnosis	At relapse
AML	23	42
ALL	33	48
Myeloma	42	69
Lymphomas	14	52
Ovarian cancer	15	47
Breast cancer	0–50	30–85
Retinoblastoma	20	100

AML, acute myeloid leukaemia; ALL, acute lymphoblastic leukeamia.

assessment of Pgp using rhodamine efflux (Table 3). The study shows that increased Pgp expression correlates with increased dye/drug efflux from leukaemia cells and both of these inversely correlate with likelihood of inducing remission. Del Poeta et al (1996) looked at survival in patients with acute myeloid leukaemia and found that patients had inferior survival if their disease was positive for Pgp. This applied equally in younger and elderly patients (Table 4).

The initial studies therefore pointed to a potentially major role for Pgp in causing clinical resistance and raised the intriguing possibility that overcoming or modulating Pgp would improve effectiveness of anticancer therapy. However, unless Pgp expression is modulated selectively in malignant tissues only, it is likely that normal tissue Pgp function will also be significantly affected and this could potentially increase treatment related toxicity.

TABLE 3 Correlation between Pgp expression, efflux and rate of CR

Pgp expression	CR rate (%)	Dye/drug efflux	CR rate (%)
Negative	71	Negative	62
Low	54	Low	59
Intermediate	36	Intermediate	43
High	31	High	33

CR, complete remission.

TABLE 4   Potential mechanisms of drug resistance in malignant cells

Mechanism	Effect	Drugs
Drug efflux pumps	Pgp, MRP — remove drug from within cell	Anthracyclines, vinca alkaloids, etoposide, taxanes
Decreased drug uptake	Changes in lipid membrane composition	Methotrexate, nitrogen mustard, melphalan, cisplatin
Tubulin mutations	Alter sensitivity to taxanes/ chemotherapy	Taxanes
Altered drug target	Changes in levels of target enzymes or alteration in target	Methotrexate, anti-metabolites, topoisomerase inhibitors
Subcellular redistribution	Altered drug binding	
Apoptosis	Decreased ability to undergo apoptosis: Bcl2, p53, Fas antigen	Alkylating agents, cisplatin, etoposide
Detoxification	Glutathione and associated enzymes bind to drug	Cisplatin, alkylating agents
DNA repair	Repair damage induced by chemotherapy	Anthracyclines, alkylating agents, cisplatin

Normal tissue expression of Pgp

High levels of Pgp expression are seen in the adrenal cortex, kidney, liver, placenta, colon, small bowel, brain (blood–brain barrier), testes, pancreas and haemopoietic precursor cells (Fojo et al 1987, Goldstein et al 1989, Ro et al 1990). Adrenal medulla, trachea, lung and prostate show moderate expression; skin, muscle, heart, spleen, oesophagus, stomach, ovary, spinal cord and bone marrow have low levels of Pgp. Diverse functions have been ascribed to Pgp, including steroid transport in the adrenal cortex, excretion of carcinogens, xenobiotics, bilirubin and drugs in the biliary tract and kidney, and as a barrier to toxic substances in the brain, placenta and testes (Lum & Gosland 1995). Thus the potential disruption of these normal functions have to be taken into account when planning to modulate Pgp, particularly for prolonged periods. For example, modulating Pgp may result in hyperbilirubinaemia, and points to a physiological role for Pgp in bilirubin transportation.

Use of Pgp modulators in oncology

Before considering specific Pgp modulators and clinical trials in oncology, it would be useful to review the general principles that governed early studies.

Some of the earliest modulators (first generation) were agents that were in clinical use and were found to have a general mild Pgp modulating ability. Examples are verapamil, cyclosporin and tamoxifen. The advantages with these agents were the general familiarity with longer-term use and knowledge of chronic toxicity. Limitations were the lack of specificity of action, poor therapeutic ratio and possibility of pharmacokinetic interaction with other drugs (particularly with agents such as cyclosporin). These agents were subsequently combined in different schedules with cyclical chemotherapy to see if the anticancer effect of chemotherapy could be enhanced.

Second- and third-generation Pgp modulators were designed specifically to modulate Pgp and therefore are considerably better at Pgp modulation *in vitro* and *in vivo*. The therapeutic ratios are therefore generally better, with significant Pgp reversal/modulation being feasible at clinically achievable doses. Table 5 summarizes drug levels needed for Pgp reversal and puts these in context of achievable levels using appropriate drug dosing.

Clinical trials

Establishing that a promising novel agent has clinical value is a lengthy process, which has to take a drug that has generally not been used in humans to a stage where it can be compared with the standard of care in a randomized Phase III study. The picture is further complicated when looking at Pgp modulators as the agents alone do not have therapeutic value (but may have significant toxicity) and

TABLE 5   Drug levels needed for reversal of multidrug resistance

Drug	*[MDR reversal]* $\mu g/ml$	*Level achieved in patients* $\mu g/ml$	*Drug dose*
Verapamil	6–10	1–2	180 mg/m^2
Tamoxifen	10	7	200–700 mg (N = 20 mg)
Toremifene	10	7.8 (2.5–15)	780 mg/day × 3
Cyclosporin A	2–4	2	
PSC 833	0.5–2	1–4	20 mg/kg per day
Dexverapamil	6–10	2	
GG918	0.05–0.1	0.1–0.5	50–100 mg qid
LY335979	60 nM (0.1–0.5)	0.5–1	480 mg/m^2 per day Tox: 1500–2800
VX710	0.5–2.5	1.3–7.8	18–120 mg/m^2
MoAB MRK16	10		

therefore have to be combined with other therapeutic agents such as chemotherapy. The initial step in clinical development of these agents is to demonstrate that the modulator can be administered safely with manageable toxicity. Once this is determined, the Pgp modulator can be used in combination with other Pgp substrates, to improve the therapeutic efficacy of the latter. The toxicity seen with Pgp modulator trials can also be predicted to a certain extent. Specificity of the modulator is of major importance and therefore significant toxicities were predictable particularly with first generation modulators such as verapamil (cardiac toxicity) or cyclosporin (immunosuppression). In general, second- and third-generation agents are much more specific and therefore non-specific toxicity is minimized. As was previously mentioned, toxicity is also dependent on the normal distribution of Pgp in the body. In this regard, class effects such as ataxia and hyperbilirubinaemia were often seen as the limiting toxicities with many agents. Although ataxia is a class effect seen with many Pgp modulators, its mechanism of action is poorly understood and presumed to be secondary to the blood–brain barrier being breached.

The process of establishing objective evidence of therapeutic value in cancer treatment will be illustrated with the clinical development of a novel non-immunosuppressive cyclosporin analogue, PSC 833 (Valspodar, Novartis Pharmaceuticals, Hanover, NJ).

PSC 833 is a highly lipophilic, oral semisynthetic non-immunosuppressive cyclosporin D analogue that can modulate MDR activity with low toxicity *in vitro* and *in vivo* (Twentyman & Bleehen 1991, Boesch et al 1991a, Simon et al 1998). PSC 833 has a high binding affinity for Pgp at concentrations that can readily be achieved in blood, and it has been shown to occupy the Pgp molecule for longer durations than cyclosporin A (CsA) (Smith et al 1998, Sonneveld et al 1996). Unlike CsA, which binds to both Pgp and cyclophilin (the latter accounting for its immunosuppressive effects), PSC 833 binds only to Pgp. In toxicology studies, PSC 833 is not immunosuppressive, nephrotoxic or cytotoxic. PSC 833 has been shown in *in vitro* models to be approximately 10-fold more potent than CsA in its ability to inhibit Pgp. Cell viability studies suggest that MDR reversal in highly resistant cell lines can be achieved at PSC 833 concentrations of 1000–2000 ng/ml (Boesch et al 1991a,b, Keller et al 1992, Kornblau et al 1997). PSC 833 completely reversed resistance of MDR-CHO, MDR-P388, and MDR-LoVo cells to four different anticancer drugs (vincristine, doxorubicin, daunorubicin and etoposide) at concentrations ranging from 31.6 ng/ml to 1000 ng/ml (Boesch et al 1991a, Keller et al 1992, te Boekhorst et al 1992). PSC 833 has no effect in sensitizing MDR-negative resistant cell lines or in altering sensitivities of resistant cell lines to anticancer drugs such as platinum analogues that are not known to be substrates for Pgp (Boesch et al 1991b). *In vivo* studies using MDR-P388 (murine monocytic leukaemia cell line) tumour-bearing mice showed two- to threefold increases in survival times when PSC 833 doses of 25–50 mg/kg orally were used to pre-treat animals 4 h prior to receiving doxorubicin i.p. compared with doxorubicin alone. Oral paclitaxel, when administered to mice at a dose of 10 mg/kg along with 50 mg/kg of oral PSC 833, showed a tenfold increase in AUC (area under the concentration curve) compared to controls that received the same dose of paclitaxel alone. Furthermore, the oral bioavailability of paclitaxel was increased 10-fold by the concomitant administration of PSC 833 (van Asperen et al 1997). Phase I/II studies of PSC 833 in conjunction with a wide range of anticancer drugs that are also Pgp substrates have shown the ability to achieve safe and consistent blood concentrations of PSC 833 that are above the *in vitro* threshold for MDR reversal (Simon et al 1998, Giaccone et al 1994, Thiessen et al 1994).

PSC 833 affects the pharmacokinetics of anticancer drugs that are Pgp substrates. In Phase I studies, the mean decreases in clearance of doxorubicin and etoposide were 29–33% and 40%, respectively. The most likely explanation for this is inhibition by PSC 833 of the physiological function of Pgp in the distribution and elimination of these agents (Lum et al 1992, 1994, Bartlett et al 1994, Erlichman et al 1993, 1994). Cytotoxic drugs that are substrates for Pgp therefore require dose reduction when administered concurrently with PSC 833. In Phase I trials of PSC 833 in combination with 3 h and 24 h paclitaxel, the recommended Phase II dose of paclitaxel was 70 mg/m^2, representing a 60% dose reduction from the commonly employed 175 mg/m^2 dose of paclitaxel (Fracasso et al 1995, Collins et al 1995).

The initial clinical development of PSC 833 established the safety and tolerability of administering this agent by itself, starting at a low dose and gradually escalating to the maximum tolerated dose (MTD). During this initial phase, pharmacology studies help determine the optimal way of administering the PSC 833, looking at different formulations, timing of therapy and impact of food/drink on its absorption (for oral formulation). Data available on 61 patients with advanced solid tumours treated with PSC 833 at 5 mg/kg four times daily demonstrated that reversible ataxia and dysmetria, suggestive of possible cerebellar dysfunction, were common side effects and were the dose-limiting toxicities. 67% of patients experienced grade 1 or 2 reversible ataxia, while an additional 8% experienced reversible grade 3 ataxia. The ataxia was maximal several hours after oral dosing, thus suggesting a peak concentration effect (Fisher et al 1994). While the aetiology of the ataxia is unknown, it is hypothesized that this may be the result of Pgp inhibition at the blood–brain barrier. Reversible hyperbilirubinaemia, though not dose-limiting, was also a frequent occurrence and was felt to be due to the inhibition of Pgp in cells lining the bile canaliculi (Fracasso et al 1995, Collins et al 1995, Hausdorff et al 1995, Covelli 1996, Boote et al 1996, Pearce & Israel 1993).

Once the therapeutic dose was established in single agent Phase I studies, additional Phase I combination studies were initiated, using the MTD of PSC 833, with gradually escalating doses of chemotherapy, the latter generally being a Pgp substrate, such as doxorubicin or paclitaxel. These studies confirmed that the clearance of the Pgp substrate was reduced, indicating that the Pgp modulator was exerting a biological effect, the result being a reduction in the dose of chemotherapy that would be equitoxic to the MTD of the chemotherapy alone. Administration of PSC 833 resulted in predictable reduction of the clearance of concomitantly administered chemotherapeutic agents and an increase in the area under the curve of the same drug. The MTD of the concomitantly administered chemotherapeutic drugs was reduced by 40–60%, illustrated in Table 6, with substrate chemotherapeutic agents such as daunomycin, mitoxantrone, etoposide and paclitaxel. Obviously, the hope and expectation was that the reduced clearance of Pgp substrate chemotherapy would go hand in hand with prolonged exposure and hence improve clinical efficacy.

The doses established in these combination Phase I studies were subsequently used in Phase II trials looking for efficacy and to demonstrate proof of principle that Pgp modulation could overcome drug resistance. For example, one design was to take patients with ovarian cancer who had either not responded to paclitaxel or progressed whilst on this agent (thus establishing resistance), and subsequently re-challenge patients to paclitaxel plus a PSC 833. Proof of principle showing Pgp modulation could overcome drug resistance would be established if patients clinically responded to the combination. This trial, reported by Fracasso et al (2001), showed that some patients whose disease was resistant to paclitaxel did respond to the combination of paclitaxel and PSC 833, increasing enthusiasm to incorporate PSC 833 into additional chemotherapeutic first line regimens.

The next and potentially final confirmatory step in the development of PSC 833 led to randomized Phase III trials comparing the new active combination with modulator with standard therapy. This can be illustrated with the clinical trial strategy used for first line therapy of advanced ovarian cancer. Standard therapy

TABLE 6   The effects of PSC 833 on the maximum tolerated doses (MTDs) of various chemotherapeutic drugs

Cytotoxic drug	MTD without PSC 833	MTD with PSC 833
Daunomycin	45 mg/m^2	35 mg/m^2
Mitoxantrone	6 mg/m^2	4.5 mg/m^2
Etoposide	80 mg/m^2	30 mg/m^2
Paclitaxel	175 mg/m^2	80 mg/m^2

for this disease is with combination chemotherapy with paclitaxel (dose 175 mg/ m^2) and carboplatin. A Phase I trial of the combination of PSC 833, paclitaxel and carboplatin was completed and reported by Patnaik et al (2000). This confirmed that the equitoxic dose of paclitaxel is 81 mg/m^2 when PSC 833 is added is to the combination, with no change in carboplatin dose. A randomized clinical trial comparing these two regimens has now been conducted in advanced ovarian cancer, and the final results are awaited. At present, we still do not have any confirmed evidence to verify that addition of a Pgp modulator to initial chemotherapy improves the outcome of therapy.

In summary, trials have shown that Pgp modulators can potentially increase drug effect at lower chemotherapy concentrations. However, the development has been directed at maximizing short term, cyclical administration of chemotherapy and the modulator studies have been designed around chemotherapy schedules. It may be time for novel designs but there are scant data from chronic dosing for these second and third generation modulators.

Limitations to use of Pgp modulation in oncology

There are several cautionary points that have to kept in mind when considering other potential roles for Pgp modulation, summarized below:

- The therapeutic window may be narrow for Pgp modulation.
- The agents may change pharmacology of other drugs.
- The modulators may affect drug metabolism, particularly through cytochrome P450 effects.
- Multiple resistance mechanisms that are now recognized in cancer cells will limit efficacy of even the most potent Pgp modulator.

Resistance to cytotoxic agents may be intrinsic or acquired. There are several forms of multidrug resistance identified in tumours, including elevated levels of Pgp and the multidrug resistance-associated protein (MRP1), both members of the ATP-binding cassette (ABC) transmembrane protein family (Allen et al 1999). Lung resistance protein (LRP), and atypical MDR (mediated through altered expression of topoisomerase II) have also been implicated in multidrug resistance (Allen et al 1999, Nooter & Stoter 1996, Loe et al 1996, Izquierdo et al 1996, Nitiss & Beck 1996). The recently identified ABC gene *BCRP/MXR/ABCP* may also contribute to resistance to drugs such as doxorubicin, mitoxantrone and topotecan which is independent of Pgp or MRP1 (Allen et al 1999). The relative contributions of each mechanism of multidrug resistance in clinical tumours is complex and there are likely to be many unidentified or poorly understood mechanisms which have yet to be elucidated.

Many other second- and third-generation Pgp modulators have been developed and are in various stages of clinical trials in oncology. Several of these share similar dose-limiting toxicities, particularly ataxia. Of necessity, the designs of these clinical trials are dependent on and revolve around standard chemotherapy schedules, with Pgp modulators being used as an adjunct. Thus the majority of, if not all, clinical trials with Pgp modulators have been cyclical, and the schedules based on the standard and established chemotherapy protocols. There is therefore little information about more chronic dosing schedules in humans and this may be a significant challenge when attempting to extrapolate from these studies to neurology.

References

Allen JD, Brinkhuis RF, Wijnholds J, Schinkel AH 1999 The mouse *Bcrp1/Mxr/Abcp* gene: amplification and overexpression in cell lines selected for resistance to topotecan, mitoxantrone, or doxorubicin. Cancer Res 59:4237–4241

Arceci RJ 1993 Clinical significance of P-glycoprotein in multidrug resistance malignancies. Blood 81:2215–2222

Bartlett NL, Lum BL, Fisher GA et al 1994 Phase I trial of doxorubicin with cyclosporine as a modulator of multidrug resistance. J Clin Oncol 12:835–842

Boesch D, Gaveriaux C, Jachez B, Pourtier-Manzanedo A, Bollinger P, Loor F 1991a In vivo circumvention of P-glycoprotein-mediated multidrug resistance of tumor cells with SDZ PSC 833. Cancer Res 51:4226–4233

Boesch D, Muller K, Pourtier-Manzanedo A, Loor F 1991b Restoration of daunomycin retention in multidrug-resistant P388 cells by submicromolar concentrations of SDZ PSC 833, a nonimmunosuppressive cyclosporin derivative. Exp Cell Res 196:26–32

Boote DJ, Dennis IF, Twentyman PR et al 1996 Phase I study of etoposide with SDZ PSC 833 as a modulator of multidrug resistance in patients with cancer. J Clin Oncol 14:610–618

Campos L, Guyotat D, Archimbaud E et al 1992 Clinical significance of multidrug resistance P-glycoprotein expression on acute nonlymphoblastic leukemia cells at diagnosis. Blood 79:473–476

Collins HL, Fisher GA, Hausdorff J 1995 Phase I trial of paclitaxel in combination with SDZ PSC 833, a multidrug resistance modulator. Proc Am Soc Clin Oncol 14:A406

Covelli A 1996 SDZ PSC 833 investigator's brochure. Sandoz Pharma, Basel

Dalton WS 1993 Drug resistance modulation in the laboratory and the clinic. Semin Oncol 20:64–69

Del Poeta G, Stasi R, Aronica G et al 1996 Clinical relevance of P-glycoprotein expression in *de novo* acute myeloid leukaemia. Blood 87:1997–2004

Dorr RT, Liddil JD, Trent JM, Dalton WS 1987 Mitomycin C resistant L1210 leukemia cells: association with pleiotropic drug resistance. Biochem Pharmacol 36:3155–3120

Epstein J, Xiao HQ, Oba BK 1989 P-glycoprotein expression in plasma-cell myeloma is associated with resistance to VAD. Blood 74:913–917

Erlichman C, Moore M, Thiessen JJ et al 1993 Phase I pharmacokinetic study of cyclosporin A combined with doxorubicin. Cancer Res 53:4837–4842

Erlichman C, Moore M, Thiessen J et al 1994 A phase I trial of doxorubicin (DOX) and PSC 833, a modulator of multidrug resistance (MDR). Anticncer Drugs 5:A97

Fisher GA, Halsey J, Hausdorff J et al 1994 A phase I study of paclitaxel (Taxol®) in combination with SDZ PSC 833, a potent modulator of multidrug resistance (MDR). Anticancer Drugs 5:A99

Fojo AT, Ueda K, Salmon DJ, Poplack DG, Gottesman MM, Pastan I 1987 Expression of a multidrug resistance gene in human tumors and tissues. Proc Natl Acad Sci USA 84:265–269

Ford IM, Hait WN 1990 Pharmacology of drugs that alter multidrug resistance in cancer. Pharmacol Rev 2:156–199

Fracasso PM, Fisher GA, Wiehl JG et al 1995 Phase I trial of paclitaxel and SDZ PSC 833 in patients with solid tumors. Proc Am Soc Clin Oncol 14: A1585

Fracasso PM, Brady MF, Moore DH et al 2001 Phase II study of paclitaxel and valspodar (PSC 833) in refractory ovarian carcinoma: a gynecologic oncology group study. J Clin Oncol 19:2975–2982

Giaccone G, Linn SC, Catimel G et al 1994 SDZ PSC 833 in combination with doxorubicin: A phase I and pharmacologic study in solid tumors. Anticancer Drugs 5:A98

Goldstein LJ, Galski H, Fojo A et al 1989 Expression of a multidrug resistance gene in human cancers. J Natl Cancer Inst 81:116–124

Hausdorff J, Fisher GA, Halsey J et al 1995 A phase I trial of etoposide with the oral cyclosporin SDZ PSC 833, a modulator of multidrug resistance (MDR). Proc Am Soc Clin Oncol 14:A407

Herweijer H, Sonneveld P, Baas F, Nooter K 1990 Expression of mdr1 and mdr3 multidrug-resistance genes in human acute and chronic leukemias and association with stimulation of drug accumulation of cyclosporine. J Natl Cancer Inst 82:1133–1140

Izquierdo MA, Scheffer GL, Flens MJ, Schroeijers AB, van der Valk P, Scheper RJ 1996 Major vault protein LRP-related multidrug resistance. Eur J Cancer 32A:979–984

Keller RP, Altermatt HJ, Nooter K et al 1992 SDZ-PSC 833, a non-immunosuppressive cyclosporine: its potency in overcoming P-glycoprotein-mediated multidrug resistance of murine leukemia. Int J Cancer 50:593–597

Kornblau SM, Estey E, Madden T et al 1997 Phase I study of mitoxantrone plus etoposide with multidrug blockade by SZ PSC-833 in relapsed or refractory acute myelogenous leukemia. J Clin Oncol 15:1796–1802

Loe DW, Deeley RG, Cole SPW 1996 Biology of multidrug-resistance in tumor cells. Eur J Cancer 32A:945–957

Lum BL, Gosland MP 1995 MDR expression in normal tissues. Pharmacologic implications for the clinical use of P-glycoprotein inhibitors. Hematol Oncol Clin North Am 9:319–336

Lum BL, Kaubisch S, Yahanda AM et al 1992 Alteration of etoposide pharmacokinetics and pharmaocodynamics by cyclosporine in a phase I trial to modulate multidrug resistance. J Clin Oncol 10:1635–1642

Lum BL, Fisher GA, Hausdorff J et al 1994 The effect of oral SDZ PSC 833 on the pharmacokinetics (PK) of etoposide (E) during a phase I trial to modulate multidrug resistance. Anticancer Drugs 5:A102

Nitiss LJ, Beck WT 1996 Anti-topoisomerase drug action and resistance. Eur J Cancer 32A:958–966

Nooter K, Stoter G 1996 Molecular mechanisms of multidrug resistance in cancer chemotherapy. Pathol Res Pract 192:768–780

Pastan I, Gottesman M 1987 Multiple-drug resistance in human cancer. N Engl J Med 316:1388–1393

Patnaik A, Warner E, Michael M et al 2000 Phase I dose-finding and pharmacokinetic study of paclitaxel and carboplatin with oral valspodar in patients with advanced solid tumors. J Clin Oncol 18: 3677–3689

Pearce T, Israel R 1993 PSC 833 investigator's brochure. Sandoz Pharmceutical, East Hannover, NJ

Riordan JR, Ling V 1985 Genetic and biochemical characterization of multidrug resistance. Pharmacol Ther 28:51–75

Ro J, Sahin A, Ro JY, Fritsche H, Hortobagyi G, Blick M 1990 Immunohistochemical analysis of P-glycoprotein expression correlated with chemotherapy resistance in locally advanced breast cancer. Hum Pathol 21:787–791

Simon N, Dailly E, Combes O et al 1998 Role of lipoproteins in the plasma binding of SDZ PSC 833, a novel multidrug resistance-reversing cyclosporin. Br J Clin Pharmacol 45:173–175

Smith A J, Mayer U, Schinkel AH, Borst P 1998 Availability of PSC 833, a substrate and inhibitor of P-glycoproteins, in various concentrations of serum. J Natl Cancer Inst 90:1161–1166

Sonneveld P, Marie J-P, Huisman C et al 1996 Reversal of multidrug resistance of SDZ PSC 833, combined with VAD (vincristine, doxorubicin, dexamethasone) in refractory multiple myeloma. A phase I study. Leukemia 10:1741–1750

te Boekhorst PAW, van Kapel J, Schoester M, Sonneveld P 1992 Reversal of typical multidrug resistance by cyclosporin and its non-immunosuppressive analogue SDZ PSC 833 in Chinese hamster ovary cells expressing the *mdr*1 phenotype. Cancer Chemother Pharmacol 30:238–242

Thiessen J J, Erlichman C, Moore M J et al 1994 The pharmacokinetics and bioavailability of a new chemosensitizer, SDZ PSC 833, in patients with advanced bladder cancer. Anticancer Drugs 5:A101

Twentyman PR, Bleehen NM 1991 Resistance modification by PSC 833, a novel non-immunosuppressive cyclosporin. Eur J Cancer 27:1639–1642

van Asperen J, van Tellingen O, Sparreboom A et al 1997 Enhanced oral bioavailability of paclitaxel in mice treated with the P-glycoprotein blocker SDZ PSC 833. Br J Cancer 76:1181–1183

Willman CL 1997 The prognostic significance of the expression and function of multidrug resistance transporter proteins in acute myeloid leukaemia: studies of the Southwest Oncology Group Leukemia Research Program. Semin Hematol 34:25–33

DISCUSSION

Sander: Do you know why Pgp modulators seem to have CNS side effects?

Oza: No. One of the revelations to me was how little is known about the CNS side-effects.

Sander: They may be telling you something.

Oza: Absolutely. This effect has been seen with several different Pgp modulators. PSC 833 causes significant ataxia in humans and a similar toxicity in animal studies. We don't know what is actually causing this.

Sander: How different are those drugs, chemically?

Newman: They represent a variety of different structural classes.

Sander: It is interesting that they all have a common CNS side effect profile.

Oza: Earlier in our discussions we touched on the fact that one of the Pgp modulators has significant effects on opiates, potentially causing toxicity. Co-administered opiates or endogenous opiates may be responsible for some of the central toxicity, but this doesn't explain all the unco-ordination and ataxia.

Brinkmann: These side effects may not be drug related but drug action related. They may be letting other drugs into the brain.

Newman: I have heard that in Pgp knockout mice there is ataxia with some Pgp inhibitors. Is this true?

Bates: Not at clinical doses.

Ling: Is dose escalation something people think about when treating epileptic patients? Is it part of the development of anti-epileptic drugs?

Sander: Yes. There is a dose–response with increasing dose; this is probably the case for most drugs. Part of the development is to do dose ranging studies.

Ling: Is the concept of the maximum tolerated dose inherent to the epilepsy field?

Sander: We do this as well. We try to escalate doses in development until toxicity is seen in patients.

Oza: I guess the difference is that we always treat at the sub-toxic dose up-front, whereas you have better-defined therapeutic windows with most of your anticonvulsants.

Bates: The definitions of toxicity are different, too.

Pirmohamed: Could you say something about the specificity of PSC 833 with regard to other transport pumps? For example, your data showing that it causes hyperbilirubinaemia suggest that it is interacting with liver bile salt export pumps.

Oza: There may be an overlap with other types of pumps, but it seems to be fairly specific for Pgp. It was thought that the hyperbilirubinaemia may be related to that overlap. I don't think it has been specifically addressed in terms of toxicity.

Wood: It is also a potent inhibitor of cytochrome P450 3A4 (CYP3A4). This probably accounts for a lot of the toxicity that has been seen. This is an important issue here; many of these drugs are also CYP3A4 substrates. You would almost certainly have to use one of the less P450 inhibiting drugs.

Oza: In terms of most of the modulators, trying to get information on long-term studies was very difficult. Most of the animal toxicology focused on sub-chronic studies of two weeks: there was very little beyond two weeks.

Wood: Is anyone still developing oral therapy? I thought most had been dropped.

Newman: OC 144-093 is highly orally bioavailable in humans. We are going ahead with oral. Even in the situation where a cancer drug is being given intravenously, it would be preferable to give additional compounds orally.

Wood: Not necessarily. One of the attractions of giving the drug intravenously may be that it doesn't influence the oral bioavailability of the other drugs. In theory it may be better to give the drug intravenously to influence intracellular concentrations with fewer effects on oral bioavailability and less need to adjust the dose of other drugs. It appears that this drug given intravenously doesn't affect enteric Pgp function.

Newman: If you don't inhibit the cytochrome Ps, and if you are giving paclitaxel intravenously, it should be safe to give your Pgp inhibitor orally. Oral administration is easier than intravenous.

Wood: If the ataxia was due to increased absorption of some endogenous substance that doesn't normally get absorbed or have access to the CNS, oral Pgp inhibition might produce different effects.

Newman: We see ataxia after either oral or i.v. administration, so it is not due to something else in the gut.

Sander: In epilepsy we might get a drug that, overall, has modest results. But within a certain group of patients, some have no response, some get worse and others show a striking response to the drug. With your chemotherapy reagents, do you find some patients that do much better than others?

Oza: It depends on the malignancy that is being treated and the chemotherapeutic agents being used. For example, with ovarian cancer there is usually a first-line responsiveness of about 70%. The majority of patients respond reasonably well to chemotherapy. Only a quarter will respond really well, and 50% will have a partial response. The remaining patients will show complete resistance to the first-line treatment agents. These patients are then re-challenged with the same drug in conjunction with the modulator. We don't know whether giving the modulator up-front will be better in the long run, and whether this improved responsiveness overall. This was the point of the phase III studies, which we don't yet have the results from. There were two aims with these studies. One was to look at Pgp modulation and overcoming drug resistance. The second was to see whether giving the Pgp modulator up-front will reduce the amount of resistance in the long term. We don't know whether that strategy has been effective or not.

Sander: So there might be some people who show a striking response.

Oza: Yes. Response has been clearly defined. In the quarter of patients who show a strong response a portion show a complete response (complete resolution of all disease) and there are some who have a partial response (their disease goes down by more than 50%).

Ruetz: It is still difficult to quantify and state clearly that the tumour is positive or negative for Pgp, particularly in solid tumours. What you showed here for the intrinsic resistance, the studies go from 10–80%. It makes it difficult to state clearly that you can reverse Pgp and increase efficacy of your drug.

Oza: The studies have been in a variety of different tissues. One of the things that we touched on earlier was overexpression of Pgp. In some of these studies, when it has been put down as overexpression of Pgp, it is very much like beauty being in the eye of the beholder: it is hard to know what overexpression is. There is no standard. In some of the smaller studies overexpression of Pgp has been recorded in over 80% of patients. However, this has not been audited by someone independently, and it would be interesting to see what the overlap is. This is why most of these studies involve a range or an average from different studies.

Wood: Although I agree that the first-generation inhibitors were much less potent and specific than the second and third generation drugs, it also true that the first generation drugs must have worked *in vivo*. The verapamil/digoxin fractions were Pgp mediated. These interactions were all seen *in vivo* in humans. This being the case, do you think it is possible that there might be data on the role of verapamil in epilepsy? You would expect to see some effect. We have shown that in humans quinidine can increase the effectiveness of loperamide, even though it is not a pure Pgp inhibitor. Given that people discovered the digoxin fractions some 30 years ago, we should still be able to see an effect *in vivo*.

Sander: Verapamil and nifedipine are 'last-ditch' drugs. They have no sustained effect. My experience with verpamil is modest. With nifedipine and nimodipine occasionally we see temporary improvement in patients.

Löscher: The idea there is not to inhibit Pgp but to add another mechanism, which is blocking Ca^{2+} channels.

Sander: That was the idea at the time.

Löscher: Verapamil does not penetrate into the brain much. This is why no one has tried using it.

Vezzani: Is it known whether these inhibitors of Pgp can permeate the brain when administered persistently? If you think about their use in association with AEDs, we should be thinking about a compound that not only blocks the pumps in the blood–brain barrier but also one that permeates the brain. We have seen that Pgp expression is increased in glia and neurons inside the brain itself. Unless we are sure that the inhibitor gets into the brain, negative results don't tell us anything relevant.

Wood: We know that. We have done experiments with the Xenova compound (XR 9576) in which we have given mice Imodium, the anti-diarrhoeal drug which has gastrointestinal but not central opiate effects. When the Xenova compound is also given it produces analgesia with the Imodium through Pgp inhibition. Similarly, if Imodium is given to people and Pgp is inhibited, this causes respiratory depression. With HIV protease inhibitors, you can modulate Pgp and increase or decrease HIV protease inhibitor access to the CNS. The evidence that you can modulate both drug effect and access is quite good.

Abbott: That's in the normal brain, where Pgp is predominantly on the luminal side of the brain endothelium. If there is an intact barrier which can only be penetrated by lipophilic agents, and Pgp expression increases on other cells in the brain, will it be possible to deliver anti-Pgp agents to those cells? I don't think this has been established for some of the second-generation Pgp inhibitors, although if they move rapidly through lipid membranes, they would be expected to get in.

Newman: We are going to have to find the right animal models and try it.

Ruetz: We are back at the question of whether the toxicity with this reversal agent in the brain is due to the fact that we are inhibiting the Pgp at the blood–brain barrier, or inhibiting another Pgp in the brain which causes the toxicity.

Gene expression profiling of epothilone A-resistant cells

Peter Atadja, Yan Yan-Neale, Harry Towbin, Frank Buxton and Dalia Cohen

Functional Genomics, Novartis Corporation, Summit, NJ 07901, USA

Abstract. In the current study, we isolated sublines of the human breast adenocarcinoma cell line MDA 435 that exhibited increasing resistance to epothilone A, a microtubule-stabilizing cytotoxic agent. The resistant cells did not express P glycoprotein or multidrug resistance-associated protein (MRP) which are known mediators of multidrug resistance (MDR). Two groups of epothilone A-resistant cells were selected: cells which exhibited low resistance to both epothilone A and Taxol, and cells which exhibit low resistance to Taxol but high resistance to epothilone A. cDNA microarrays of epothilone A-resistant and Taxol-resistant cells were utilized to further characterize epothilone A resistance. Hierarchical clustering of genes according to their levels of expression indicated that the majority of genes which were highly expressed in epothilone A-resistant cells but not in taxol-resistant MDR cells encode known interferon-inducible proteins. Genes whose expression increased with increasing epothilone A resistance include microtubule-associated GTPases, cytoskeletal proteins, cell signalling proteins and a drug metabolising enzyme. The majority of the genes that were repressed in both epothilone A- and Taxol-resistant cells encode proteins regulating cellular growth signalling mechanisms.

2002 Mechanisms of drug resistance in epilepsy: lessons from oncology. Wiley, Chichester (Novartis Foundation Symposium 243) p 119–136

A major obstacle to the effective treatment of cancer is the intrinsic or acquired resistance to chemotherapeutic agents. One form of drug resistance, known as multidrug resistance (MDR), is a phenomenon whereby cells that acquire resistance to certain cytotoxic drugs generally demonstrate cross-resistance to other, sometimes structurally and functionally unrelated drugs. Several mechanisms that mediate MDR have been identified. P glycoprotein (Pgp) is a known mediator of MDR. However, failure to completely sensitize some drug resistant tumours to chemotherapy using Pgp-reversing agents suggests the existence of multiple mechanisms of cancer drug resistance. Selecting resistant cells to non-Pgp substrates would reveal novel mechanisms of resistance.

Epothilones A and B are macrolide polyketides that were isolated in a screening programme for antifungal metabolites from myxobacteria and were found to exhibit cytotoxic activity (Bollag et al 1995). Epothilones, like Taxol, have the ability to arrest cells in mitosis, bind directly to tubulin and microtubules, cause formation of bundles of intracellular microtubules in non-mitotic cells and induce the formation of hyperstable tubulin polymers (Bollag et al 1995, Ojima et al 1999, Muhlradt & Sasse 1997, Kowalski et al 1997). However, in contrast to Taxol, epothilones A and B do not appear to be substrates for Pgp and they retain high toxicity against Pgp-expressing multidrug-resistant cancer cell lines (Bollag et al 1995). Since the epothilones are not Pgp substrates, generation and characterization of epothilone-resistant cells may be helpful for identifying novel drug resistance mechanisms.

In the present study, we generated sublines of the breast adenocarcinoma cell line MDA-MB-435 that exhibit increasing resistance to epothilone A. Epothilone A-resistant cell lines did not express the major drug efflux proteins Pgp or multidrug resistance-associated protein (MRP), and exhibited a very limited cross resistance with Taxol and epothilone B. As a first step to elucidate the mechanism of resistance to epothilone A, we analysed gene expression changes in epothilone A-resistant cell lines. Potential mediators of epothilone A resistance have been identified.

Materials and methods

Selection of epothilone-resistant cells

MDA 435 cells were seeded (1×10^6 cells per plate) and allowed to grow in drug-free media to about 80% confluence. Growth of the cells was then continued in media containing 10 nM of epothilone A over 5 weeks (with frequent media changes). Twelve epothilone A-resistant colonies emerged. Individual resistant colonies were isolated and successively expanded in 12 wells, 6 wells, 25 cm and 75 cm plates. One out of the 12 resistant colonies expanded well and was designated as an epothilone A-resistant cell line (EA10 cells). EA10 cells were maintained in media containing 10 nM epothilone A. Further selection of more resistant cells from EA10 cells yielded cells resistant to 20 nM (EA20), 40 nM (EA40), 60 nM (EA60) or 150 nM (EA150) epothilone A.

MTS growth inhibition assays

Approximately 4000 cells per well were seeded in 96 well plates and incubated at 37 °C for 72 h with decreasing order of drug concentration. Growth inhibition was analysed using the CellTiter 96TM MTS assay (PROMEGA). Absorbance was quantitated with a Thermomax Microplate Reader (Molecular Devices, CA). Cells grown without drug for 24 h were used as growth control in determining the drug concentration resulting in 50% inhibition of cell growth (IC_{50}). Six assays were done per drug per plate.

Western immunoblotting

Plasma membrane proteins were extracted as previously described (Georges et al 1991, Archinal-Mattheis et al 1995). Equal amount of proteins were electrophoresed by SDS-PAGE, transferred onto PVDF membranes (Millipore) and probed with monoclonal antibodies against Pgp and MRP.

RNA isolation and northern blotting

Total RNA and polyA RNA isolation from the various cell lines were done by the RNAeasy and oligotex protocols (Qiagen) respectively, as described by the manufacturer. Labelling of polyA RNA and hybridization of microarray chips were done by Incyte Pharmaceuticals (Palo Alto, CA). For Northern blotting, $10\,\mu g$ of total RNA was electrophoresed over 1% agarose gel, transferred onto nylon membrane and hybridized with ^{33}P-labelled probes synthesized from expressed sequence tag (EST) clones ordered from Genome Systems Inc. (St Louis, MO). Detection and quantification of Northern blot signals were done by phosphoimaging.

Results

Generation of epothilone A-resistant cells

MDA 435 breast adenocarcinoma cells were incubated in the presence of 10 nM of epothilone A for 5 weeks. Although majority of the cells died, several clones survived the drug selection. Each clone was further expanded in media containing 10 nM epothilone A but only one clone expanded well resulting in a resistant cell line named EA10. EA10 cells served as founder cells for the selection of cells with higher epothilone A resistance that were maintained in the presence of 20 nM (EA20), 40 nM (EA40), 60 nM (EA60) or 150 nM (EA150) of epothilone A, respectively.

Two potential mechanisms of resistance in epothilone A-resistant cells

The MTS assay was used to determine the concentration (IC_{50}) of drug required to inhibit the growth of 50% of MDA-MB-435, EA10, EA20, EA40, EA60 and EA150 cells. As shown in Table 1, the IC_{50} of epothilone A in EA10 and EA20 increased 4.5-fold and sevenfold, respectively, over sensitive MDA-MB-435 cells. However, the IC_{50} of epothilone A was similar in EA20 ($IC_{50}=28+3$) and

TABLE 1 IC_{50} values of epothilone A, epothilone B and Taxol compared in MDA-MB-435, EA10, EA20, EA40, EA20, EA40, EA60 and EA150 cells

Drug	MDA-MB-435 IC_{50}/nM	EA10 IC_{50}/nM	EA20 IC_{50}/nM	EA40 IC_{50}/nM	EA60 IC_{50}/nM	EA150 IC_{50}/nM
EpoA	4.0+1.8	18.0+3.8	28.0+3.0	36.0+2.0	82.1+1.5	>1000
EpoB	2.1+0.8	2.9+1.4	6.2+2.9	7.8+3.5	10+4.2	15+3.1
Taxol	7.5+3.0	13.0+3.1	22.0+4.0	23.0+4.0	27+3.1	34+2.6

EpoA, epothilone A; EpoB, epothilone B. The values are a mean of three separate experiments+SEM.

EA40 ($IC_{50}=36+2$) cells, although EA40 cells were selected in twice the concentration of epothilone A that was used to select EA20. Further selection with 60 nM or 150 nM epothilone A resulted in 15-fold and > 100-fold increases in the IC_{50} of epothilone A in EA60 and EA150 cells respectively over parental cells. Interestingly, as shown in Fig. 1, all epothilone A-resistant cells also exhibited a low resistance to Taxol. However, selection with 60 nM (EA60) and 150 nM (EA150) of epothilone A, while resulting in a substantial increase in IC_{50} of epothilone A, did not produce a concormitant increase in resistance to Taxol. Therefore at least two potential mechanisms of epothilone A resistance might exist. A lower epothilone A resistance mechanism that is cross-resistant to Taxol and a higher, epothilone A specific resistance mechanism.

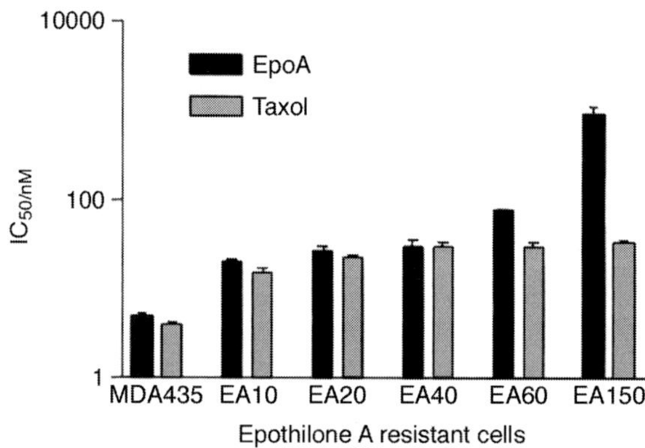

FIG. 1.   Epothilone A-resistant cells exhibit two mechanisms of resistance. Bar chart showing IC_{50} of epothilone A and Taxol in parental and epothilone A-resistant cells. EA10, EA20 and EA40 showed equivalent resistance to epothilone A and Taxol. EA60 and EA150 showed similar resistance to Taxol as EA10, EA20 and EA150 but exhibited increased resistance to epothilone A.

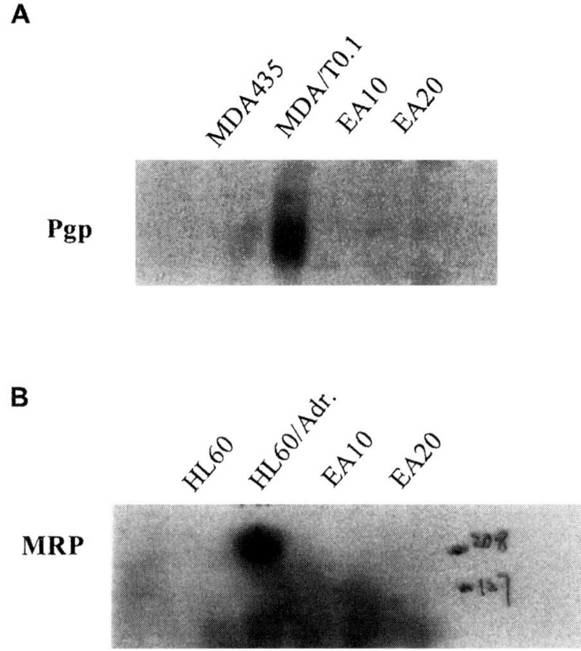

FIG. 2.   Pgp and MRP are not expressed in epothilone A-resistant cells. Plasma membranes from MDA-MB-435, MDA/T0.1, HL60, HL60/ADR EA10, EA20 and HL60 cells were prepared by differential centrifugation. Equal amounts of protein from (A) MDA-MB-435, MDA/T0.1, EA10 and EA20 cells or (B) HL60, HL60/ADR, EA10 and EA20 cells were electrophoresed by SDS-PAGE, transferred onto nylon membranes and immunostained with antibodies against Pgp or MRP.

Resistance to epothilone A is not mediated by Pgp or MRP

The best characterized mechanisms of resistance to anticancer drugs are those mediated by the multidrug transporters Pgp and MRP, and cells that over-express these transporters are usually resistant to a wide variety of drugs. Pgp and MRP are plasma membrane ATP-dependent pumps that efflux a large variety of cytotoxic drugs out of the cell, resulting in a phenomenon referred to as multidrug resistance (MDR). In Pgp-mediated MDR, increased resistance is associated with increased expression of Pgp. To determine whether epothilone resistance might be mediated by Pgp and/or MRP, the levels of expression of these drug transporters were compared in sensitive, epothilone A-resistant and Taxol-resistant MDR cells by western immunoblotting. As shown in Fig. 2, the Taxol-selected multidrug-resistant MDA/T0.1 cells and the Adriamycin-selected multidrug-resistant HL60 cells expressed Pgp and MRP, respectively. However, these transporters were not detectable by Western blotting of plasma membrane lysates of low epothilone A-resistant cells (EA10 or EA20) that were found to be cross-resistant to Taxol.

Expression profiling of epothilone A resistance-associated genes

To determine whether changes in gene expression might underlie epothilone A-specific resistance, we analysed genes differentially expressed in epothilone A-resistant cell lines using Incyte human Unigem V DNA microarray chips. cDNA synthesized from parental MDA435 cells were hybridized in pairwise combinations with cDNA from the low epothilone A-resistant EA40 or from the high epothilone A-resistant EA150 cells. To compare specific gene expression changes in epothilone A-resistant cells to expression changes in Taxol selected MDR cells, we hybridized cDNA synthesized from MDA/T0.1 cells (selected from the same parental cell line as the epothilone A-resistant cells) in pairwise combination with cDNA from parental MDA435 cells. Hybridization and scanning of the chips were done at the Incyte Pharmaceuticals facility in Palto Alto, CA.

On the basis of analyses from multiple experiments, genes that were differentially expressed >threefold were considered as true changes. Of the 7800 cDNAs spotted on each chip, 4000 spots produced signals above background, of which only about 1% changed >threefold in EA150, EA40 and MDA/T0.1 cells. The low percentage of genes that were differentially expressed suggests that global changes did not occur during drug selection.

Identification and functional classification of
genes specifically expressed in EA150 or MDA/T0.1 cells

Hierarchical clustering methods were used to classify the differentially expressed genes according to their levels of expression in the resistant cells. The results illustrated in Figs 3 and 4 show gene clusters and functional classes of genes that changed in EA150 or MDA/T0.1 cells. Further classification of the differentially expressed genes according to their functional annotation in Genbank indicated that, as shown in Table 2, a large percentage of the genes overexpressed in the epothilone A-resistant cells encode known interferon-inducible genes. Specifically, the interferon pathway that induces the expression of the major histocompatibility class II (HLA II in human) genes was activated in the epothilone A-resistant cells but not in the multidrug-resistant MDA/T0.1 cells. In addition, genes encoding cytoskeletal proteins, growth factors and other growth signalling proteins, proteins involved in lipid and RNA metabolism, transcription and chromatin structure-related proteins, as well as proteins involved in drug metabolism were up-regulated in EA150 cells (Fig. 3, Table 2).

A

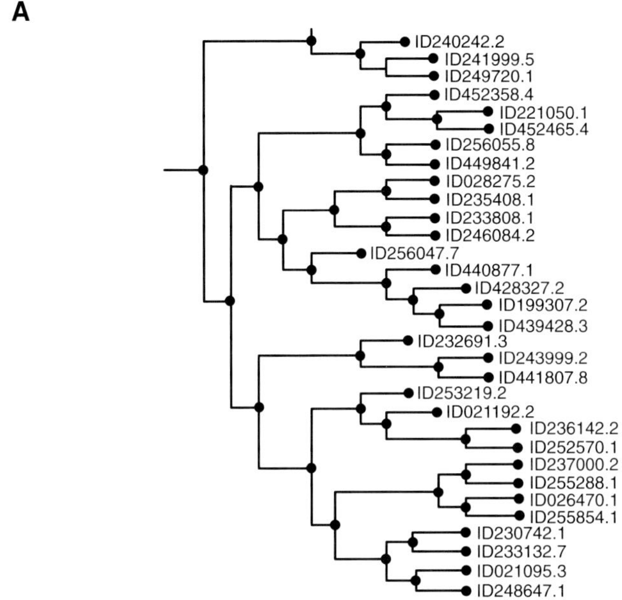

B

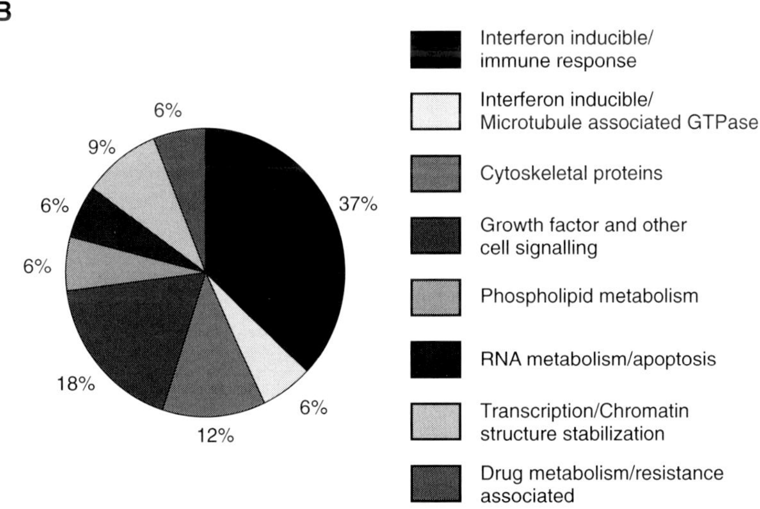

FIG. 3. Cluster of genes specifically up-regulated in EA150 cells. (A) Illustration of genes upregulated in EA150 cells clustered hierarchically based on their fold overexpression. (B) A pie chart representing genes overexpressed in EA150 cells. Genes were grouped according to their known biochemical functions. 37% of genes specifically expressed in EA150 cells encode interferon-inducible genes.

A

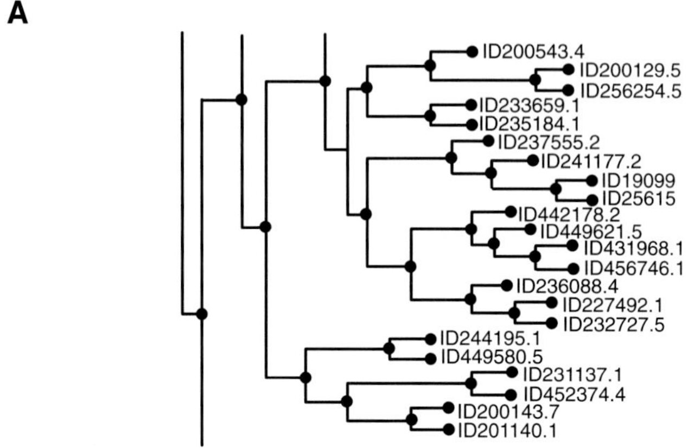

B

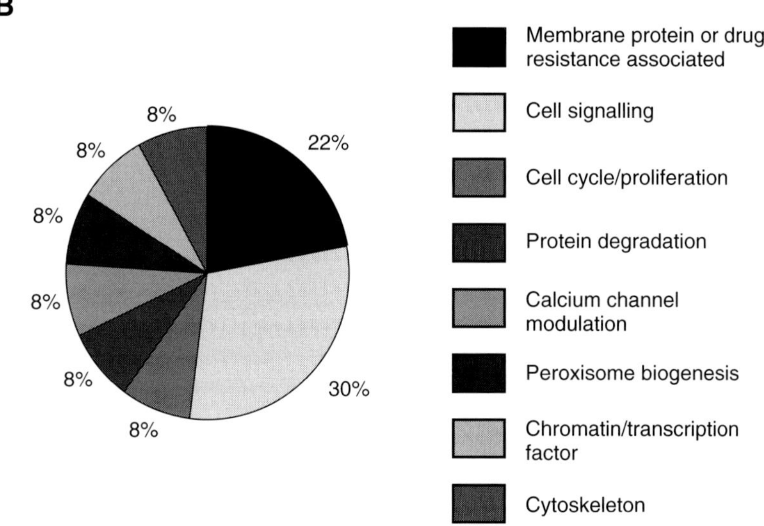

FIG. 4.   Cluster of genes specifically up-regulated in MDA/T0.1 cells. (A) Illustration of genes up-regulated in MDA/T0.1 clustered hierarchically based on their fold overexpression. (B) A pie chart representing genes overexpressed in MDA/T0.1 cells. Genes were grouped according to their known biochemical functions.

In accordance with the observation that EA150 cells exhibited an epothilone A-specific resistance mechanism, genes up-regulated only in the highly resistant EA150 cells were identified and listed in Table 3. The EA150-specific genes encode the interferon-inducible microtubule-associated GTPases Mx and p44,

TABLE 2   Genes up-regulated in EA150 cells but not in MDA/T0.1 cells

Gene	Biochemical function
HLA II γ chain	Interferon inducible/ immune response
HLA II DP 1 α chain precursor	
HLA II DR α chain precursor	
HLA II DR $\beta 5$	
HLA II DQ $\beta 1$	
HLA II DP $\beta 1$	
IFN regulatory factor 7	
IFNα-induced 11.5 kDa	
IFN-inducible 56 kDa	
IFN-inducible protein 1–8U	
IFN-induced leucine zipper	
IFN-inducible protein 9–27	
Mx resistance 1	Interferon-inducible microtubule-associated GPTase
IFN-inducible microtubular aggregate protein p44	
α tubulin	Cytoskeletal protein
Troponin T1	
β sarcoglycan A3b	
WASP interacting protein	
Integrin $\alpha 6$	Growth factor and other cell signalling
Integrin $\beta 3$	
Human follistatin gene	
Early growth response protein	
Arg/Abl interacting protein	
Human Cyr61	
Human lysophospholypase analogue	Phospholipid metabolism RNA metabolism/apoptosis
Tryptophanyl tRNA synthetase	
Zinc finger protein 151	Transcription/chromatin structure stabilization
RNA polymerase elongation factor ELL2	
Transcription factor AREB6	
Xenobiotic epoxide hydrolase	Drug metabolism/ resistance associated

HLA, human leukocyte antigen; IFN, interferon.

TABLE 3   Genes specifically up-regulated in EA150 but not in low epothilone A-resistant or in MDA/T0.1 cells

Gene product	Biochemical function
Mx resistance 1	Interferon-inducible microtubule-associated
IFN-iducible microtubular aggregate protein p44	GTPase
Troponin T1	Cytoskeletal protein
β sarcoglycan A3b	
Integrin β3	Cellular signalling
Human follistatin gene	
Xenobiotic epoxide hydrolase	Drug metabolism

IFN, interferon.

the cytoskeletal proteins troponin T1 and β sarcoglycan, the signalling proteins integrin β3 and follistatin, as well as the human xenobiotic epoxide hydrolase. As expected, the gene encoding Pgp was overexpressed in MDA/T0.1 cells but not in the epothilone-resistant cells (Table 4). Regarding genes down-regulated in the resistant cells, ~50% of changes in EA150 or MDA/T0.1 encode growth signalling proteins (Fig. 5, Table 5).

Discussion

Development of resistance to chemotherapeutic agents is a major hurdle during anticancer therapy. One major mechanism of drug resistance is increased efflux of drugs from cancer cells, mediated by the plasma membrane pump Pgp (Gottesman et al 1996). However, inability to completely cure resistant tumours with Pgp inhibitors suggests that other clinically relevant resistance mechanisms exist and elucidation of such mechanisms may reveal novel targets for drug discovery.

In the current study, we selected cells resistant to epothilone A, a natural product that, like Taxol, stabilizes microtubule polymerization and possesses potent cytotoxic activity (Casazza et al 1996). As a first step to elucidate the mechanism of epothilone A resistance, we used DNA microarrays to identify differentially expressed genes. The majority of genes up-regulated in low and high epothilone A-resistant cells were found to encode interferon-inducible proteins, several of which belong to the HLA class II family. However, the fact that neither increased expression of interferons nor their receptors were observed in epothilone A-resistant cells indicated that if interferon signalling events are involved in epothilone A resistance, then these are likely to be further downstream of the receptor. Constitutive expression of HLAII genes requires the transcription factor CIITA (Mach 1999, Boss 1997) and occurs only in

TABLE 4   Genes up-regulated in MDA/T0.1 cells

Gene product	*Relevance to biochemical/biological pathway*
Human Pgp MDR1	Membrane protein/drug resistance/
Human MDR3	extracellular matrix
Aggrecan	
Cell surface glycoprotein A15	
Tenascin C	
AHNAK nucleoprotein	Growth factor and other cellular cell growth
Human phospholipase C	signalling
G protein γ11	
Human secreted cyclophilin-like protein	
RII-a subunit of PKA	
AKAP120	
Cdc7-related kinase	
mRNA for mitotic kinesin-like protein SCYLP	
Mpp5	
mRNA for tob family	
PRC1	
Proteasome subunit HC9	Protein degradation
HMGIC	Chromatin/transcription
Sorcin CP-22 mRNA	Ca^{2+} channel modulation
Human collagen α	Structural protein/cytoskeletal
PEX1	Peroxisome biogenesis

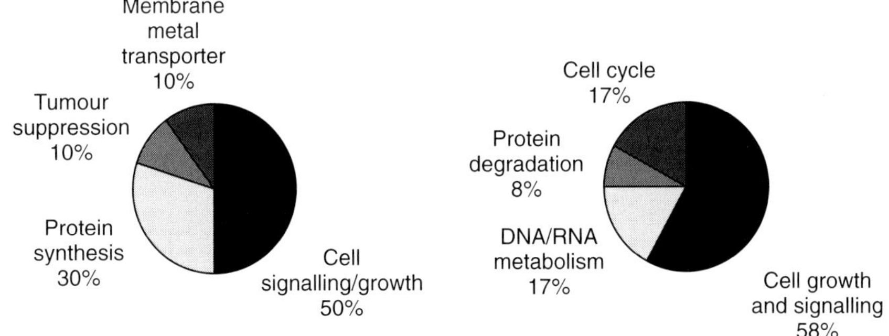

FIG. 5.   >50% of genes down-regulated in E150 or MDA/T0.1 cells encode cell signalling proteins. A pie chart representing genes down-regulated in MDA/T0.1 cells. Genes were grouped according to their known biochemical functions.

TABLE 5   Genes repressed in EA150 cells or MDA/T0.1 cells

Gene product	*Relevance to biochemical/ biological pathway*
Pigment epithelium-derived factor	Cell signalling/growth/survival
Mitogen-responsive DOC2 protein	
Neuronal membrane glycoprotein M6b	
Prostacyclin stimulating factor	
Ocular albinism type 1 related	
Met protooncogene	
EDDR1 tyrosine kinase	
Novel glucocorticoid receptor-associated protein	
Integral membrane protein E16	
OX-2 Membrane glycoprotein precursor	
Glycogenin 2γ mRNA	Energy metabolism
Phosphoglycerate kinase 1	
Ornithine decarbolase 1	Polyamine biosynthesis/Cell proliferation
Spermidine/spermine N1-acetyl transferase	
Ring finger protein FXY	Spans the X–Y chromosome pseudoautosomal boundary
mRNA for JM5 protein	Renal function
Shab-related K^+ channel α subunit (KCNS3)	Ion channel function
Growth arrest specific protein 1	Cell cycle arrest
Human Toll protein homologue	Immune response
VESPR	Axon guidance
mRNA for testican	Ca^{2+} binding proteoglycan

immune cells such as dendritic and activated B cells (Steimle et al 1994, Chang et al 1994). However, CIITA was not found overexpressed on the chips hybridized with epothilone A-resistant cells.

Two interferon-inducible genes whose expression increased with increasing epothilone A resistance encode the microtubule associated GTPase p44 and Mx protein, respectively (Honda et al 1990, Takahashi et al 1990, Haller et al 1998, Staeheli & Pavlovich 1991). p44 is a microtubule-associating protein (MAP), whose GTPase activity is activated by association with microtubules (Honda et al 1990, Takahashi et al 1990). The biological function of p44 is not known. However, it is usually found in microtubule clusters. Mx protein, whose up-regulation in EA150 was confirmed by Western blotting, belongs to the dynamin superfamily of large GTPases, and is known to interfere with the intracellular synthesis of negative-strand RNA viruses, leading to viral resistance (Honda et al

1990). Like p44, Mx and other dynamins also associate with microtubules and their GTPase activities were recently found to be stimulated 75-fold by association with microtubule polymers (Haller et al 1998, Staeheli & Pavlovich 1991). However, p44 and Mx proteins were not previously shown to be involved in anticancer drug resistance: because GTP binding is important for microtublule polymerization, and cytotoxicity of epothilones is mediated by stabilization of microtubules, increased association of p44 and/or Mx GTPases with microtubules might decrease local GTP concentration, leading to depolymerization and resistance to epothilone A. Moreover, kinesin, which like the dynamins is also a microtubule associated motor protein, was recently found to be involved in survival against certain anticancer drugs (Shpetner & Vallee 1992, Urrutia et al 1997). Other cytoskeletal proteins, Troponin T1 and β sarcoglycan which were overexpressed only in EA150 cells and α tubulin and vimentin which were overexpressed in EA40 and EA150, may also play a role in epothilone A resistance. Since α tubulin is a component of the microtubules, the molecular target of epothilones, and aberrant expression of tubulins was previously shown to be associated with anticancer drug resistance (Vallee & Gee 1998), up-regulation of α tubulin may contribute to epothilone resistance. Furthermore, cytoskeletal alterations in the multidrug-resistant breast cancer MCF7R cell line were found to be accompanied by increased expression of vimentin (Kavallaris et al 1997).

Drug-metabolizing enzymes may also play a role in epothilone A resistance. In this regard, the human xenobiotic epoxide hydrolase was identified among the microarray hits as overexpressed in EA150 cells but not EA40 nor MDA/T0.1 cells. Since the epoxide moeity in epothilones was found to be required for the cytotoxic activity of the drug (Bollag et al 1995), increased activity of epoxide hydrolase might decrease epothilone A activity, leading to resistance. The vast majority of the other non-interferon inducible EA150 hits encode cell surface, extracellular matrix and cellular signalling proteins. In addition to the known involvement of cell surface transporters in drug resistance, cell–cell adhesion mechanisms have also been reported to contribute directly or indirectly to anticancer drug resistance (St Croix & Kerbel 1997, Damiano et al 1999, Axenovich et al 1998).

References

Axenovich SA, Kazarov AR, Boiko AD, Armin G, Roninson IB, Gudkov AV 1998 Altered expression of ubiquitous kinesin heavy chain results in resistance to etoposide and hypersensitivity to colchicine: mapping of the domain associated with drug response. Cancer Res 58:3423–3428

Archinal-Mattheis A, Rzepka RW, Watanabe T et al 1995 Analysis of the interactions of SDZ PSC 833 ([3′-keto-Bmt]-Val2]-cyclosporine), a multidrug resistance modulator, with P-glycoprotein. Oncol Res 7:603–610

Bollag DM, McQueney PA, Zhu J et al 1995 Epothilones, a new class of microtuble-stabilizing agents with a taxol-like mechanism of action. Cancer Res 55:2325–2333

Boss JM 1997 Regulation of transcription of MHC II genes. Curr Opin Immunol 9:107–113

Casazza AM, Fairchild CR 1996 Paclitaxel (Taxol): mechanisms of resistance. Cancer Treat Res 87:149–171

Chang CH, Fontes JD, Peterlin M, Flavell RA 1994 Class II transactivator (CIITA) is sufficient for the inducible expression of major histocompatibility complex class II genes. J Exp Med 180:1367–1374

Damiano JS, Cress AE, Hazlehurst LA, Shtil AA, Dalton WS 1999 Cell adhesion mediated drug resistance (CAM-DR): role of integrins and resistance to apoptosis in human myeloma cell lines. Blood 93:1658–1667

Georges E, Zhang JT, Ling V 1991 Modulation of ATP and drug binding by monoclonal antibodies against P-glycoprotein. J Cell Physiol 148:479–484

Gottesman MM, Pastan I, Ambudkar SV 1996 P-glycoprotein and multidrug resistance. Curr Opin Genet Dev 6:610–617

Haller O, Frese M, Kochs G 1998 Mx proteins: mediators of innate resistance to RNA viruses. Rev Sci Tech 17:220–230

Honda Y, Kondo J, Maeda T et al 1990 Isolation and purification of a non-A, non-B hepatitis-associated microtubular aggregates protein. J Gen Virol 71:1999–2004

Kavallaris M, Kuo DYS, Burkhart CA et al 1997 Taxol-resistant epithelial ovarian tumors are associated with altered expression of specific beta-tubulin isotypes. J Clin Invest 100:1282–1293

Kowalski RJ, Gianakakou P, Hamel E 1997 Activities of the microtubule-stabilizing agents epothilones A and B with purified tubulin and in cells resistant to paclitaxel (Taxol®) J Biol Chem 272:2534–2541

Mach B 1999 Regulating the regulator. Science 285:1367

Muhlradt PF, Sasse F 1997 Epothilone B stabilizes microtubuli of macrophages like taxol without showing taxol-like endotoxin activity. Cancer Res 1997 57:3344–3346

Ojima I, Chakravarty S, Inoue T et al 1999 A common pharmacophore for cytotoxic natural products that stabilize microtubules Proc Nat Acad Sci USA 96:4256–4261

Shpetner HS, Vallee RB 1992 Dynamin is a GTPase stimulated to high levels of activity by microtubules. Nature 355:733–735

St Croix B, Kerbel RS 1997 Cell adhesion and drug resistance in cancer. Curr Opin Oncol 9:549–556

Staeheli P, Pavlovic J 1991 Inhibition of Stomatitis virus mRNA synthesis by human MxA protein. J Virol 65:4498–4501

Steimle V, Siegrist CA, Mottet A, Lisowska-Grospierre B, Mach B 1994 Regulation of MHC class II expression by interferon-gamma mediated by the transactivator gene CIITA. Science 265:106–109

Takahashi K, Kitamura N, Shibui T et al 1990 Cloning, sequencing and expression in *Escherichia coli* of cDNA for a non-A, non-B hepatitis-associated microtubular aggregates protein. J Gen Virol 71:2005–2011

Urrutia R, Henley JR, Cook T, McNiven MA 1997 The dynamins: redundant or distinct functions for an expanding family of related GTPases? Proc Natl Acad Sci USA 94:377–384

Vallee RB, Gee MA 1998 Make room for Dynein. Trends Cell Biol 8:490–494

DISCUSSION

Ling: When you reverse with PSC 833, is Taxol resistance reversed?

Atadja: Yes, but not completely.

Ling: But the epothilone does not reverse at all.

Atadja: No, the epothilone resistance is not reversed. When the MDA/TO.1 cells selected with Taxol were tested with PSC 833, there was reversal. But in the epothilone A-resistant cells, PSC 833 has no effect at all. This means that there is another Taxol-related mechanism involved in the low-grade epothilone A resistance other than Pgp.

Scheper: In the list of interferon γ inducible genes you showed, I didn't see class I molecules. Are they missed out, or aren't they included in the chip?

Atadja: They were on the chip. The expression of the interferon-inducible genes was changed so highly that they eclipsed a lot of the other genes that were up-regulated. Less than threefold up-regulation was not of interest; the inducible genes we concentrated on were changed above threefold and class I genes were not among them.

Scheper: In the chip, did you have MRP1–7 and BCRP?

Atadja: Yes, but their expression wasn't induced. We looked specifically for MRP1 and MDR1. Aquaporin was up-regulated slightly. This was the only channel protein that we saw. LRP was up-regulated about threefold.

Pirmohamed: Can I ask about epoxide hydrolase: was it microsomal or cytosolic epoxide hydrolase?

Atadja: Microsomal.

Pirmohamed: Did your chip contain the glutathione transferases?

Atadja: Yes. We might have seen some marginal changes in glutathione transferases, but not a lot.

Sander: Was it a surprise to see these interferon-inducible genes coming out at such a high frequency?

Atadja: To me it was a surprise, because interferons are usually supposed to induce apoptosis or inflammation. Although I saw these interferon-inducible genes coming up I noticed that interferon itself was not up-regulated, nor was its receptor. There is probably something along the interferon signalling pathway that got constitutively up-regulated. We also know that these epithelial cell lines don't usually express these MHC class II genes. They are not immune cell lines.

Ling: Do you see a quantitative correlation of the epoxide hydrolase gene expression with the increase in drug resistance?

Atadja: Yes. The interferon-inducible GTPases and epoxide hydrolases were among the few that increased with increasing resistance.

Ling: Have you checked the epoxide hydrolase enzyme activity in these cells?

Atadja: We haven't looked at this.

Ling: It could be a simple thing — in crude material you have the substrate so you can see it convert.

Atadja: We tried getting the inhibitor of epoxide hydrolase, so we could see whether inhibiting the enzyme would make cells more sensitive. But we didn't succeed in obtaining it.

Ling: In your understanding, chemically, could the epoxide hydroxylase cause resistance to Taxol?

Atadja: No, not to taxol. Taxol doesn't have an epoxide group.

Pirmohamed: Is your epoxide metabolized by microsomal epoxyhydrolase? Have you shown this?

Atadja: No, we haven't done the metabolic studies. The only correlation we have is that its expression is not increased in the low-resistance cells, only in the high-resistance cells which appear to have epothilone A-specific resistance mechanisms.

Ling: Could the epoxide hydroxylase explain all the resistance other than that to Taxol? Could the set of interferon-inducible genes have nothing to do with resistance at all?

Atadja: It is possible that epoxide hydrolase could explain the resistance. However, the interferon-inducible GTPases are also highly expressed in the EA150 cells.

Newman: Did you try treating the parental cell line with a non-toxic dose of interferon to see whether that induces epothilone resistance?

Atadja: Yes, and it doesn't.

Newman: If this is the case, you could use that with a microarray to eliminate most of your suspects.

Atadja: We did that, and it didn't work. We know that the interferon receptor is not up-regulated. We didn't see a signal for interferon receptor on our chips. The question is, even if you add a lot of the interferon, if the receptor is not there you won't see anything. But it may be different if you have something that is intracellular. For example, there is a transcription factor, STAT3, which mediates interferon signalling. If STAT3 were constitutively switched on by selection of the resistant cell lines (it normally isn't), then you can imagine a scenario where interferon-inducible genes could be up-regulated without the upstream effects of interferon.

Brinkmann: I have a question about the comparability of those cells. You mentioned the cells get sick by doing the selection. In our experience, even when the selection is taken away, the cells are not really happy. Frequently they grow more slowly and appear different under the microscope. Many of these genes could have been just the effect of comparing happy cells with unhappy cells.

Atadja: Growth regulatory/cell cycle genes also change in the epithilone-resistant cells. But the cells looked happy under the microscope!

Sisodiya: I was fascinated by your paper, and also a little intimidated: there seem to be so many mechanisms of drug resistance. I have been focusing on Pgp, but there are clearly many other mechanisms. I don't want to draw a parallel between cancer and epilepsy too closely, but there are other things going on in epilepsy: it isn't necessarily a question of membrane excitability and ion channels. We know that many of the developmental pathologies that cause epilepsy involve microtubular dysfunction, for example, that may be persistent into adulthood. If this is the case, the question is how many mechanisms of drug resistance in oncology are recognized *in vitro*, and how many of these have some clinical role? If we are going to look at drug resistance in epilepsy, this may become a huge issue.

Bates: That is the $64 million question. We don't know the answer. It frequently seems that the more you look, the more you find. In oncology we reasoned that Pgp would be defined as important if we could prove that by modulating it, patients responded. Even this paradigm hasn't succeeded. We haven't been able to prove that Pgp is important with modulation. Add to all of the potential mechanisms that Dr Atadja has brought up through use of the gene array methodology, those that have been identified by individual experimentation. We know that in experimental models you can have drug resistance through decreased uptake, increased efflux, drug metabolism and survival pathways. These are general categories, and within each one there is an enormous variety of possibilities. Right now we don't have any way of overcoming drug metabolism or inhibiting a survival pathway, so a pragmatic approach is to focus on transporters.

Ling: But before the pendulum swings too far, I would point out that even though we are 'intimidated' by the amount of data that a chip array can generate, it is important to remember that not every change on a chip is relevant.

Atadja: You have to look at patterns: how the expression follows the phenotype. And you have to use educated guesses with respect to what the genes encode and are probably doing. The chip is just a starting point that suggests some possible directions to go in.

Bates: You made the point that 99% of genes aren't changed. This is also remarkable.

Ruetz: You don't know that. We are looking here at endpoints, and we have no idea whether there are crucial changes in genes within 30 min which then return to normal levels. The whole thing is very complicated. You can take a dish of cultured cells and treat with a low dose for a long period, or you can do a short treatment with a high dose. These both give different resistance patterns. One has to consider what type of resistance is induced in the clinic. It depends on how you treat.

Atadja: This touches on the issue of acquired versus intrinsic resistance. Perhaps 1% of the cancer cells already have a mutation, and it is just when you treat the 99% that the 1% reveals itself as resistant. Or is the drug inducing the change in gene expression that is now manifesting itself as resistance?

Bates: That is a good point, because epilepsy treatment won't be selecting cells. You can just look at what chronic exposure to these drugs induces. This simplifies the problem a bit.

Scheper: With the human genome project nearing completion, it seems that there is a limited number of pumps available. There may be as many as 30 or 40 pumps, but I would be surprised if there were many more than this.

Atadja: Putting all the 40 or so ABC transporters on a chip would form a closed system where we could look for changes in specific genes. However, one has to first identify and clone the genes.

Scheper: In this case it is still plausible that one of these 30–40 pumps may be seriously involved but it hasn't yet been included on the chip. Furthermore, those chips concentrate on the mRNA level; protein levels may be seriously different. You might still consider taking your cell line, injecting it into mouse and screen for a monoclonal antibody that discriminates your resistant and sensitive cell lines.

Varadi: You have illustrated beautifully here that what you pick up with your chips are probably multiple resistance genes. Is this correct?

I also want to comment on Rik Scheper's point. Exactly the same approach was used a couple of years ago to identify the important cholesterol efflux genes. Instead of doing traditional positional cloning, they made a hybridization filter for the different ABC transporters and looked at which of these are up-regulated upon cholesterol loading in macrophages, and then down-regulated very fast. They thought that these genes were good candidate genes. Within a matter of weeks they could identify the Tangier disease gene, which encodes most probably a cholesterol efflux pump. There are two contrasting approaches. The first is the one you suggested. The second is to suppose that for multiple resistance, learning the lesson from cholesterol-transport genes, the multiple resistance genes are most probably transporters, and you just focus on those. There are probably other types of resistance where you can find specific resistance genes by using chip technology.

Atadja: I don't know whether epothilone-resistant cells are yet displaying multidrug resistance. They probably have other compounds that they might exhibit resistance to. But the epothilone-resistant cells are still sensitive to vincristine, Taxol and a few other chemotherapeutic drugs tested.

Brinkmann: You cannot make the general conclusion that multiple resistance genes must be transporters. If you look in the tumour field for apoptosis genes, it is possible to induce apoptosis by many different drugs. If there is an apoptosis-resistance gene it would cover a whole series of pathways.

Bates: I understood him to mean anti-epilepsy drugs: to set up a model and see whether any of these transporters are altered, as with the cholesterol-inducible genes. This could be done in a cell line model.

Ling: Microarray technology is clearly a powerful tool, but we recognize that by itself it cannot answer many questions. It doesn't take the place of a sharply asked question.

Imaging of P glycoprotein function *in vivo* with PET

N. H. Hendrikse and W. Vaalburg

PET Center, University Hospital of Groningen, PO Box 30001, 9700 RB Groningen, The Netherlands

Abstract. P glycoprotein (Pgp) is expressed on cell membranes of various organs in the body, such as the capillary endothelial cells of the brain. Furthermore, Pgp can also be expressed on the cell membrane of tumour cells. Because of Pgp-mediated efflux, tissue levels of several Pgp substrates are lower than in Pgp-negative tissues. Drug levels in Pgp-expressing organs may be increased by modulation of this Pgp-facilitated transport with several compounds, such as cyclosporin A. Up to now, the presence of drug efflux pumps in tissues could only be examined at the mRNA and protein level. However, this gives no insight into the important question of the functionality of these drug efflux pumps. Information about the transport function of Pgp and the effect of modulating this function may improve the therapeutic treatment of these patients. Positron emission tomography (PET) gives us a unique opportunity to study non-invasively (patho)physiological dynamic processes *in vivo*. We have therefore developed and validated a method for studying Pgp-mediated transport and its modulation *in vivo* with PET.

2002 Mechanisms of drug resistance in epilepsy: lessons from oncology. Wiley, Chichester (Novartis Foundation Symposium 243) p 137–148

Drug efflux pumps such as P glycoprotein (Pgp) are involved in the transport of (endo)toxic compounds out of the body (Higgins 1992, Cordon-Cardo et al 1990). Pgp also plays a clinically relevant role in the extrusion of therapeutic drugs from Pgp-expressing tissues into the blood, leading to an inadequate pharmacological response. To solve this problem, modulation of drug efflux may be part of a successful therapeutic treatment. Therefore, insight in the physiological transport function of Pgp in tissues such as the brain and also in tumours is important.

In this paper we focus on Pgp expression and its function, especially in the brain and in tumours. Furthermore, we describe visualization of the transport function and its modulation *in vivo* with positron emission tomography (PET).

The blood–brain barrier

The blood–brain barrier (BBB) consists of endothelial cells lining the capillaries in the brain. It is considered as an important barrier to drug transport into the brain.

In contrast to the endothelium in other tissues, the endothelial cells in the brain are closely interconnected by tight junctions. Furthermore, the BBB contains very few fenestrations and pinocytosis is virtually absent. Consequently, only very small hydrophilic molecules can enter the brain by diffusion via tight junctions (Abbott & Revest 1991, Rubin & Staddon 1999). Other molecules can only pass through the BBB via endothelial cells. To pass through endothelial cells, a molecule has to be lipophilic. There is a strong relationship between a molecule's lipophilicity and its ability to enter the brain (see Fig. 1). However, there are several molecules which, on the basis of their lipophilicity, would be expected to cross the BBB, for which very little brain uptake is observed. It now appears that Pgp in the BBB is a major factor explaining the low uptake of such lipophilic drugs into the

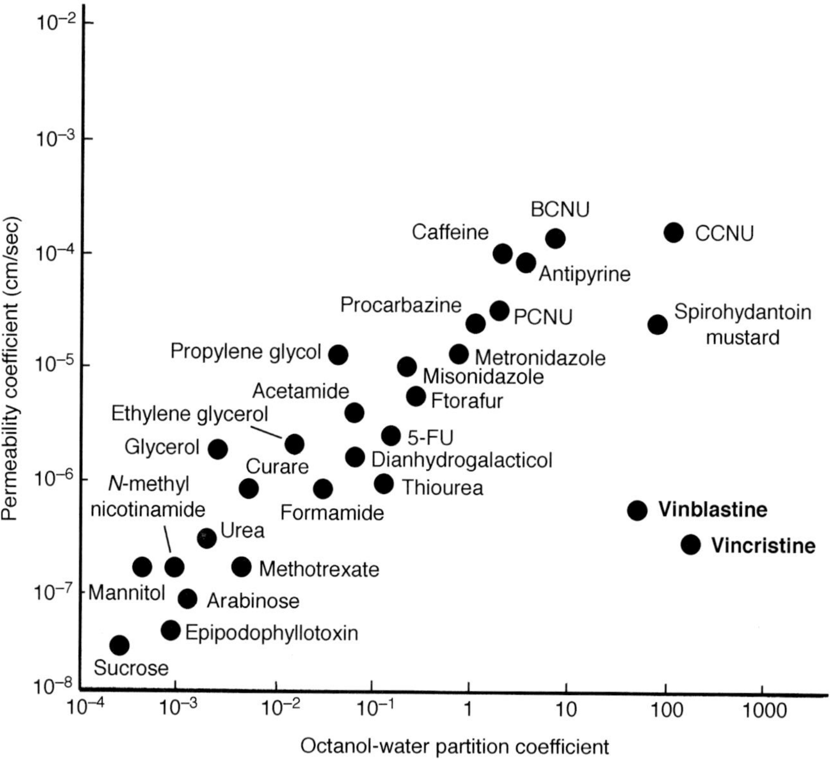

FIG. 1.   Relationship between the LogP value of several substrates and their permeability across capillaries in the brain (Levin 1980). It is clear that there is a strong correlation between LogP value and the brain permeability. However, the permeability of vinblastine and vincristine is much lower than could be expected from their LogP value, which can be explained by transport out of the brain by Pgp.

brain. For the purpose of studying the physiological function of Pgp in the brain, *Mdr1a*(−/−) Pgp knockout mice have been developed by Schinkel et al (1994). Disruption of the *Mdr1a* gene results in the absence of Pgp, especially in the BBB, in these animals. Results obtained with radiolabelled Pgp substrates in this unique *in vivo* model are described below.

Pgp

One of the efflux pumps involved in multidrug resistance (MDR) is Pgp. This protein belongs to the ATP binding cassette (ABC) superfamily of membrane transporters (Higgins 1992). In humans, two closely related genes, *MDR1* and *MDR3*, encode highly homologous Pgps.

It has been suggested that Pgp substrates enter the cell by passive diffusion and subsequently bind to the drug efflux pump in the bilayer or on the cytoplasmic side of the cell membrane.

Pgp is expressed in cell membranes of various organs in the body, such as the renal proximal tubule, the biliary membrane of hepatocytes, the adrenal gland, the apical membrane of intestinal epithelial cells, and the capillary endothelial cells of the brain and the testes (Cordon-Cardo et al 1990, Tsuij et al 1992).

Several structurally unrelated drugs, such as Ca^{2+} channel blockers (e.g. verapamil), immunosuppressives (e.g. cyclosporin A), chemotherapeutics (e.g. doxorubicin) and HIV protease inhibitors (e.g. saquinavir), are transported by Pgp. Other examples are presented in Table 1.

Although increased levels of Pgp are likely to contribute to MDR in at least some tumour types and also in the brain, it has become evident that another drug efflux pump is involved, namely the multidrug resistance-associated protein (MRP) (Cole et al 1992).

Positron emission tomography

To study the Pgp function *in vivo*, several invasive techniques, like Northern blotting and PCR (for detection of mRNA), and immunohistochemistry and Western blotting (for detection of the gene product) are now available. However, due to ethical limitations, tumour biopsies are often hard to obtain. Furthermore, these methods give no insight in the dynamic function of Pgp. PET offers the possibility of probing the physiological function of Pgp in humans *in vivo*. PET can provide information on drug transport over the BBB via Pgp. For PET studies, a radiopharmaceutical, often a pharmacologically active compound, is labelled with a positron-emitting radionuclide or isotope. After purification and pharmaceutical quality control, the radiopharmaceutical is administered to humans or experimental animals. Because of the short physical

TABLE 1   Substrates of the Pgp drug efflux pump

Cytotoxic agents	Doxorubicin
	Daunorubicin
	Paclitaxel
	Vincristine
	Vinblastine
	Etoposide
	Actinomycin D
HIV1 protease inhibitors	AZT
	Ritanovir
	Saquinavir
	Indinavir
Anti-emetics	Loperamide
	Domperidone
	Ondansetron
Opioids	Morphine
	Fentanyl
Cardiovascular drugs	Verapamil
	Quinidine
	Digoxin
Immunosuppressive drugs	Cyclosporin A
	Dexamethasone
	Tacrolimus
Pgp modulators (experimental drugs)	PSC 833
	S 9788
	GF 120918
	LY 335979
	RU 486
	Trifluoperazine
Others	Propyl-bis-acridone
	Progesterone
	Bilirubin
	Phenytoin
	Ivermectin
	Megestrol acetate

half-lives of the isotopes (varying from 2 min to 110 min), the preparation and
purification of a positron-emitting pharmaceutical is a major challenge. After
being emitted from the atomic nucleus, the positron travels 2–5 mm and
subsequently combines with an electron. The total mass of the particles is then

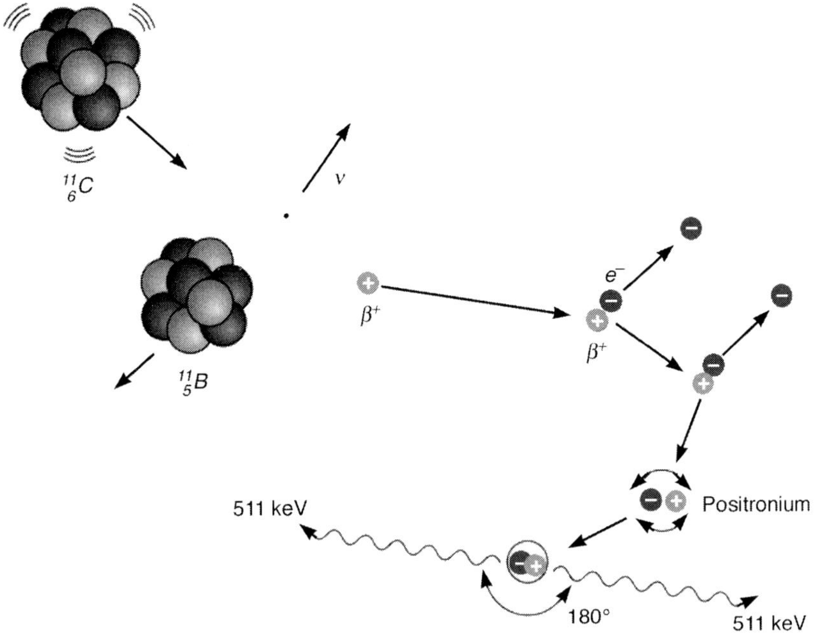

FIG. 2.   This schematic represents a positron-emitting (β^+) radioisotope. A positron is an anti electron, i.e. a particle with the same mass as an electron but the opposite charge. Such positrons originate during the decay of the nuclei of specific radioisotopes. After travelling a few millimetres through the body, a positron meets an electron. Both particles are then annihilated, producing two γ quanta with the same energy (511 keV) but in opposite directions (180°). The γ quanta leave the body and are detected by a PET scanner. Detection information is fed into a computer and converted to an image.

converted into two photons (511 keV), which are emitted in opposite (180°) directions (annihilation) (see Fig. 2). Due to their high energy, the photons leave the body and are detected simultaneously by two opposite detectors of the PET camera (coincidence detection). The PET data provide quantitative information about the biodistribution of radioactivity *in vivo* as a function of time.

Imaging Pgp transport *in vivo* with PET

Radiolabelled MDR-associated cytostatic agents can be used to study drug efflux pumps *in vivo*. One example is colchicine, a Pgp substrate which is a naturally occurring alkaloid (Ford & Hait 1990). Mehta et al (1992) studied the biodistribution of [^{3}H]colchicine in mice xenografted with Pgp-negative and Pgp-positive human neuroblastoma tumours (Mehta et al 1992). The pharmacokinetics of colchicine are possibly favourable for PET studies due to their limited metabolism (Hunter & Klaassen 1975). Using [^{14}C]colchicine, the colchicine distribution and metabolism were studied (Mehta et al 1994). *In vivo* uptake of [^{14}C]colchicine in tumour-bearing mice demonstrated that activity in sensitive tumours was twice as high as in resistant tumours at 60 min after [^{14}C]colchicine injection. The biodistribution of [^{14}C]colchicine in tumour-bearing mice was also studied with whole body quantitative autoradiography. The accumulation in sensitive tumours was twice as high as in resistant tumours (Mehta et al 1996). This study suggests that it is feasible to image Pgp functionality in tumours with [^{11}C]colchicine and PET. However, biodistribution studies in the tumour-bearing mice showed a relatively high uptake of radioactivity in the liver and intestine, due to detoxification of colchicine via the bile (Hunter et al 1975). This makes radiolabelled colchicine less useful for monitoring Pgp drug efflux in abdominal tumours.

In our institute, we prepared [^{11}C]verapamil and [^{11}C]daunorubicin to study Pgp function non-invasively (Elsinga et al 1996). *In vitro* experiments in ovarian carcinoma cell lines (A2780) and its Pgp overexpressing counterpart (A2780AD) demonstrated that the accumulation of [^{11}C]daunorubicin and [^{11}C]verapamil were respectively 16-fold and fivefold increased in A2780 as compared to 2780AD and the accumulation of [^{11}C]daunorubicin was increased in A2780AD cells after addition of unlabelled verapamil (Hendrikse et al 1998a).

Subsequently, the Pgp function in the BBB and the effects of a modulator on this function were imaged in *Mdr1a*-disrupted mice (*Mdr1a$^{-/-}$* mice) and wild-type mice (*Mdr1a$^{+/+}$* mice). *Ex vivo* biodistribution studies revealed 9.5-fold higher [^{11}C]verapamil levels in the brain and 3.4-fold higher levels in the testes of *Mdr1a$^{-/-}$* mice than in *Mdr1a$^{+/+}$* mice. The [^{11}C]verapamil levels were dose-dependently increased by the Pgp blocker cyclosporin A in *Mdr1a$^{+/+}$* mice. No modulating effects of cyclosporin A were found in the *Mdr1a$^{-/-}$* mice. Positron camera data showed lower [^{11}C]verapamil levels in the brain of *Mdr1a$^{+/+}$* mice than in *Mdr1a$^{-/-}$* mice. Time–activity curves demonstrated that [^{11}C]verapamil accumulation in the brain of *Mdr1a$^{+/+}$* mice was increased by cyclosporin A to levels comparable with those in *Mdr1a$^{-/-}$* mice, indicating that reversal of Pgp mediated efflux can be monitored by PET (Hendrikse et al 1998b).

We also studied Pgp transport of [^{11}C]verapamil and [^{11}C]daunorubicin in a two-sided tumour-bearing rat. Rats were inoculated with GLC$_4$ cells in one flank and with the *MDR1*-transfected Pgp-overexpressing subline GLC$_4$/Pgp in the other flank. Biodistribution studies demonstrated higher accumulation of [^{11}C]verapamil and [^{11}C]daunorubicin in GLC$_4$ than in the GLC$_4$/Pgp tumours. The decreased accumulation of radioactivity in the GLC$_4$/Pgp tumours could be completely reversed by cyclosporin A. *In vivo* data of [^{11}C]verapamil kinetics and the modulating effects of cyclosporin A showed that Pgp function and its reversal can be visualized non-invasively with a positron camera (Hendrikse et al 1999).

Implications for CNS-active drugs

Due to Pgp expression in the BBB, the brain uptake of several clinically and moderately lipophilic drugs is low. For instance, several CNS-active drugs such as anti-epileptics (phenytoin) (Lazarowski et al 1999, Schinkel et al 1996) and HIV protease inhibitors (saquinavir, indinavir) (Kim et al 1998, Shiraki et al 2000, Choo et al 2000) interact with Pgp. Therefore Pgp overexpression might be a mechanism underlying drug therapy resistance in epileptic and AIDS patients. Furthermore, co-administration of other Pgp substrates (dexamethasone, cyclosporin A) may improve drug delivery to the brain (Friedenberg et al 1993, Weber et al 1995). However, neurotoxicity is seen in some cases of co-medication. This has often been described for transplantation patients, where central neurotoxicity may occur after treatment with dexamethasone and cyclosporin A (Weber et al 1993, Bertrand et al 1992). Besides Pgp, MRP has recently been found in the BBB (Regina et al 1998, Seetharaman et al 1998, Huai-Yun et al 1998, Kusuhara et al 1998). Therefore, novel insights in the pathophysiology and in the pharmacology of drugs would be gained if the Pgp and MRP functions in the BBB could be visualized and quantified with a non-invasive imaging technique such as PET. When the function of drug efflux pumps in the BBB can be measured quantitatively, a modulator can be administered in a dose which is just high enough to inhibit transport. The concentration of clinically relevant CNS drugs could be increased in the brain. In this way, measurement of the function of drug efflux pumps in the BBB can improve therapeutic treatment in the CNS.

References

Abbott N J, Revest PA 1991 Control of brain endothelial permeability. Cerebrovasc Brain Metab Rev 3:39–72

Bertrand Y, Capdeville R, Balduck N, Philippe N 1992 Cyclosporin A used to reverse drug resistance increases vincristine neurotoxicity. Am J Hematol 40:158–159

Choo EF, Leake B, Wandel et al 2000 Pharmacological inhibition of P-glycoprotein transport enhances the distribution of HIV-1 protease inhibitors into brain and testes. Drug Metab Dispos 28:655–660

Cole SP, Bhardwaj G, Gerlach JH et al 1992 Overexpression of a transporter gene in a multidrug-resistant human lung cancer cell line. Science 258:1650–1654

Cordon-Cardo C, O'Brien JP, Boccia J, Casals D, Bertino JR, Melamed MR 1990 Expression of the multidrug resistance gene product (P-glycoprotein) in human normal and tumor tissues. J Histochem Cytochem 38:1277–1287

Elsinga PH, Franssen EJF, Hendrikse NH et al 1996 Carbon-11-labeled daunorubicin and verapamil for probing P-glycoprotein in tumors with PET. J Nucl Med 37:1571–1575

Ford JM, Hait WM 1990 Pharmacology of drugs that alter multidrug resistance in cancer. Pharmacol Rev 42:155–199

Friedenberg WR, Anderson J, Wolf BC, Cassileth PA, Oken MM 1993 Modified vincristine, doxorubicin, and dexamethasone regimen in the treatment of resistant or relapsed chronic lymphocytic leukemia. An Eastern Cooperative Oncology Group study. Cancer 71:2983–2989

Hendrikse NH, De Vries EGE, Fluks E, Van der Graaf WTA, Vaalburg W, Franssen EJF 1998a P-glycoprotein mediated kinetics in tumor bearing rats with carbon-11-daunorubicin and positron emission tomography. Proc Am Assoc Cancer Res 39:488

Hendrikse NH, Schinkel AH, De Vries et al 1998b Complete *in vivo* reversal of P-glycoprotein pump function in the blood–brain barrier visualized with positron emission tomography. Br J Pharmacol 124:1413–1418

Hendrikse NH, De Vries EGE, Eriks-Fluks E et al 1999 A new *in vivo* method to study P-glycoprotein transport in tumors and the blood–brain barrier. Cancer Res 59:2411–2416

Higgins CF 1992 ABC transporters: from microorganisms to man. Annu Rev Cell Biol 8:67–113

Huai-Yun H, Secrest DT, Mark KS et al 1998 Expression of multidrug resistance-associated protein (MRP) in brain microvessel endothelial cells. Biochem Biophys Res Commun 243:816–820

Hunter AL, Klaassen CD 1975 Biliary excretion of colchicine. J Pharmacol Exp Ther 192:605–617

Kim AE, Dintaman JM, Waddell DS, Silverman JA 1998 Saquinavir, an HIV protease inhibitor, is transported by P-glycoprotein. J Pharmacol Exp Ther 286:1439–1445

Kusuhara H, Suzuki H, Naito M, Tsuruo T, Sugiyama Y 1998 Characterization of efflux transport of organic anions in a mouse brain capillary endothelial cell line. J Pharmacol Exp Ther 285:1260–1265

Lazarowski A, Sevlever G, Taratuto A, Massaro M, Rabinowicz A 1999 Tuberous sclerosis associated with MDR1 gene expression and drug-resistant epilepsy. Pediatr Neurol 21:731–734

Levin VA 1980 Relationship of octanol/water partition coefficient and molecular weight to rat brain capillary permeability. J Med Chem 23:682–684

Mehta BM, Rosa E, Fissekis JD, Bading JR, Biedler JL, Larson M 1992 *In vivo* identification of tumor multidrug resistance with [^{3}H]colchicine. J Nucl Med 33:1373–1377

Mehta BM, Rosa E, Biedler JL, Larson SM 1994 *in vivo* uptake of carbon-14-colchicine for identification of tumor multidrug resistance. J Nucl Med 35:1179–1184

Mehta BM, Levchenko A, Rosa E et al 1996 Evaluation of carbon-14-colchicine biodistribution with whole-body quantitative autoradiography in colchicine-sensitive and -resistant xenografts. J Nucl Med 37:312–314

Regina A, Koman A, Piciotti M et al 1998 Mrp1 multidrug resistance-associated protein and P-glycoprotein expression in rat brain microvessel endothelial cells. J Neurochem 71:705–715

Rubin LI, Staddon JM 1999 The cell biology of the blood–brain barrier. Annu Rev Neurosci 22:11–28

Schinkel AH, Smit JJM, Van Tellingen O et al 1994 Disruption of the mouse mdr1a P-glycoprotein gene leads to a deficiency in the blood–brain barrier and to increased sensitivity to drugs. Cell 77:491–502

Schinkel AH, Wagenaar E, Mol CA, Van Deemter L 1996 P-glycoprotein in the blood–brain barrier of mice influences the brain penetration and pharmacological activity of many drugs. J Clin Invest 97:2517–2524

Seetharaman S, Barrand MA, Maskell L, Scheper RJ 1998 Multidrug resistance-related transport protein in isolated human brain microvessels and in cells cultured from these isolates. J Neurochem 70:1151–1159

Shiraki N, Hamada Y, Yasuda K, Fujii J, Arimori K, Nakano M 2000 Inhibitory effect of human immunodeficiency virus protease inhibitors on multidrug resistance transporter P-glycoproteins. Biol Pharm Bull 23:1528–1531
Tsuij A, Terasaki T, Takabatake Y et al 1992 P-glycoprotein as drug efflux pump in primary cultured bovine brain capillary endothelial cells. Life Sci 51:1427–1437
Weber DM, Dimopoulos MA, Alexanian R 1993 Increased neurotoxicity with VAD-cyclosporin in multiple myeloma. Lancet 341:558–559
Weber DM, Dimopoulos MA, Sinicrope F, Alexanian R 1995 VAD-cyclosporine therapy for VAD-resistant multiple myeloma. Leuk Lymphoma 19:159–163

DISCUSSION

Löscher: How good is the resolution of your technique? Is it possible to see more than just the whole brain in small animals such as mice?

Hendrikse: The clinical camera has a resolution of 3 mm, so studies in animals are possible, but it is on the borderline. It would be better to do studies in animal PET scanners that have a resolution of 1 mm.

Ling: What are the limitations in terms of the compounds that can be imaged?

Hendrikse: Due to the short half-life of ^{11}C, of about 20 min, we have to prepare the compounds near the camera and patient. Verapamil is relatively simple, and it took us about a year to get enough activity to do a patient study. Now we are trying to measure cytostatic drugs that will be useful in the clinic. However, it is not simple to prepare and develop these drugs.

Ling: What are the challenges with the 50 or so anti-epileptic drugs?

Hendrikse: I think we have to just choose one drug. It is currently impossible to prepare and radiolabel 50 drugs, and test them all.

Deisz: A technical question: has verapamil in some way been changed by the radiolabelling?

Hendrikse: No, we only replaced a ^{12}C with an ^{11}C. Nothing changes in the molecular structure.

Löscher: How robust is the labelling? Is it possible that the ^{11}C is also incorporated in a metabolite of the parent compound?

Hendrikse: We did some metabolite studies in the animals, in both tumour and brain tissue. In the time frame of the experiments (1 h) we didn't see metabolism of the compound. More than 90% was present as parent compound.

Wijnholds: Verapamil binds to Pgp, but the off-rate is probably different to that of other drugs. It may be that verapamil is transported relatively slowly by Pgp.

Hendrikse: This might be due to the high lipophilicity of verapamil. It has a logP value of more than 5, and the literature suggests that most optimal Pgp substrates have a logP of 2–2.5. I think the slow efflux of verapamil that we measure with the camera is due to its high lipophilicity.

Ling: Does the environment in which these molecules find themselves affect the PET signal? In other words, if the molecule is in dense tissue as opposed to the lipid bilayer, does this affect the quantitation or imaging quality at all?

Hendrikse: No. It is difficult to discriminate the localization of the radioactivity, though.

Ling: From a practical perspective, what would your advice be in terms of using PET rather than other more traditional medical imaging techniques?

Hendrikse: The disadvantage of PET is that there are relatively few PET centres in the world. If a PET facility is available, I would try to label a radiopharmaceutical and test in the presence of different modulators at different concentrations.

Wood: Is there an absolute number—some proportion of the drug that is mediated by Pgp so that you can see it against background? Take the two extremes. For a drug that is 0% excreted by Pgp, it will enter the tissue and be present at high concentrations, independently of whether Pgp is modulated. At the other extreme is a drug that is 100% removed from the cell by Pgp. This will be exquisitely sensitive to modulation. But it seems to me there must be some percentage between these two where the discrimination begins to break down.

Hendrikse: The quantity of activity is not important, but the signal:noise ratio is. Our experience is that a signal:noise ratio of two is enough for quantitative studies.

Wood: Take, for example, the lung: would it be hard to show the role of Pgp in that tissue with such a high background level?

Hendrikse: That's difficult to answer. In the patient studies, it might be problematic to measure tumour kinetics quantitatively in a small tumour. However, with a big, bulky tumour mass in the thorax, measuring quantitative Pgp kinetics in the tumour is less problematic, due to less background disturbance.

Ling: How many patients have you looked at so far? Have you looked at the normal organs and tissues, and how much variation do you see among 'normal' individuals? Is it possible to compare individuals in a quantitative way?

Hendrikse: So far we have looked at six patients, and there is high inter-individual variability. To test the concept further we are looking in lung transplantation patients before and after transplant. Before transplantation we give verapamil and scan the brain. After transplantation they get a high dose of cyclosporin and dexamethasone, which are immune system modulators. We then give these patients another verapamil scan. Thus we can compare the patients with themselves, although there are a lot of problems: transplantation of the lungs may change the pharmacokinetics. I agree with you that to overcome the heterogeneity of the quantitative data, we have to compare the patients with themselves. We hope that we can do this in the future, in tumour patients before and after chemotherapy.

Bates: How do you explain the high level of lung uptake? Can you extrapolate that to say that some modulators might be higher in lung and others might be higher in liver, for example? Is this a possibility?

Hendrikse: I don't have a good explanation for the enhanced lung uptake. The literature suggests that there are amine receptors present in the lungs. Verapamil has a similar structure to amines. It is possible that these drugs bind to the amine receptors, and when you inject intravenously the first passage is through the lung. Several drugs, including some antidepressants, are especially taken up by the lung.

Deisz: What would a scan from a leg look like compared to the lung? The lungs obviously have the least amount of tissue per volume. Could this contribute to the relatively small signal?

Hendrikse: I haven't done the calculations.

Bates: What about liver uptake of verapamil after treatment with a modulator? With Sestamibi we saw marked liver retention.

Hendrikse: We didn't measure that because the region of interest is only 11 cm. The tumour was located higher in the thorax, so I don't know about the liver.

Wood: It seems to me that there are two different questions in play and we are not addressing them directly. One is tissue localization of the drug, which in this case is verapamil, on which there is a lot of information. Verapamil and related drugs are highly taken up by tissues such as the lung and are then released. This is not necessarily through a Pgp-related mechanism. The first question is if you just look at imaging of the verapamil, you'll measure drug uptake in tissue. This isn't very different from the first studies in animals in which drug companies injected radiolabelled drugs and analysed different tissues. The second experiment, which is the critical one here, is how this changes specifically when you give a selective Pgp modulator. The point I was trying to grapple with earlier is that it seems that if the initial binding is high, and most of that is not in a tissue mediated by Pgp, then your ability to detect Pgp modulation will be very small. The strength of Sestamibi is that relatively little uptake is seen until Pgp is inhibited, at which time there is a lot of uptake. The background noise is relatively small. Here you are seeing a lot of uptake without any inhibition, which would make me suspicious that it will be hard to get high sensitivity.

Hendrikse: We have to try to find a radiopharmaceutical that shows less non-specific binding. Furthermore, we need to know that it is a Pgp substrate. Then we will be able to study Pgp function *in vivo* in patients.

Newman: The background that you found in the brains in the mouse experiments looked pretty good. The effect of cyclosporin on the verapamil levels in the brains of the mice seemed quite convincing. This might be a useful model.

Wood: The cyclosporin may be inhibiting metabolism. It seems to me that there is some number there that we haven't got to grips with. It must be dependent on the background uptake. We know a lot about uptake of drugs into tissue, and most of these data came long before we thought about pumps.

Abbott: We have tended to assume that any drug that is a Pgp substrate would show a great difference in brain penetration between the Pgp knockout animal and the wild-type, reflecting the strong influence of Pgp on brain penetration. For ivermectin the ratio is ~ 80 (Schinkel et al 1994), whereas for doxorubicin it is much less (~ 3) (van Asperen et al 1997). Thus it is not a simple matter to predict how brain concentrations of Pgp substrate drugs will be affected by changes in Pgp expression on the brain endothelium, or indeed on other cells in the brain.

Hendrikse: In the *ex vivo* data I showed, we measured a ratio of 12. With the camera the ratio was two. This might be due to partial volume problems, because we measured small animals with a big clinical camera.

The clinicians are interested in drugs that are used in the treatment of patients. For example, it would be useful to test phenytoin in epileptic patients in order to work out its pharmacokinetics. When we measure Pgp pharmacokinetics with non-clinically used drugs, the next question is whether we can translate these data to the cancer patients. We prefer to label drugs that are used clinically.

Abbott: It may be that if you weren't restricted to cancer patients there would be some other therapies for which there would be good markers. For example, morphine, which has low penetration.

References

Schinkel AH, Smit LLM, Van Tellingen O et al 1994 Disruption of the mouse *mdr*1a P-glycoprotein gene leads to deficiency in the blood–brain barrier and to increased sensitivity to drugs. Cell 77:491–502

van Asperen J, Mayer U, Tellingen O van, Beijnen JH 1997 The functional role of P-glycoprotein in the blood–brain barrier. J Pharm Sci 86:881–884

Animal models of drug-resistant epilepsy

Wolfgang Löscher

Department of Pharmacology, Toxicology, and Pharmacy, School of Veterinary Medicine, Bünteweg 17, 30559 Hanover, Germany

Abstract. It is not known why and how epilepsy becomes drug resistant in 20–30% of patients, while other patients with seemingly identical seizure types can achieve control of seizures with medication. An animal model of epilepsy allowing selection of pharmacoresistant and pharmacosensitive subgroups of animals would be a valuable tool to study mechanisms of pharmacoresistance and to develop more effective treatment strategies. Only a few models are available which mimic patterns of drug resistance in humans with epilepsy. One model seems to be particularly interesting: amygdala-kindled rats. In this model in Wistar rats, animals which do not respond to repeated or chronic administration of anti-epileptic drugs (non-responders) can be separated from animals in whom anti-epileptics are effective (responders). Hence, pharmacoresistant subgroups of kindled rats provide a unique tool to study why seizures become intractable, particularly because pathophysiological processes in these resistant rats can be directly compared with those of kindled rats that respond to treatment. By using this model, we have recently shown that both the individual genetic background and kindling-induced processes determine whether a rat becomes a responder or a non-responder to anticonvulsant treatment after kindling. We are currently studying the cellular mechanisms underlying the development of drug-resistant kindled seizures.

2002 Mechanisms of drug resistance in epilepsy: lessons from oncology. Wiley, Chichester (Novartis Foundation Symposium 243) p 149–166

In most patients with epilepsy the prognosis for seizure control is very good. However, a significant proportion of individuals with epilepsy suffer from pharmacoresistant epilepsy, despite early treatment and an optimum daily dosage of an adequate anti-epileptic drug (AED) (Regesta & Tanganelli 1999). Thus, there is a clear need for new drugs or new strategies of therapeutic management. Although surgical treatment of epilepsy may be an alternative if AEDs fail, surgery for epilepsy might not be needed if we knew more about ways to prevent medical intractability or if we had more effective and less toxic AEDs.

The majority of epileptic patients with intractable seizures despite treatment with one of the major AEDs will not improve by alternative monotherapy or combination drug therapy, even if the recently marketed novel AEDs are employed. We do not know why and how epilepsy becomes an intractable disorder in such patients. The fact that two patients with seemingly identical seizure types may dramatically differ in their response to the same AED (i.e. one patient becoming controlled and the other patient being refractory), indicates that there may be interindividual pathophysiological differences, but the nature of these differences is not known (Regesta & Tanganelli 1999). Attempts to study pathophysiological factors that may be important for intractability of seizures in brain biopsy samples from pharmacoresistant epileptic patients undergoing surgical treatment of epilepsy are hampered by the lack of suitable control tissue. Thus, an animal model of epilepsy allowing selection of subgroups of animals with pharmacoresistant and pharmacosensitive seizures could be a valuable tool to study why and how seizures become intractable and to develop more effective treatment strategies.

Two models seem to be particularly interesting in this regard: epileptic dogs with different types of spontaneous recurrent seizures and amygdala-kindled rats (Löscher 1997). In both models, animals which do not respond to repeated or chronic administration of AEDs (non-responders) can be separated from animals in whom AEDs are effective (responders). Unfortunately, the dog model has several inherent logistical problems, such as the high prime and maintenance costs of epileptic dogs in the numbers necessary for selection of pharmacoresistant subgroups (Löscher 1997). The kindling model of temporal lobe epilepsy (TLE), one of the most frequent types of intractable epilepsy (Regesta & Tanganelli 1999), does not share these limitations with the dog model. Hence, pharmacoresistant subgroups of kindled rats provide a unique tool to study why seizures become intractable, particularly because pathophysiological processes in these resistant rats can be directly compared with those of kindled rats which respond to treatment. In the following, the development of this animal model and its use in unravelling how epilepsy becomes intractable will be described in more detail.

Identification of pharmacoresistant kindled rats

Kindling refers to the phenomenon that animals chronically implanted with a stimulation electrode in one structure of the limbic system or other brain areas (the amygdala being among the most responsive structures) develop focal and secondarily generalized seizures of increasing severity and duration upon a period of electrical stimulation with an initially subconvulsive current. Since its introduction by Goddard et al (1969) kindling has become one of the most widely used animal models of epilepsy, particularly because the mechanisms involved in kindling are thought to be relevant for development of TLE, the most common and difficult-to-treat type of epilepsy in adults.

We first proposed amygdala kindling as a model to investigate intractable epilepsy in 1986 (Löscher 1986, Löscher et al 1986). This proposal was based on several lines of evidence. Among the most important factors indicating a poor prognosis of epilepsy are the site of the primary epileptogenic focus and the period of time over which the patient experiences repetitive seizures without treatment. Since kindling involves a progressive potentiation of seizure susceptibility as well as a functional change in secondary brain sites, due to repetition of partial seizures, kindling may provide a powerful model to investigate the question why epilepsy becomes intractable. By directly comparing standard AEDs in the amygdala-kindling model and the standard maximal electroshock seizure (MES) test in age-matched female Wistar rats, we found that kindled seizures were less sensitive to anticonvulsant treatment than primarily generalized seizures as produced in the MES test. Furthermore, in the kindling model focal seizure stages were found to be much less responsive to AEDs than secondarily generalized seizures, which is consistent with clinical experience. We proposed therefore that search for novel compounds with high potency in the kindled amygdaloid seizure model may be a promising strategy in the development of new AEDs for patients with intractable epilepsy (Löscher 1986, Löscher et al 1986, Löscher & Schmidt 1988).

In follow-up studies in the amygdala-kindling model, using female rats of the Wistar outbred strain, we found that the individual response of fully kindled rats to phenytoin differs: kindled seizures in some animals consistently respond and others never respond to phenytoin (Rundfeldt et al 1990). This finding was systematically explored by determining the effect of phenytoin on the threshold for induction of after-discharges (ADT), i.e. the threshold for induction of focal seizure activity in kindled rats. Phenytoin was repeatedly tested in large groups of fully kindled rats in order to prove the reproducibility of its effect on ADT in individual animals. In a first study with 52 female kindled rats (Löscher & Rundfeldt 1991), phenytoin reproducibly increased the ADT in 21% ('phenytoin responders'), induced variable effects (i.e. an increase in one trial but no increase in another trial, or vice versa) in 58% (variable responders), and failed to increase the ADT in another 21% of kindled rats ('phenytoin non-responders'). The difference in response to phenytoin between responders and non-responders was dramatic in that average ADT increases induced by phenytoin in responders at plasma concentrations of 25–30 $\mu g/ml$ were between 400% and more than 1000% above individual predrug control values, whereas no increase or even slight decreases in ADT were determined in non-responders at the same phenytoin plasma concentration range. Interestingly, phenytoin responders and non-responders did not differ in kindling acquisition or the severity and duration of their fully kindled seizures. In other words, there was no prognostic measure by which it could be predicted that a given kindled rat would respond or not respond to treatment with phenytoin.

In a subsequent prospective study, we investigated whether the original finding of phenytoin-resistant and non-resistant kindled animals was reproducible among another group of 68 fully amygdala-kindled rats (Löscher et al 1993). Phenytoin was tested four times in each fully kindled animal at intervals of at least 5 days. Twelve percent of the rats were non-responders, another 12% were responders, and the remaining animals were variable responders. Thus, we could reproduce the original finding, although the frequency of responders and non-responders differed between the two studies. Since all rats had had the same number of kindled seizures before phenytoin application, the difference in sensitivity to phenytoin between responders and non-responders was certainly not due to the period of time over which the animals had experienced repetitive seizures without treatment. We concluded that kindled rats with phenytoin resistance are a unique resource for the investigation of mechanisms of drug resistance in epilepsy, particularly because pathophysiological processes in phenytoin-resistant rats can be directly compared with those of kindled rats which reproducibly respond to this drug (Löscher & Rundfeldt 1991, Löscher et al 1993).

In recent years, we have repeated the selection of phenytoin responders and non-responders in female Wistar rats several times, using either phenytoin or its prodrug fosphenytoin for selection. Average data from more than 200 rats show a consistent anticonvulsant response to phenytoin in only 16% of the animals, no anticonvulsant response in 23%, and a variable response in the remaining 61% (Löscher 1997). An example for a selection of these subgroups is shown in Fig. 1.

Pharmacoresistant kindled rats as a tool to evaluate AEDs

Following the identification of phenytoin-resistant kindled Wistar rats, most clinically available AEDs were tested in these animals. Results are shown in Table 1. Except the novel drug levetiracetam, all AEDs were significantly less efficacious or not efficacious at all in phenytoin non-responders compared to phenytoin responders, demonstrating that the phenytoin resistance of a subgroup of kindled Wistar rats extends to various other old and new AEDs. This reflects the clinical situation because most epileptic patients who are refractory to one AED are also resistant to other AEDs, including newly developed drugs (Regesta & Tanganelli 1999). Whether levetiractam has advantages in this respect remains to be determined.

Mechanisms of drug resistance in kindled rats

Various factors that could be important for our finding of pharmacoresistant subgroups of amygdala-kindled Wistar rats have been studied since the first description of this model (Löscher 1997, Ebert et al 1999). These studies have

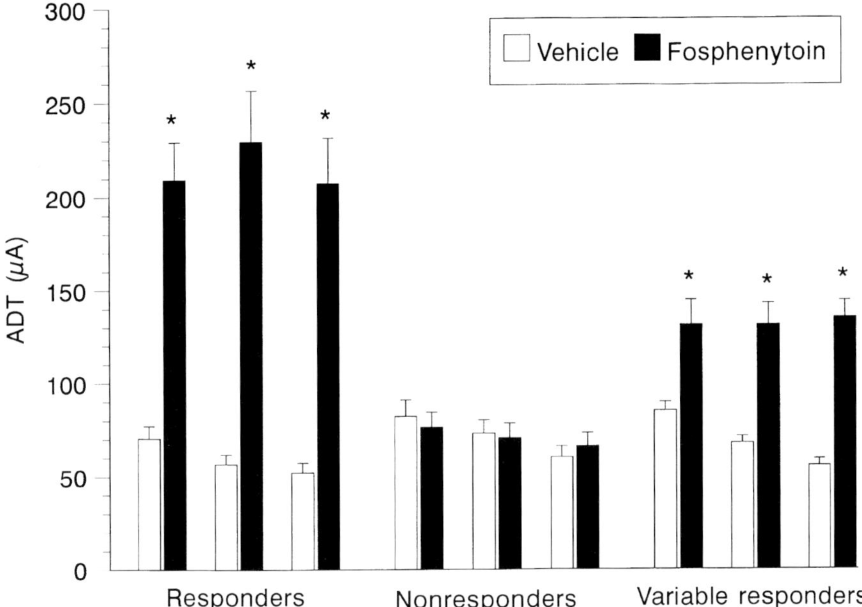

FIG. 1   Average increases in after-discharge threshold (ADT) after treatment with the phenytoin prodrug fosphenytoin in 80 amygdala-kindled Wistar rats. Fosphenytoin was i.p. injected at 83.5 mg/kg (equivalent to 50 mg/kg phenytoin) and ADT and phenytoin plasma levels were determined after 1 h. This experiment was repeated twice in each rat at intervals of 1 week. Control recordings after vehicle injection were done 4 days before each drug trial in the same rats. After the drug trials, animals were grouped according to their response in phenytoin responders ($n=25$), non-responders ($n=17$), and variable responders ($n=38$). Responders showed an anticonvulsant effect (i.e. an increase in ADT) after fosphenytoin in each trial, non-responders did not show any effect, and variable responders showed inconsistent effects (e.g. a response in one trial but no response in the next trial), so that ADT increases of variable responders as a group are below ADT increases in responders. Data are shown as mean ADT ± SEM; significance of differences between ADT in control and drug trials in each group is indicated by asterisk ($P < 0.0001$). The phenytoin plasma levels did not differ significantly between groups (not illustrated). (Data are from Ebert et al 2000).

shown that pharmacoresistance is not due to differences in the location of the kindling electrode in the amygdala, drug pharmacokinetics, seasonal variations in drug response, or the sex of the animals, i.e. phenytoin non-responders could also be selected from male Wistar rats.

One likely explanation for phenytoin non-responders could be genetic differences in general susceptibility to phenytoin's pharmacodynamic effects between the two subgroups of kindled rats. However, two observations argued against this possibility. In contrast to the dramatic difference in anticonvulsant response, the level of adverse effects such as ataxia induced by phenytoin in

TABLE 1 Anticonvulsant efficacy of old and new anti-epileptic drugs in kindled Wistar rats selected by their response to phenytoin into non-responders and responders

Drug	*Loss of anticonvulsant efficacy against focal seizures in non-responders (in % compared to responders)*	*Reference*
Phenytoin	100	Löscher and Rundfeldt 1991
Carbamazepine	51	Löscher and Rundfeldt 1991
Phenobarbital	85	Löscher et al 1993
Valproate	79	Löscher et al 1993
Vigabatrin	46	Löscher et al 1993
Lamotrigine	60	Ebert et al 2000
Felbamate	75	Ebert et al 2000
Topiramate	61	Reissmüller et al 2000
Gabapentin	52	Löscher et al 2000a
Levetiracetam	No loss of efficacy	Löscher et al 2000a

responders and non-responders did not differ (Löscher & Rundfeldt 1991). Furthermore, when the effect of phenytoin on the MES threshold was determined in kindled rats, both responders and non-responders showed the same significant increase in this threshold for primarily generalized seizures, thus demonstrating that the difference in susceptibility to the anticonvulsant effect of phenytoin was restricted to focal kindled seizures (Löscher & Rundfeldt 1991).

Although the observations on adverse effects and MES threshold described above seem to argue against involvement of genetics in response differences of kindled rats to phenytoin, they are not sufficient to exclude genetic differences between individual rats of the Wistar outbred population used for the kindling experiments. In this respect, it is also interesting to note that, in different strains of mice, sublines were described which differed in their sensitivity to the depressant but not anticonvulsant effects of benzodiazepines (Gallaher & Crabbe 1991), thus demonstrating that genetic factors can affect only one out of several pharmacodynamic effects of a drug. For a closer examination of the possible involvement of genetics in the differential effects of phenytoin found in kindled rats, we therefore undertook breeding studies with phenytoin responders and non-responders, using male and female Wistar rats (Ebert & Löscher 1999). Altogether, four generations of kindled Wistar rats were studied. The data suggest that the ability to respond or not to respond to phenytoin is genetically determined, although it does not follow a simple scheme of inheritance (Ebert & Löscher 1999).

The involvement of genetics in the differing drug sensitivity in responders and non-responders selected from kindled Wistar rats was substantiated by a study in which we selected phenytoin responders and non-responders in six other outbred and inbred rat strains, Sprague-Dawley, Wistar-Kyoto, Lewis, Fischer 344, ACI and Brown Norway (Cramer et al 1998, Löscher et al 1998). The only strain in which non-responders could be selected was Brown Norway. However, in contrast to Wistar outbred rats, no responders could be selected in the Brown Norway strain, so that Wistar rats were the only strain allowing selection of both non-responders and responders. All subsequent experiments were thus done in the Wistar strain.

Besides genetics, another possible explanation for development of different pharmacosensitivity in kindled rats would be the kindling process itself. Epileptic patients often initially respond to an AED, but this effect may be lost with increasing duration of the disease, i.e. when epilepsy becomes chronic. To address the influence of kindling on the anticonvulsant response to phenytoin, we tested phenytoin's anticonvulsant effect before and after kindling in the same rats. Following kindling, rats were repeatedly tested with phenytoin to allow subgroup selection. Unexpectedly, in rats which were responders after kindling, phenytoin exerted no significant anticonvulsant effect before kindling, while kindled non-responders were very sensitive to phenytoin before kindling (Löscher et al 2000b). This study indicates that kindled phenytoin non-responders become non-responders through the kindling process (i.e. kindling induced brain alterations), whereas kindled responders are rats in which kindling enhances the efficacy of phenytoin compared to the prekindling state. In view of the results of our recent breeding studies in Wistar rats (Ebert and Löscher 1999), the genetic background of an individual rat seems to determine whether it becomes a responder or non-responder by limbic epileptogenesis.

Which kindling-induced brain alterations could determine whether a rat becomes a responder or non-responder to an AED such as phenytoin? We currently concentrate on two possibilities which are described in the following.

Does kindling change the cellular targets of anti-epileptic drugs?

It has been proposed that the mechanisms underlying pharmacoresistance in TLE most likely involve the functional and morphological changes developing in regions such as the hippocampus in the course of the disease (Heinemann et al 1994). Drugs of primary choice for treatment of TLE such as phenytoin or carbamazepine are thought to act via modulation of voltage-activated Na^+ and Ca^{2+} channels (DeLorenzo 1995, Macdonald 1999). It was previously shown that the properties of these channels change in the hippocampus of patients with therapy-refractory TLE (Beck et al 1997, 1998, Reckziegel et al 1999), which could explain the loss of therapeutic efficacy of major AEDs. Indeed, Wadman and colleagues found an impaired modulation of sodium current inactivation by carbamazepine in hippocampal neurons from patients with pharmacoresistant TLE that was associated with hippocampal sclerosis (Vreugdenhil et al 1998). A similar reduction in carbamazepine's effect on Na^+ channels was also determined in hippocampal CA1 neurons of kindled rats (Vreugdenhil & Wadman 1999). However, the reduction in carbamazepine's effect was only transient in kindled rats (Vreugdenhil & Wadman 1999). Furthermore, carbamazepine is a very potent and efficacious anticonvulsant in kindled rats (Albertson et al 1984, Löscher et al 1986, Hönack & Löscher 1989) so that the transiently reduced carbamazepine response of Na^+ channels described in the hippocampus of kindled rats by Vreugdenhil & Wadman (1999) is not associated with any resistance to the drug's anticonvulsant effect *in vivo*.

However, as shown by our experiments in amygdala-kindled Wistar rats, individual kindled rats differ in their response to AEDs, which could be due to differences in the sensitivity of cellular targets of such drugs. To directly address the possibility that neuronal Na^+ currents in the hippocampus play a crucial role in the pharmacoresistance of TLE, we selected amygdala-kindled rats with respect to their *in vivo* anticonvulsant response to phenytoin into responders and non-responders and then compared phenytoin's effect on voltage-activated Na^+ currents in CA1 neurons (Jeub et al 2001). Furthermore, in view of the potential role of Ca^{2+} current modulation in the anticonvulsant action of phenytoin, the effect of phenytoin on high-voltage-activated Ca^{2+} currents was studied in CA1 neurons. Electrode-implanted but not kindled rats were used as sham controls for comparison with the kindled rats. In all experiments, the interval between last kindled seizure and ion channel measurements was at least 5 weeks. In kindled rats with *in vivo* resistance to the anticonvulsant effect of phenytoin (phenytoin non-responders), *in vitro* modulation of Na^+ and Ca^{2+} currents by phenytoin in hippocampal CA1 neurons did not differ to any extent from respective data obtained in phenytoin responders, i.e. phenytoin resistance was not associated with a changed modulation of the Na^+ or Ca^{2+} currents by this drug. Compared to sham controls, phenytoin's inhibitory effect on Na^+ currents was significantly reduced by kindling, with no difference between the responder and non-responder subgroups. These findings cast doubt on the previous hypothesis that pharmacoresistance is related to a reduced pharmacological sensitivity of Na^+ or Ca^{2+} currents.

Does kindling change the brain uptake of AEDs?

In view of the fact that a patient being resistant to one AED is often resistant to other AEDs, even drugs with different mechanisms, it seems unlikely that functional changes at target sites for AEDs (e.g. voltage-dependent Na^+ channels) underlie pharmacoresistance. A more likely explanation to account for medical intractability is that AEDs do not reach sufficiently high brain levels despite adequate plasma levels within the 'therapeutic range'. Tishler et al (1995) were the first to report that brain expression of the multiple drug resistance gene (*MDR1*), which encodes the multidrug transporter P glycoprotein (Pgp), is markedly increased in the majority of patients with medically intractable epilepsy. In line with enhanced *MDR1* expression, immunohistochemistry for Pgp showed increased staining in capillary endothelium and astrocytes (Tishler et al 1995). This group also proposed that Pgp may play a clinically significant role by limiting access of AEDs to the brain parenchyma, so that increased *MDR1* expression may contribute to the refractoriness of seizures in patients with pharmacoresistant epilepsy.

However, until now it is not known whether AEDs are transported to any significant extent by Pgp in the brain. Pgp is thought to constitute a defence mechanism limiting brain accumulation of naturally occurring toxins and xenobiotics (Silverman 1999, Fromm 2000, Spector 2000). In the brain, Pgp is thought to be primarily located in the luminal cell membrane of endothelial cells of the blood–brain barrier (BBB) and is involved in transferring certain drugs back into blood after they have entered endothelial cells from the blood, thus limiting penetration of such drugs into brain parenchyma (Spector 2000). In Mdr1a knockout mice, in which the Mdr1a Pgp isoform is absent in the BBB, various drugs reach markedly higher brain levels compared to normal mice, but brain levels of the AED phenytoin are not different from controls (Schinkel et al 1996). However, in a kidney epithelial cell line transfected with *Mdr1a* cDNA, phenytoin was transported, which could be blocked by the Pgp inhibitor PSC 833 (Schinkel et al 1996). Tishler et al (1995) found that intracellular phenytoin levels in a *MDR1*-expressing neuroectodermal cell line were only one quarter that in *MDR1*-negative cells, suggesting that Pgp significantly contributes to cell export of phenytoin. This is substantiated by recent *in vivo* experiments in rats in which we demonstrated that extracellular concentrations of phenytoin in the brain could be markedly enhanced by Pgp inhibitors such as PSC 833 (Potschka et al 2000). We are currently studying whether the expression of Pgp is enhanced by kindling and whether differences in Pgp expression exist between phenytoin responders and non-responders in kindled Wistar rat populations.

Conclusions

Pharmacoresistant epilepsy represents a challenge for both experimental and clinical research to gain new insights and perspectives of its mechanisms in order to improve future rational management approaches. Phenytoin-resistant kindled rats are the first animal model of pharmacoresistant epilepsy that can be used to study mechanisms of drug resistance and to develop more efficacious AEDs. It is hoped that further investigation and exploitation of this model may contribute to our understanding of the processes through which epilepsy becomes intractable. Furthermore, this model should be added to the late preclinical phases of AED development in order to prove at a relatively early stage whether a new drug exhibits advantages towards standard AEDs in drug resistant seizure types.

References

Albertson TE, Joy R, Stark LG 1984 A pharmacological study in the kindling model of epilepsy. Neuropharmacology 23:1117–1123

Beck H, Steffens R, Heinemann U, Elger CE 1997 Properties of voltage-activated Ca^{2+} currents in acutely isolated human hippocampal granule cells. J Neurophysiol 77:1526–1537

Beck H, Steffens R, Elger CE, Heinemann U 1998 Voltage-dependent Ca^{2+} currents in epilepsy. Epilepsy Res 32:321–332

Cramer S, Ebert U, Löscher W 1998 Characterization of phenytoin-resistant kindled rats, a new model of drug-resistant partial epilepsy: comparison of inbred strains. Epilepsia 39:1046–1053

DeLorenzo RJ 1995 Phenytoin: mechanisms of action. In: Levy RH, Mattson RH, Meldrum BS, Dreifuss FE, Penry JK, Hessie BJ (eds) Antiepileptic drugs, 4th edn. Raven Press, New York, p 271–282

Ebert U, Löscher W 1999 Characterization of phenytoin-resistant kindled rats, a new model of drug-resistant partial epilepsy: influence of genetic factors. Epilepsy Res 33:217–226

Ebert U, Rundfeldt C, Lehmann H, Löscher W 1999 Characterization of phenytoin-resistant rats, a new model of drug-resistant partial epilepsy: influence of experimental and environmental factors. Epilepsy Res 33:199–215

Ebert U, Reissmüller E, Löscher W 2000 The new antiepileptic drugs lamotrigine and felbamate are effective in phenytoin-resistant kindled rats. Neuropharmacology 39:1893–1903

Fromm MF 2000 P-glycoprotein: a defense mechanism limiting oral bioavailability and CNS accumulation of drugs. Int J Clin Pharmacol Ther 38:69–74

Gallaher EJ, Crabbe JCJ 1991 Genetics of benzodiazepines, barbiturates, and anesthetics. In: Crabbe JCJ, Harris RA (eds) The genetic basis of alcohol and drug actions. Plenum Press, New York, p 253–277

Goddard GV, McIntyre DC, Leech CK 1969 A permanent change in brain function resulting from daily electrical stimulation. Exp Neurol 25:295–330

Heinemann U, Draguhn A, Ficker E, Stabel J, Zhang CL 1994 Strategies for the development of drugs for pharmacoresistant epilepsies. Epilepsia 35:S10–S21

Hönack D, Löscher W 1989 Amygdala-kindling as a model for chronic efficacy studies on antiepileptic drugs: experiments with carbamazepine. Neuropharmacology 28:599–610

Jeub M, Beck H, Siep E et al 2001 Effect of phenytoin on sodium and calcium currents in hippocampal CA1 neurons of phenytoin-resistant kindled rats. Neuropharmacology, in press

Löscher W 1986 Experimental models for intractable epilepsy in nonprimate animal species. In: Schmidt D, Morselli PL (eds) Intractable epilepsy: experimental and clinical aspects. Raven Press, New York, p 25–37

Löscher W 1997 Animal models of intractable epilepsy. Prog Neurobiol 53:239–258

Löscher W, Rundfeldt C 1991 Kindling as a model of drug-resistant partial epilepsy: selection of phenytoin-resistant and nonresistant rats. J Pharmacol Exp Ther 258:483–489

Löscher W, Schmidt D 1988 Which animal models should be used in the search for new antiepileptic drugs? A proposal based on experimental and clinical considerations. Epilepsy Res 2:145–181

Löscher W, Jäckel R, Czuczwar SJ 1986 Is amygdala kindling in rats a model for drug-resistant partial epilepsy? Exp Neurol 93:211–226

Löscher W, Rundfeldt C, Hönack D 1993 Pharmacological characterization of phenytoin-resistant amygdala-kindled rats, a new model of drug-resistant partial epilepsy. Epilepsy Res 15:207–219

Löscher W, Cramer S, Ebert U 1998 Selection of phenytoin responders and nonresponders in male and female amygdala-kindled Sprague-Dawley rats. Epilepsia 39:1138–1147

Löscher W, Reissmüller E, Ebert U 2000a Anticonvulsant efficacy of gabapentin and levetiracetam in phenytoin-resistant kindled rats. Epilepsy Res 40:63–77

Löscher W, Reissmüller E, Ebert U 2000b Kindling alters the anticonvulsant efficacy of phenytoin in Wistar rats. Epilepsy Res 39:211–220

Macdonald RL 1999 Cellular actions of antiepileptic drugs. In: Eadie MJ, Vajda FJE (eds) Antiepileptic drugs. Pharmacology and therapeutics. Springer-Verlag, Berlin, p 123–150

Potschka H, Wirth U, Löscher W 2000 P-glycoprotein mediated transport of phenytoin: relevance to pharmacoresistant epilepsy? Soc Neurosci Abstr 26:1782

Reckziegel G, Beck H, Schramm J, Urban BW, Elger CE 1999 Carbamazepine effects on Na+ currents in human dentate granule cells from epileptogenic tissue. Epilepsia 40:401–407

Regesta G, Tanganelli P 1999 Clinical aspects and biological bases of drug-resistant epilepsies. Epilepsy Res 34:109–122

Reissmüller E, Ebert U, Löscher W 2000 Anticonvulsant efficacy of topiramate in phenytoin-resistant kindled rats. Epilepsia 41:372–379

Rundfeldt C, Hönack D, Löscher W 1990 Phenytoin potently increases the threshold for focal seizures in amygdala-kindled rats. Neuropharmacology 29:845–851

Schinkel AH, Wagenaar E, Mol CA, van Deemter L 1996 P-glycoprotein in the blood-brain barrier of mice influences the brain penetration and pharmacological activity of many drugs. J Clin Invest 97:2517–2524

Silverman JA 1999 Multidrug-resistance transporters. Pharm Biotechnol 12:353–386

Spector R 2000 Drug transport in the mammalian central nervous system: multiple complex systems. A critical analysis and commentary. Pharmacology 60:58–73

Tishler DM, Weinberg KT, Hinton DR, Barbaro N, Annett GM, Raffel C 1995 *MDR1* gene expression in brain of patients with medically intractable epilepsy. Epilepsia 36:1–6

Vreugdenhil M, Wadman WJ 1999 Modulation of sodium currents in rat CA1 neurons by carbamazepine and valproate after kindling epileptogenesis. Epilepsia 40:1512–1522

Vreugdenhil M, van Veelen CW, van Rijen PC, Lopes da Silva FHL, Wadman WJ 1998 Effect of valproic acid on sodium currents in cortical neurons from patients with pharmaco-resistant temporal lobe epilepsy. Epilepsy Res 32:309–320

DISCUSSION

Meldrum: All the data you presented concern the ADT. If you instead do a supramaximal stimulation and measure just the clinical manifestation, do you get the same phenomenon?

Löscher: Not with phenytoin. In our experimental paradigm, phenytoin increases ADT but does almost nothing on seizure severity or other parameters recorded at ADT current. But please remember that we don't use a fixed stimulus; instead we increase ADT until we have a seizure. This situation may be rather artificial, but it allows us to quantitate the level of the effect. Again, phenytoin has no effect on seizure severity under these conditions. There are other drugs, such as carbamazepine, that do both: they increase ADT and decrease seizure severity and duration at ADT. The non-responders also show a lowered response in terms of seizure severity and duration to carbamazepine. The same is true for valproate and phenobarbitone, which show an almost 100% loss of efficacy.

Meldrum: That is a curious pharmacological differentiation, in comparison with the human drug resistance.

Löscher: If you do the same experiment, using a fixed electrical stimulus that is 20% above the focal seizure threshold, then in the responders all the drugs block all seizure activity. But we do not allow this because we increase the ADT until the animals show seizure. Of course, you can recalculate from the ADT determination what the situation would be if you stopped the stimulus at 20% above threshold. The information coming out from this is the same: we have these two subgroups. This allows us to have a more quantitative measure.

Sander: If you pretreat the rats with phenytoin, do you still see the same results?

Löscher: Yes, but this was only one dose. It was not easy to do, because we had to avoid kindling. Because we wanted to avoid kindling, it was only possible to test them once. Otherwise, the pre-testing would kindle them. One acute dose of phenytoin before kindling does not change kindling. The half-life in rats is two hours, so phenytoin is gone after 4 h.

Sander: Do you know of any drug that delays or protects from kindling?

Löscher: There are a number of drugs that do this. It is an interesting topic, because these days everyone is looking for antiepileptogenic drugs that prevent epilepsy. The interesting thing is that both phenytoin and carbamazepine do not retard kindling, and you know that as a clinician these two drugs have been used for many years after events such as head trauma, to prevent traumatic epilepsy. Hence, they are not efficacious to prevent kindling in this paradigm, and controlled clinical trials have shown that these drugs cannot prevent human epilepsy either. Other drugs, such as valproate, phenobarbitone and NMDA antagonists, are effective in inhibiting kindling. It is interesting that these are two sides of the same coin. In fully kindled rats, drugs such as phenytoin or carbamazepine are highly efficacious, but they cannot retard kindling. Other drugs, such as NMDA antagonists, are very efficacious in retarding kindling, but they are poor drugs once the rats are fully kindled. Then there are other drugs still, such as valproate, which do both. By using this model it is possible to separate three categories of drugs.

Sills: Can you demonstrate subgroups of responders and non-responders to other AEDs in the Wistar kindled rat?

Löscher: We tried to do this. All the new drugs were initially tested in patients resistant to the old drugs. Even though the overall picture is frustrating, some patients react to these new drugs. We used topiramate, which is one of the novel AEDs and did the selection in kindled rats again. We found phenytoin non-responders that were topiramate responders and vice versa.

Sills: You were doing these experiments on animals that had previously been treated with phenytoin. Have you performed any similar experiments with other AEDs in previously untreated naïve animals?

Löscher: No. I should add that this model is a nightmare. As I showed you, we have only 10–20% non-responders, so we have to test a lot of animals in order to end up with 8–10 rats. Everyone is asking us for these rats, but it is very time consuming to produce them. I am dreaming of a rat strain in which a higher proportion are non-responders. The second disadvantage is these are outbred rats, so it is not possible to do back-crossing. On the other hand, if we had used inbreds we probably would never have seen this phenomenon of responders and non-responders.

Vezzani: Can you select between the two populations by stimulating other brain areas, after having kindled the amygdala? For example, if you do focal stimulation in the hippocampus, do you still discriminate between the two groups?

Löscher: I would guess that we could, although we haven't tried this. We do a lot of studies on networks in these brains. For instance, if the hippocampus is taken away from amygdala-kindled rats, they are still fully kindled. There is still the same reaction to the stimulus. The same is true in an experiment where you start to kindle the animals via the amygdala and then the amygdala is removed, and the stimulation is continued from another brain site. The animals remain to be fully kindled. We see a functional and structural change in a network of regions. The primary focus, the amygdala, is not the only focus. You have to remember that if you do a temporal lobe resection in temporal lobe epilepsy patients, most of these patients are not seizure free. They still need anticonvulsant drugs. The difference between this state and the situation before surgery is that now 70–80% of the patients can be successfully treated. In other words, by removing the primary focus you have changed the patient into a responder. But many of these patients still have spontaneous seizures if they are not treated. There is a network phenomenon occurring here, which gives us the opportunity to manipulate one region in this network.

Deisz: I'm glad you mentioned the difference between anticonvulsant and anti-epileptic drugs. In this context, the data by Halonen et al (1996) should be mentioned. These authors provided evidence that tiagabine prevents seizures, neuronal damage and memory impairment in an animal model of status epilepticus. These features would make tiagabine an ideal antiepileptic drug. On the other hand, the large synaptic potentials in acute slices from epilepsy surgery tissue are only marginally reduced by tiagabine, which may indicate that the anticonvulsant potency is limited.

Sander: This brings up the issue that we might be taking the wrong approach with our models. Kindling is a very interesting: it is the nearest we have to chronic partial epilepsy. But you don't see kindling on a day-to-day basis in patients.

Löscher: At least two clinical observations suggest that kindling is possible in humans (for review see Sato et al 1990). First, treatment of pain in patients with repeated periodic electrical stimulation through depth electrodes implanted in the thalamus resulted in the development of partial seizures and secondarily generalized seizures during the course of treatment in a number of patients. Second, recurrent spontaneous seizures have developed in schizophrenic patients who had received repeated electroconvulsive therapy. For instance, Naoi (1959) reported 35 cases with spontaneous epileptic seizures out of 172 patients with schizophrenia who had been treated with electroconvulsive therapy more than 50 times.

Sander: I accept that you could put electrodes there, but this is not the way that nature works. Do you know a clinical situation in which you see the development of kindling?

Löscher: Please remember that most of the current popular models of epilepsy are status epilepticus models: they induce status epilepticus either by electrical means or by drugs such as kainate. After a period of three weeks or so, epilepsy then develops and spontaneous seizures begin. I can do the same thing in the kindling model if I apply around 70 stimuli to the amygdala on one day. Then after two weeks, there are spontaneous recurrent seizures in the animals. My current interpretation is that status epilepticus is nothing other than a kindling phenomenon. There is a massive induction of a series of seizures over a short time, which then after a latency period (that may be as long as a year in humans) results in chronic brain alterations, culminating in epilepsy. We have been doing some work on this hypothesis, because if this is true, it would explain a lot. It is a pity that no one is looking at head trauma models or stroke models in terms of the development of epilepsy. It might be very similar: the initial event creates something that gives abnormal firing of neurons on a prolonged basis. This then could induce functional alterations culminating in epilepsy. We are now studying status models, for instance inducing status epilepticus by pilocarpine, and then taking the rats when they have spontaneous seizures and looking at whether there are responders or non-responders in the rats with spontaneous seizures. We have finished a study with levetiracetam that showed that it is possible to select responders and non-responders in such a situation. This is probably closer to the clinical picture.

Sander: Have you seen this with other drugs?

Löscher: We have just started this with levetiracetam.

Sander: It would be interesting to see how other drugs behave in this experiment.

Löscher: Now we can test the rats that do not react to one drug with other drugs.

Newman: I am curious whether anyone feels that the microdialysis method might be one of the better approaches for looking at uptake of AEDs into the brain.

Löscher: We have just begun cooperating with clinical scientists to think about a situation where you could do such experiments in a clinical setting. Clinicians already use microdialysis during epilepsy surgery. These probes have been increasingly miniaturized. Normally, they combine a recording electrode with the microdialysis probe. We now have the first three patients in whom microdialysis was used during surgery in the tissue which is then resected by the surgeon. This allows us to determine the anticonvulsant drug that has been given earlier, both during surgery in the microdialysis fluid and then afterwards in the whole tissue. This gives us a comparison between extracellular and intracellular levels in the same patient.

Abbott: You have shown functional evidence for some Pgp-mediated effect on your system. Do you know where the relevant Pgp is? Is it in neurons or glia?

Löscher: In the rat brain, we have found Pgp by immunohistology primarily in the endothelial cells of the blood–brain barrier. In our rat preparations we also see antibody staining of Pgp in astroglia under normal situations, but it is still too premature to speak about the kindling-induced changes. One problem is that in the so-called focal tissue we have is partially destroyed by the electrodes. This is a problem.

Bates: What antibody are you using for rat Pgp?

Löscher: It is C219 in combination with the antibody Mdr-Ab-1. We started our Pgp studies with simple experiments that involved taking a model, such as maximal electroshock-induced seizures (which can be done in mice without any kindling), and combining the Pgp inhibitor with another drug. Unfortunately, we did not see any clear effects of Pgp inhibitors under these conditions.

Schmutz: The development of tolerance may be another mechanism responsible for drug resistance. You mentioned this briefly. Could you elaborate on this work in kindled animals?

Löscher: My impression is that there are two different populations of resistant patients. One population is resistant from the beginning. If the clinician starts treatment, there is no reaction to the drug. In most of those patients, the second drug will also have no effect. However, there is another subpopulation of patients who react to the drugs initially but then efficacy is lost during subsequent treatment. There are two possible explanations for this second population. One is that there is a progression of the disease during the treatment. In other words, the pathophysiology of the disease changes under anticonvulsant treatment. The other possibility, which seems to be ignored by most clinicians, is that the drug itself loses efficacy. In animal experiments, there is a loss of efficacy upon chronic treatment of experimental animals with many anticonvulsant drugs. Many clinicians don't like the word tolerance at all, but if you ask them about side effects, they all agree that there is tolerance to side effects. This is what you normally see in patients: the side effects are higher at the beginning of treatment than after a couple of weeks. This is tolerance. If I talk about loss of anticonvulsant efficacy, no one understands what I mean. As a simple pharmacologist, it is difficult for me to understand why the side effects should be reduced during chronic treatment but not the anticonvulsant effects. In animals this is not the case: there is often a decrease of anticonvulsant efficacy with most drugs and a corresponding decrease in side effects. Very often the decrease in side effects is more marked in animal models than the loss of anticonvulsant activity. One problem, which might be a problem for clinical trials, is that most anticonvulsant drugs are not given at a high dose from the beginning. Initially, low doses are used and then the patients are titrated to higher doses. Tolerance in animal models occurs within the first 2–4 weeks and then the anticonvulsant effect is relatively stable. In the clinical setting you may not see this, because the development of tolerance, if it is the same in patients as in animal models, is in the first couple of weeks when the titration is taking place. Thus you will never pick up this loss of efficacy. The only drugs where clinical tolerance is established are the benzodiazepines. With some patients there is a total loss of anti-epileptic efficacy that cannot be overcome by increasing the dose.

Sander: There is a different time span. For quite a number of patients, whatever drug is tried they do well for a short period. Then, a few weeks later, they return to their former state. But then with benzodiazepines 50–60% of these patients will develop tolerance 8–10 months later. And with vigabatrin, tolerance develops over an even longer period of some two years. What is the explanation for the differences in timing here?

Löscher: Different mechanisms. We also see this in animals. The duration of the development of tolerance depends on the category of drugs tested. Even within the benzodiazepines, there are some where tolerance develops in a matter of days and others where it takes months. This is explained by the intrinsic efficacy at the receptor sites and affinity for receptors. And, of course, this is all set in different genetic backgrounds. Take benzodiazepines. If you have 10 patients with epilepsy and you treat them with clobazam, some of them remain on the drug for years without any tolerance. Others lose efficacy. It must be the genetic background that is responsible.

Sander: With vigabatrin you can stop treatment and re-start it, but it never works again. The same occurs with drugs that show a shorter time for resistance to develop. With the benzodiazepines, in contrast, if you stop treatment and restart it some weeks later, you have a good response for more-or-less the same period as you did initially. Why is this?

Löscher: With benzodiazepines it is the resetting of receptor sensitivity.

Sisodiya: Isn't it possible that this is a bit like the epotholide story that we heard about earlier? Another mechanism for tolerance (or loss of effect with time), apart from the two that you have already discussed, is that there are other drug resistance mechanisms that are being selected out as time goes on. The different times taken for resistance to show are because of the time it takes for this mechanism to become effective.

Löscher: What we have just started to do is to treat animals chronically with either phenytoin or phenobarb, and then look at the expression of Pgp in the blood-brain barrier. There was some indication that phenobarb overexpresses Pgp in other tissues.

Andermann: The tolerance to clobazam, which is the best anticonvulsant among the benzodiazepines, occurs in our hands in about 30%. This is very different from the person who eventually develops tolerance to every antiepileptic agent. It is probably due to a very different mechanism. It is interesting that the tolerance to side effects seems to be unrelated to the tolerance to anti-epileptic effects. To some extent the personality has a lot to do with what patients will tolerate and what they won't. The perception of their epilepsy also has a role. Topiramate is a good example. The side effects may be severe, and there are some people who cannot tolerate it. Others tolerate it very well. People with epilepsy will often accept a level of memory loss and speech impediment because of the beneficial seizure control of the anti-epileptic medication. It is important to look at the various aspects of drug tolerance, and neurologists don't always do this. The obverse approach to increasing the dose is that taken by a senior neurologist who worked in Kentucky when Dilantin was first introduced. Because the patients were not particularly likely to be compliant, he used to treat them with high doses of phenytoin from the start until they became ataxic, at which point he would reduce the dose. No one else has been able to do this because it is well known that people will never remember who controlled their seizures, but will always remember who intoxicated them.

Kwan: What we are dealing with here is the interplay between disease itself and the drugs. I want to echo Dr Löscher's point that the drugs might be doing something to the disease itself, such as inducing Pgp or other drug resistance mechanisms. We sometimes forget that drugs do actually stop the seizures. We are also forgetting the possibility that seizures cause the neuronal changes that we are all aware of: perhaps by stopping the seizures we are modifying the disease itself. This could be why we don't see the tolerance. If you look at the AED withdrawal studies, those patients were seizure free for a period without AEDs and only about 20–30% relapsed. Clearly, in some patients there are dynamic changes in the neurobiology.

References

Halonen T, Nissinen J, Jansen JA, Pitkänen A 1996 Tiagabine prevents seizures, neuronal damage and memory impairment in experimental status epilepticus. Eur J Pharmacol 299: 69–81

Naoi T 1959 Electroencephalographic study of the electric convulsive treatment. Psychiatr Neurol Jpn 61:871–894

Sato M, Racine RJ, McIntyre DC 1990 Kindling: basic mechanisms and clinical validity. Electroencephalogr Clin Neurophysiol 76:459–472

Drug resistance in epilepsy: human epilepsy

S. M. Sisodiya*, W.-R. Lin†, B. N. Harding‡, M. V. Squier§ and M. Thom†

*Epilepsy Research Group, University Department of Clinical Neurology, †Department of Neuropathology, Institute of Neurology, and ‡Department of Neuropathology, Institute of Child Health, University College London, Queen Square, London, and §Department of Neuropathology, Radcliffe Infirmary, Oxford, UK

Abstract. The basis of drug resistance in human epilepsy is not understood. Parallels with resistance in cancer suggest that drug resistance proteins may have a role. To examine this possibility, we have studied human brain tissue containing pathologies capable of causing refractory epilepsy. Using immunohistochemistry for P glycoprotein (Pgp) and multidrug resistance-associated protein 1 (MRP1), we examined both pathological tissue and control tissue. We demonstrate expression of Pgp and MRP1 in glia from cases of malformation of cortical development studied both before and after the onset of epilepsy, as well as in cases of hippocampal sclerosis and dysembryoplastic neuroepithelial tumours. In one particular type of malformation, we also demonstrate that dysplastic neurons express MRP1. The pattern of immunolabelling suggests overexpression is concentrated particularly around vessels in most of the pathologies. The timing shows that expression may be constitutive in some pathologies. These findings suggest that drug resistance proteins may contribute to drug resistance in refractory epilepsy.

2002 Mechanisms of drug resistance in epilepsy: lessons from oncology. Wiley, Chichester (Novartis Foundation Symposium 243) p 167–179

Epilepsy is resistant to drug treatment in about one-third of cases overall (Sander 1993). The proportion of cases resistant to drug treatment varies with the specific cause or syndromic diagnosis. A higher proportion of subjects with epilepsy due to hippocampal sclerosis (HS), malformations of cortical development (MCD) and dysembryoplastic neuroepithelial tumours (DNTs) are likely to have refractory epilepsy.

Most patients resistant to drug treatment do not become seizure-free with any of a broad range of antiepileptic drugs (AEDs). AEDs have a range of postulated antiepileptic actions, but tend to be physically similar: for example, most AEDs in current use are planar and lipophilic (Levy et al 1995). These phenomena suggest the involvement of non-specific mechanisms of resistance, such as P glycoprotein (Pgp) and multidrug resistance-associated protein 1 (MRP1). The normal human brain is protected by both Pgp and MRP1, which contribute to the blood–brain and blood–CSF barriers (Schinkel 1999, Wijnholds et al 2000). In normal human brain, Pgp is found only in the vicinity of blood vessels, most probably on endothelial cell membranes, whilst MRP1 is found only in the choroid plexus epithelium (Rao et al 1999). A number of preliminary reports have documented brain overexpression of Pgp or MRP in refractory epilepsy. Tishler et al (1995) demonstrated Pgp overexpression histologically in glia in brain tissue from patients with refractory epilepsy. Using cell lines overexpressing Pgp *in vitro*, they showed that phenytoin is a Pgp substrate, making Pgp overexpression a plausible cause of drug resistance. Lazarowski et al (1999) showed Pgp overexpression in resected epileptogenic tissue from a case of tuberous sclerosis.

As an essential first step in the further analysis of the possible contribution of drug resistance proteins Pgp and MRP1 to drug resistance in epilepsy, we undertook a histological study of Pgp and MRP1 expression in three common causes of refractory epilepsy: malformations of cortical development (MCD), dysembryoplastic neuroepithelial tumours (DNTs) and hippocampal sclerosis (HS).

Methods

Tissue

We studied formalin-fixed paraffin-embedded human brain tissue from neuropathological archives. The study was approved by the Joint Ethics Committee of the Institute of Neurology and the National Hospital for Neurology and Neurosurgery. All tissue was surplus to diagnostic requirements.

Sections with epileptogenic pathology from surgical resections had ideal fixation conditions, suffering no significant preresection hypoxia, being immersed in formalin immediately, embedded and sectioned within a week. All tissue from surgical specimens had been resected for the treatment of refractory epilepsy, all cases having been exposed to at least three antiepileptic drugs. Postmortem tissue containing pathologies with epileptogenic potential was also studied. Control tissue used was: (1) histologically-normal adjacent brain tissue from the same resection specimen, allowing control for age, sex, brain region, AED exposure and effects of seizures; (2) age-matched, histologically normal tissue from neurologically normal cases; and (3) positive control tissue (normal human liver or kidney or, as a positive disease control, breast carcinoma). We have shown that duration of fixation per se is unlikely to reduce Pgp or MRP expression (Sisodiya et al 1999).

Antibodies

For detection of MRP1, the monoclonal antibody MRPr1 (1:100 dilution; Alexis Corporation, Nottingham, UK) was used. This antibody has been well characterized (Hipfner et al 1998) and is specific for MRP1, with no reported cross-reactivity (Scheffer et al 2000). To detect Pgp expression, monoclonal antibody C494 (1:250 dilution; Alexis Corporation) was used (Beck et al 1996). In some studies, a second antibody for C494 was also used (monoclonal antibody 6/1C, BioResearch Ireland).

Immunohistochemistry

Details of protocols are given in previous publications (Sisodiya et al 1999, 2001). All sections were reviewed independently by four observers, including three neuropathologists. Blinding was not possible for neuropathology. For each antibody run, experimental sections were assessed only if positive and negative controls (obtained with omission of primary antibody) reacted as predicted.

Results

Malformations of cortical development

MCD were studied in two states: firstly, MCD found incidentally at postmortem in individuals who had never had witnessed seizures or treatment with AEDs; and secondly, brain tissue containing MCD obtained from surgical resections or postmortems from subjects who had previously had epilepsy and exposure to AEDs. Because MCD will almost always eventually cause epilepsy, the first state allowed examination of constitutive expression of drug resistance proteins, before the onset of seizure.

MCD before onset of epilepsy.   In all study samples, capillary based labelling with C494 was noted throughout the sample, serving as an internal control for this antibody. Capillary based structures (endothelium or glial end-feet) did not label in any section with 6/1C. Neurons did not label in any section. Labelling with both antibodies used to detect C494 was noted in glia from 10 of 16 cases of MCD (including cases with polymicrogyria, lissencephaly and periventricular heterotopia), whilst glia from age-matched control cases were immunoreactive with both antibodies in only 2 of 16 cases (χ^2, $P=0.003$). Immunoreactive glia were concentrated perivascularly within the malformed region and were not seen in apparently normal perilesional brain in MCD-containing brains. The one control with many immunoreactive glia had previously had chronic hypoxia.

After onset of epilepsy: focal cortical dysplasia causing epilepsy.   Focal cortical dysplasia (FCD) is the most common type of MCD. Fifteen cases of FCD were examined. In six cases, the specimens were large resections with adjacent normal cortex for comparison. All cases contained typical FCD.

Staining for MRP1 was intense on dysplastic neurons in five cases. Positive labelling of balloon cells was seen in two cases. Labelling of reactive astrocytes was seen in all cases, more pronounced in the area of dysplasia compared to the adjacent cortex. Prominent and distinctive MRP1-positive processes were seen surrounding dysplastic neurons and accentuation of labelling was seen in foot processes around vessels compared to the glial fibrillary acidic protein (GFAP). In one case, staining for MRP1 specifically highlighted discrete nodules of balloon cells in the white matter, whereas the GFAP staining in this case showed a more diffuse white matter gliosis. Immunostaining for Pgp was similar but less intense. The adjacent normal cortex, where available for study, showed markedly less immunostaining with either antibody; no normal neurons were labelled with either antibody.

Hippocampal sclerosis

Eight cases were studied. All showed typical patterns of cell loss involving CA4 and CA1 with sparing of the CA2 sector. GFAP immunostaining confirmed a marked fibrillary gliosis in CA1 and CA4 in all cases. Pgp immunostaining was confined to astrocytic cells in the hippocampus and was observed in five cases. MRP1 immunopositivity was seen in 5/8 cases, again localized to cells with the morphology of reactive astrocytes. Immunostaining was not present in the adjacent non-gliotic subiculum in any of the cases with either of the antibodies.

Dysembryoplastic neuroepithelial tumours

Eight cases of DNT were examined, all large excisions. Each case showed characteristic features of a DNT, including oligodendroglia-like cells (OLC). In all cases there was adjacent normal appearing cortex.

Positive immunostaining, to variable degrees, was noted for MRP1 and for Pgp in all cases. Immunopositive cells had the morphology of reactive astrocytes. The OLC and mature neuronal element was uniformly negative with these antibodies. Striking positivity of the processes of the astrocyte-like cells was noted, with meshworks of positive fibres within some of the nodules, encasing the OLC, and extensive labelled foot processes around the fine anastomosing capillary networks within the DNT. Within individual cases there was heterogeneity in the density of positive cells in different regions of the tumour with some nodules showing fewer labelled cells than others.

Immunoreactivity in adjacent normal cortex in all cases was restricted to subpial astrocytes and meshworks of labelled fibres. This immunoreactivity was less intense than that seen in the DNT itself. Despite evidence of moderate cortical gliosis with numerous reactive astrocytes demonstrated by GFAP immunostaining in the adjacent cortex in all cases, very few of these astrocytes labelled with either antibody.

Discussion

In pathologies that commonly cause refractory epilepsy, we have shown the presence of known potential mediators of drug resistance, Pgp and MRP1, in lesional glia and, for FCD only, in a proportion of lesional dysplastic neurons. Normal human glia are not thought to express either protein under normal conditions (Tishler et al 1995) and, as far as we can determine, normal neurons have never been reported to express either protein. Thus detection of Pgp and MRP1 in glia and neurons in HS, DNT and MCD represents their overexpression in these pathologies causing refractory epilepsy.

Immunohistochemical study of Pgp especially is complicated by the cross-reactivity of some anti-Pgp antibodies (Beck et al 1996). The antibody we used, C494, is known to cross-react with a ubiquitous mitochondrial enzyme, pyruvate carboxylase (Rao et al 1994). However, reaction against pyruvate carboxylase is unlikely to explain our findings for the following reasons: (1) though gliosis, with possible associated changes in pyruvate carboxylase, is extensive both lesionally and perilesionally, the great majority of immunostaining with C494 occurs only lesionally, and not throughout the areas of gliosis; (2) at a microscopic level, intense immunostaining with C494 is noted in thin astrocytic processes and astrocytic endfeet, where mitochondria are unlikely to be found (Peters et al 1991); and (3) on Western blotting, a band of immunoreaction with C494 is found at a molecular weight compatible with presence of Pgp; no such band is found for pyruvate carboxylase (molecular weight $\sim$ 130 kDa; Rao et al 1994). In addition, we were able in some cases to confirm the presence of Pgp by using a second antibody against a separate epitope in the Pgp molecule. Lastly, the regions of maximum immunoreaction for the two antibodies (C494 and MRPr1) overlap in all the cases examined. For MRP1, no cross-reactivity has been reported (Hipfner et al 1999a, Scheffer et al 2000). MRP1 and Pgp have only a 15% amino acid identity: the antibodies we have chosen do not cross-react with these two proteins (Hipfner et al 1998, Scheffer et al 2000). Therefore, the proteins detected in this study are likely to be Pgp and MRP1 rather than cross-reacting antigens.

Immunohistochemistry of adjacent histologically normal brain tissue in cases from each of the pathologies we have studied demonstrates that immuno-reactivity for Pgp and MRP1 is limited very largely to regions of pathology, irrespective of the extent of gliosis. Such adjacent brain tissue is of the same age, sex and brain region, and would have been exposed to the same seizure effects and drugs, and is therefore ideal control tissue. We can conclude that (1) immunohistochemically detectable overexpression is delimited by the extent of observable epileptogenic pathology, (2) overexpression need not follow seizures, drug treatment or other consequences of epilepsy and (3) some MCD have constitutive overexpression of Pgp. Overall, overexpression of drug resistance proteins in HS, MCD and DNTs is thus likely to be an intrinsic property of these pathologies, whilst in normal-appearing brain, seizures, AEDs and other effects of epilepsy need not cause overexpression, though some drugs, including phenobarbitone (Schuetz et al 1996), cellular stress and hypoxia (Vilaboa et al 2000) are known to cause overexpression in some, but not all, cell lines *in vitro* (Hipfner et al 1999b).

From our study of fixed material, we cannot determine whether the detected proteins are functionally active. Absence or inhibition of Pgp and MRP1 can lead to excessive CSF penetration of a range of molecules (Schinkel 1999, Wijnholds et al 2000), whilst overexpression of one or other protein is associated with resistance to anticancer treatment in some neurological malignancies. Pgp can transport phenytoin (Tishler et al 1995) and phenobarbitone (Schuetz et al 1996), and is also able to transport other planar lipophilic molecular structures: most current antiepileptic drugs are planar and lipophilic (Levy et al 1995). MRP1 may be able to transport valproate (Adkison et al 1995) and is known to transport drug epoxides and glucuronides, into which conjugates carbamazepine and lamotrigine are metabolized (Levy et al 1995). It is possible, therefore, that overexpressed Pgp and MRP1, in the pattern observed in our cases, might lower local CSF AED concentration and thereby reduce their antiepileptic effects. Anecdotal evidence, from incidental inhibition of Pgp in patients with epilepsy, suggests that inhibition of Pgp may improve the control of previously refractory epilepsy.

The distribution of immunostaining is intriguing. Immunoreaction appears most marked around balloon cells, dysplastic neurons and lesional vessels. Pgp contributes to the blood–brain barrier, whilst MRP1 also has a role in regulating CSF constitution (Schinkel 1999, Hipfner et al 1999b, Rao et al 1999, Wijnholds et al 2000). The cytoplasmic appearance of immunostaining may obscure any underlying membranous labelling, such localization of Pgp and MRP1 being most likely to be capable of drug export from the CSF, but the importance of intracellular activity of both proteins has also been demonstrated (Tan et al 2000).

Ours is an observational study: we cannot in this material explore the possible functional consequences of overexpression. However, this study is an essential first step in the further exploration of this field, and the results would suggest investigation of AED and AED conjugate transport capacity of Pgp and MRP1 might be worthwhile. If Pgp and MRP1 are able to transport or sequester AEDs in some form, new options might eventually be considered for the adjunctive treatment of refractory epilepsy.

Acknowledgements

This work was supported by grants from the Institute of Neurology and the National Hospital for Neurology and Neurosurgery, Glaxo-Wellcome plc through the Epilepsy Research Foundation, UK, the Patrick Berthoud Trust and University of London Central Research Fund. We wish to thank Dr G. Keir for Western blotting results and Josephine Heffernan, Steve Durr and Nick Win for technical assistance.

References

Adkison KD, Artru AA, Powers KM, Nochlin D, Shen DD 1995 Role of choroid plexus epithelium in the removal of valproic acid from the central nervous system. Epilepsy Res 20:185–192

Beck WT, Grogan TM, Willman CL et al 1996 Methods to detect P-glycoprotein-associated multidrug resistance in patients' tumors: consensus recommendations. Cancer Res 56:3010–3020

Hipfner DR, Deeley RG, Cole SP 1999b Structural, mechanistic and clinical aspects of MRP1. Biochim Biophys Acta 1461:359–376

Hipfner DR, Gao M, Scheffer G, Scheper RJ, Deeley RG, Cole SP 1998 Epitope mapping of monoclonal antibodies specific for the 190-kDa multidrug resistance protein (MRP). Br J Cancer 78:1134–1140

Hipfner DR, Mao Q, Qiu W et al 1999a Monoclonal antibodies that inhibit the transport function of the 190-kDa multidrug resistance protein, MRP. Localization of their epitopes to the nucleotide-binding domains of the protein. J Biol Chem 274:15420–15426

Lazarowski A, Sevlever G, Taratuto A, Massaro M, Rabinowicz A 1999 Tuberous sclerosis associated with MDR1 gene expression and drug-resistant epilepsy. Pediatr Neurol 21:731–734

Levy RH, Mattson RH, Meldrum BS 1995 Antiepileptic drugs. Raven Press, New York

Peters A, Palay SL, de Webster H F 1991 The fine structure of the nervous system. Oxford University Press, Oxford

Rao VV, Anthony DC, Piwnica-Worms D 1994 MDR1 gene-specific monoclonal antibody C494 cross-reacts with pyruvate carboxylase. Cancer Res 54:1536–1541

Rao VV, Dahlheimer JL, Bardgett ME et al 1999 Choroid plexus epithelial expression of MDR1 P glycoprotein and multidrug resistance-associated protein contribute to the blood-cerebrospinal-fluid drug-permeability barrier. Proc Natl Acad Sci USA 96:3900–3905

Sander JW 1993 Some aspects of prognosis in the epilepsies: a review. Epilepsia 34:1007–1016

Scheffer GL, Kool M, Heijn M et al 2000 Specific detection of multidrug resistance proteins MRP1, MRP2, MRP3, MRP5, and MDR3 P-glycoprotein with a panel of monoclonal antibodies. Cancer Res 60:5269–5277

Schinkel AH 1999 P-Glycoprotein, a gatekeeper in the blood-brain barrier. Adv Drug Deliv Rev 36:179–194

Schuetz EG, Beck WT, Schuetz JD 1996 Modulators and substrates of P-glycoprotein and cytochrome P4503A coordinately up-regulate these proteins in human colon carcinoma cells. Mol Pharmacol 49:311–318

Sisodiya SM, Heffernan J, Squier MV 1999 Over-expression of P-glycoprotein in malformations of cortical development. Neuroreport 10:3437–3441

Sisodiya SM, Lin WR, Squier MV, Thom M 2001 Multidrug-resistance protein 1 in focal cortical dysplasia. Lancet 357:42–43

Tan B, Piwnica-Worms D, Ratner L 2000 Multidrug resistance transporters and modulation. Curr Opin Oncol 12:450–458

Tishler DM, Weinberg KI, Hinton DR, Barbaro N, Annett GM, Raffel C 1995 MDR1 gene expression in brain of patients with medically intractable epilepsy. Epilepsia 36:1–6
Vilaboa NE, Galán A, Troyano A, de Blas E, Aller P 2000 Regulation of multidrug resistance 1 (MDR1)/P-glycoprotein gene expression and activity by heat-shock transcription factor 1 (HSF1). J Biol Chem 275:24970–24976
Wijnholds J, deLange EC, Scheffer GL et al 2000 Multidrug resistance protein 1 protects the choroid plexus epithelium and contributes to the blood-cerebrospinal fluid barrier. J Clin Invest 105:279–285

DISCUSSION

Schmutz: In epilepsy there is a unique opportunity to work with human tissue i.e. with tissue of epileptic patients who are drug resistant. One can do molecular biology, electrophysiology and testing of new, experimental drugs on this tissue. We should make more use of this opportunity: it may give us new insights into the problems of drug resistance in epilepsy, and may lead to development of novel drugs.

Meldrum: Seeing this association between the maldeveloped neurons and the transporter proteins, I wonder whether the oncologists could give us any developmental interpretation of the expression of these proteins. In development, when cells are sick or feel that they have bad relations with their neighbours, they tend to initiate apoptosis. But if a cell thinks it is being poisoned, is there an option that it then expresses these proteins? There must be some developmental meaning to the enhanced expression of these proteins on cells that are developing abnormally. Is this a defensive response that is universal? What you showed can't be specially related to epilepsy. The link between the abnormality of these cells and the later development of epilepsy is not obvious. It happens much later.

Sisodiya: It may well be that these are defence proteins in the broadest sense, and in some ways are a response to tissue being sick. But I am not sure how we would address this question with human tissue. It wouldn't necessarily exclude these proteins then contributing to drug resistance as an incidental but clinically important side effect.

Bates: I agree. There has been promoter work with Pgp that suggests that it can be induced by stress. Some people have theorized that there is a cassette of stress responses that includes cytochrome P450s and Pgp, and perhaps even the MRPs. There is currently work going on looking to see how these promoters might be similar to each other. The only tissue where this has clearly been shown is in the liver, where after various stresses, including surgery itself, you can see induction of Pgp in the regenerating liver.

Scheper: You can mimic this *in vitro* with leukocytes. If you take monocytes and give any type of stress signal, such as cytokines, peroxides or even DMSO (dimethylsulfoxide), these induce an overexpression of Pgp and MRP1 within 48 h. These cells then display some sort of drug resistance.

Sander: Does this resistance disappear, or is it then permanent?

Scheper: It is transient.

Bates: The cells usually die after exposure to the differentiating agents. The induction of Pgp following differentiating agents is typically true of cell types that express Pgp to begin with. In the CNS, once you work out which subtypes are likely to have Pgp expression, those are the subtypes that are more likely to get induction with stress.

Newman: In terms of insult-induced expression of Pgp, there was a report showing induction of Pgp in tumours of patients after chemotherapy (Abolhoda et al 1999). It is possible to get a direct induction of Pgp *in vivo* after insult.

Meldrum: It is not a general response to a toxic environment, because Pgp is not universally seen in an inflammatory response.

Bates: It is tissue-type specific.

Andermann: Could you say something about the medial temporal structures? Did you have the opportunity to look at tissue from patients who did well after surgery, and others who did not become seizure free?

Sisodiya: We did look at hippocampal sclerosis. We found that there was up-regulation of Pgp and MRP1. We haven't seen a clear link between those who did become seizure free and those who did not. This is an important point. There are likely to be other factors in the failure to respond to drug or surgical therapy. There may be a more extensive circuit that has not been completely resected. Perhaps other areas also express drug resistance proteins. There doesn't seem to be a clear link between good outcome and poor outcome and expression of drug resistance proteins.

Andermann: Have you looked at postmortem tissue from patients with generalized epilepsy?

Sisodiya: We haven't got much brain tissue from patients with generalized epilepsy, so we haven't looked at this.

Sander: You could argue that an episode of status epilepticus would be a major insult to the brain. You said you had some data: what do they show?

Sisodiya: We looked at the brains from individuals who died in status epilepticus, from a variety of causes. Perhaps the most interesting case was someone who had focal cortical dysplasia, which is normally a localized abnormality to some extent. In this case, the pathology was more extensive, there was status epilepticus and the patient died despite treatment with a range of intravenous anti-epileptic agents. The interesting finding from this is that whereas in the cases I showed the overexpression was really limited to the area of malformation, in the cases of status epilepticus it was much more widespread. I have no idea of the significance of this. There could be a range of issues involved. It could just be a temporal up-regulation, and if status had settled it would have declined. Or it may have been the cause of the refractory status. I don't know. I think it will take animal models to sort this out. This does suggest that if you want to treat the refractory status you need to get in quickly.

Deisz: You implied that balloon cells are crucially involved in the initiation of epileptic activity. The presence of balloon cells is indeed associated with a greater seizure frequency in cases of cortical dysplasia (Rosenow et al 1998). But these cells are not obligatory in pharmacoresistant epilepsy: in extra-temporal epilepsies only about 10% of the resected tissues showed balloon cells (Frater et al 2000). In any case, do you have any recent information about the mechanism by which balloon cells facilitate the occurrence of seizure activity, for example through certain intrinsic properties such as burst firing (e.g. Deisz 1996)? Or are they just wired weirdly?

Sisodiya: It isn't known. There is a lot of electrophysiological evidence showing that these areas are epileptogenic and the neurons are abnormal, both *in vivo* and *in vitro*.

Scheper: What is your experience with the quality of the tissue depending on the postmortem delay? This is always a problem with these sorts of studies.

Sisodiya: Most of the tissue we use is from surgical resection specimens, for which there is no delay. With the postmortem tissue, I agree; it is difficult. No one had the intention of doing this work when this tissue was originally stored, the cases of malformation were unsuspected. In most cases the delay to fixation was greater in the cases with malformation than in those cases that were the controls, which were usually from hospital postmortems. If there is an issue with molecular stability after death, I think it would work against our findings, rather than for them. For most of these tissues we do not know the delay before they were fixed.

Ling: This is quite an important issue. On the one hand I think we are creating exquisite tools with these monoclonal antibodies, but on the other hand the information we get out will only be as good as the preparation of the material. It seems to me from this discussion that it would be extremely valuable to have some real hard data as to what is expressed, at what level, and where, for a range of molecules that we think might play a role in disease. When we do work on mouse or rat brains, it is one of the most challenging tissues to stain. I was impressed with your data, but I agree with Rik Scheper that there could be pitfalls in terms of technical aspects such as sample preparation.

Deisz: In the surgical resection specimens, what was the delay between the resection and fixation?

Sisodiya: It was the postmortem cases that had an unknown delay. With the surgical resection specimens there was none. The tissue was fixed in theatre. Surgical specimens are the best to look at because there is no significant hypoxia before resection and they are fixed immediately. Most of the tissue we have looked at is surgical resection material.

Ling: With animal tissue, you can also fix it immediately. We found, for example, that with C494 there is significant background depending on the type of tissue. One way to get around this is to use small peptide epitopes to compete with the antibody. In this manner it was possible to get a clear indication of what is epitope-specific staining. For example, we observed that staining of the plasma membranes was competed by the peptides (showing specificity); cytoplasmic staining did not compete. We have no idea what the non-specific cytoplasmic staining was due to.

Bates: I would add that for Pgp it has been very difficult to get really clean samples using formalin-fixed specimens. You may have to divide up your surgical samples and do some staining with frozen sections and some with chemically fixed sections.

Pirmohamed: It is clearly crucial to determine whether Pgp and MRP1 expression is a cause of the resistance, or is just an epiphenomenon. One of the aspects that must be considered is what drugs the patients had previously been taking. Many of the drugs used in epilepsy, such as the aromatic anticonvulsants, are known to be P450 enzyme inducers. They may also induce Pgp. I wonder whether if you had a drug history, you could relate this expression. On the promoter region of Pgp there are various regulatory elements for expression of Pgp. When someone is having a seizure, there will be many stress proteins that are induced, including cytokines. In the Pgp promoter region there is an NF-κB site that interacts with cytokines. Has any work been done looking at how important this site is in inducing Pgp?

Sisodiya: I can't answer that. But with regard to the possible induction of Pgp by drugs or stress, I take your point. The rest of the brain tissue is also exposed to these drugs, and Pgp did not seem to be up-regulated. This suggests to me that there is something specific about the lesional tissue. It may have a specific potential to express Pgp; I don't know. It is not just a non-specific, widespread up-regulation. We don't know whether these drug resistance proteins do transport all the AEDs. But if we assume that they do, then does it matter what the cause of up-regulation is? It is there, and it may be causing a problem that needs to be dealt with.

Ling: In my view, the crucial issue is whether the responsive patients have the same stress as the non-responsive patients. If the responsive patients do have the same amount of stress and the same level of the transporters, then this isn't an issue.

Sisodiya: It is difficult to find out. Responsive patients don't come to surgery, so we don't get the brain tissue.

Sills: If I remember correctly, you showed some up-regulation of expression in pre-epileptic tissue. If these people were pre-epileptic, the chances are they have not been treated with AEDs, and so the up-regulation in those samples is not related to prior drug administration. If drug transporters are important in drug-resistant epilepsy, is there a possibility that, in this population, the patients are already drug-resistant before they are even epileptic?

Sisodiya: That was the hypothesis. I don't know how we would test this.

Sills: Is there an inherent drug resistance in a subset of patients that are expressing these transporters before they develop seizures?

Sisodiya: I think that is probably the case, but the only evidence is that longitudinally we know that patients who have refractory seizures tend to have this sort of pathology.

Newman: Is there any possibility that malformations induce or cause overexpression of Pgp, and that Pgp then contributes directly to epilepsy by transporting away some peptide or natural substance that is involved in regulating neural transmission?

Sisodiya: I don't know. It is interesting that other functions of Pgp were mentioned earlier. There were some that weren't mentioned, also. As I understand it, Pgp is involved in apoptosis and transport of platelet-activating factor (PAF). PAF activity can be involved in the generation of some malformations. It may be that overexpression in the early cases is not some non-specific response to tissue sickness, but has some role in the genesis of these malformations.

Brinkmann: Perhaps MDR1 is just an indicator. Liver enzymes and MDR are correlated in their expression patterns. What could happen is that the sick cells have high expression of the transcription factors and you are looking at MDR1, which is indicative of a highly active metabolic spot in the brain that doesn't belong there. This spot could produce other substances because it is metabolized in a totally abnormal way. These different substances could cause epilepsy. You are looking at MDR1, but perhaps this is just an indicator for transcription activity of metabolic enzymes. I would be looking at CYP3A4 liver enzymes.

Wood: That is an interesting hypothesis, but inducers of CYP3A4 and Pgp are not convulsants.

Brinkmann: I am just saying that this is active, and all kinds of other natural substances could be converted into something else.

Wood: I agree, but if that were true, you would expect rifampin, for example, to be epileptogenic, and it is not.

Brinkmann: The question is whether or not you get induction of Pgp in the brain in all cells.

Schmutz: Returning to the subject of up-regulation of Pgp in pre-epileptic tissue, was this seen throughout the samples?

Sisodiya: No, it seems also to be regionalized.

Schmutz: Was it seen consistently? If this is a cause of therapeutic resistance, one would have to assume that all these patients would have been resistant.

Sisodiya: We didn't see it in every case.

Andermann: As far as I know, there are no asymptomatic cases of focal cortical dysplasia from an epileptic point of view. In other disorders of cortical organization, such as polymicrogyria, for instance, there may be more variation.

Sisodiya: The pre-epileptic cases we studied were of lissencephaly, polymicrogyria and periventricular heterotopia. We didn't have any pre-epileptic focal cortical dysplasia; that would be fantastic tissue to look at. Neither did we have pre-epileptic hippocampal sclerosis.

Andermann: What about polymicrogyria?

Sisodiya: We didn't see it in every case, but we did in some cases.

Vezzani: Can you exclude the possibility that there is some subclinical epileptic activity going on in the pre-epileptic cases you studied?

Sisodiya: No. It is a possibility.

Sander: Most of these were fetal.

Sisodiya: Yes. That doesn't exclude them from having seizures.

Kwan: I have a question about your surgical cases. Is there any relationship between seizure control and level of Pgp expression? Are you able to analyse whether there is a relationship between the two? That is, is there a dose–response relationship between the duration of epilepsy and level of expression?

Sisodiya: Our work is qualitative and descriptive. We haven't started to quantitate the level of expression. But that is an interesting idea.

References

Abolhoda A, Wilson AE, Ross H, Daneberg PV, Burt M, Scotto KW 1999 Rapid activation of *MDR1* gene expression on human metastatic sarcoma after in vivo exposure to doxorubicin. Clin Cancer Res 5:3352–3356

Deisz RA 1996 A tetrodotoxin-insensitive sodium current initiates burst firing of neocortical neurons. Neuroscience 70:341–351

Frater JL, Prayson RA, Morris III HH, Bingaman WE 2000 Surgical pathologic findings of extratemporal-based intractable epilepsy: a study of 133 consecutive resections. Arch Pathol Lab Med 124:545–549

Rosenow F, Luders HO, Dinner DS et al 1998 Histopathological correlates of epileptogenicity as expressed by electrocorticographic spiking and seizure frequency. Epilepsia 39:850–856

General discussion I

Kwan: I want to describe some of the studies we have done in Glasgow. The hypothesis is that refractory epilepsy is associated with a localized over-expression of P glycoprotein (Pgp), which restricts the access of drugs to their intended site of action. To test this hypothesis we carried out two parallel sets of experiments. The first set involved gene expression studies. We measured the expression of *Mdr1a* and *Mdr1b* by quantitative RT-PCR, using an internal standard to allow absolute quantification. We looked at the distribution in different regions of normal rat brain and also a model of seizures. In the second set of studies we tried to screen whether the commonly used anti-epileptic drugs (AEDs) could be substrates for Pgp. Seven drugs were given to *Mdr1a* knockout mice and wild-type mice. We compared the brain:plasma concentration ratios in these two different genotypes. Apart from the olfactory bulbs, which seem to express a relatively low level of the Mdr1a RNA, the levels seem to be fairly uniform in the seven brain regions we looked at in normal rats. For *Mdr1b*, the situation is different: we only see an appreciable level of expression in the hippocampus. We tested the effects of seizures on the level of expression using the genetically epilepsy-prone (GEPR) rats. This is one of the animal models of epileptic seizure. These rats have an increased vulnerability for developing seizures, which can be induced by sound. These seizures appear to be initiated in the inferior colliculus of the midbrain, and then spread to the cortex to produce the phenotype of convulsion. After a single audiogenic stimulation, animals were sacrificed at four different time points and we measured the level of *Mdr1a* mRNA in different brain regions. We found an increase in the midbrain and cortex following a single seizure. The increase can be seen at 4 h and reaches a maximum at 24 h. After 7 days it has begun to decline but is still elevated.

In the knockout experiments, a single dose of each of seven drugs was given subcutaneously to *Mdr1a* knockout mice and wild-type mice. These were sacrificed 30, 60 and 240 min later, and we measured the brain:plasma concentration ratio. There was no difference in plasma levels in the knockout and wild-type mice. However, with some drugs we did see a difference in the brain:plasma ratio. For carbamazepine the brain:plasma concentration reached a higher level 30 min after injection in knockout mice than in the wild-type mice. We looked at four new drugs: vigabatrin, gabapentin, lamotrigine and topiramate. There was a significant increase in the brain:plasma concentration ratio in the knockout mice. For topiramate the brain:plasma ratio was significantly higher at 30, 60 and 240 min compared with the wild-type mice.

What does this all mean in humans? Humans only have one isoform of MDR1. Does this translate to a higher level of Pgp on a protein level? Clearly, we need more time points and pick out a range of doses to work out the temporal changes in kinetics. We need to find out whether the seizure changes we see will apply to other seizure models also.

Ling: You have used the *Mdr1a* knockout. My suspicion is that *Mdr1b* will not play such an important role. There is also a triple knockout, which the Dutch group has. It will be interesting to see what role MRP1 plays. There might be a tremendous difference in terms of the ratios.

Sander: Did I understand correctly that the levels of topiramate were much higher in the knockout than the wild-type mice?

Sills: Yes. In the knockout mice there was a higher brain concentration of topiramate than in normal mice. However, the plasma topiramate levels were essentially identical. We opted to express the results as brain:plasma concentration ratios as we were concerned that any slight variation in plasma levels might be observed as variability in brain concentrations.

Kwan: We are limited by the number of animals that we can use.

Pirmohamed: How did you quantitate the concentrations in brain and plasma?

Sills: The standard drugs were analysed by an enzyme-mediated immunoassay technique that we use for plasma concentrations in patients. The newer drugs were assayed by HPLC and, in the case of topiramate, by fluorescence polarization immunoassay.

Pirmohamed: Did you have to use a different internal standard for every drug?

Sills: Where appropriate, yes.

Vezzani: Dr Löscher has shown us data about phenytoin being a substrate for Pgp. I wonder whether it would be wise to measure the drug concentration by microdialysis and not only the tissue levels. I know this is difficult in mice. Why does phenytoin change very little in these mice if it is a substrate?

Kwan: The phenytoin data are mostly *in vitro*. Professor Schinkel, whose laboratory generated these knockout mice, has also looked at phenytoin in the *Mdr1a* knockout mouse, and he couldn't find a difference *in vivo* (Schinkel et al 1996). He suspected that this might be something to do with metabolism.

Sills: The question is really about whether we might see different effects with microdialysis as opposed to measuring tissue levels. I don't think there's much doubt about this. Ours is a simple study, employing crude techniques, designed to provide rapid answers to some basic questions. The results are, accordingly, preliminary but offer a platform for future experiments. I don't deny that the use of microdialysis might have given us clearer data. I also suspect that if we had extended the time profile of our experiments, we might have seen a greater difference in the phenytoin results. By using gross tissue measurements we are required to use sufficient doses to be able to detect the drug. With microdialysis it is possible to measure much lower concentrations. In our study, there is a possibility that, even if the drugs are substrates, we may be swamping the transporters with the amount of drug that we are using.

Bates: I am not terribly worried about the discrepancy. You do have a small difference, and you were working with a small number of animals. There are also species differences to take into account. We have already agreed that phenytoin is probably a poor Pgp substrate. The fact that it may be a Pgp substrate is verified by Wolfgang Löscher's data. If you expanded your study to 10 animals you might find that the small difference you see becomes statistically significant. The fact that you didn't get a difference in plasma also doesn't bother me, if you think about data with the knockout mice, where the orthologue for MDR1 has been deleted. For vinblastine, there is at most a twofold difference in the plasma and a 22-fold difference in the CNS, relative to the wild-type. Vinblastine is an excellent Pgp substrate.

Vezzani: I would like to describe our data showing that seizures induce Pgp protein when they are induced in otherwise normal animals. We don't use genetically modified mice but rather naïve mice that receive a convulsant drug. We injected kainic acid into mice that have been prepared with chronically implanted electrodes. Seizures were recorded by EEG analysis and were often associated with behavioural convulsions. These seizures were recorded for about 90 min. We killed the animals and measured *Mdr1a* by quantitative RT-PCR. There was a significant increase in *Mdr1a* transcript as soon as 3 h after the induction of seizure activity. This was a maximal effect: the transcript was up-regulated at about the same level for 24 h and then dropped to control levels after 72 h. Thus seizure activity *per se* can increase the expression of the protein in critical areas. This work was done of the hippocampus, which is an area involved in limbic seizures. This is a model of transient seizure activity; we are now studying whether the protein level is elevated in models of spontaneously recurring seizures. We have also looked at the expression of MRP1 in the same tissues. We haven't seen any induction in the transcript of this protein in these mice. We also addressed the possibility that prolonged anticonvulsant drug treatment could change the protein expression in brain tissue. This work was done in naïve mice. We injected phenytoin every 12 h for four consecutive days at a dose of 30 mg/kg. Then we sacrificed the animals at different time points after the last administration. At 6 h after the last phenytoin administration, the MDR1 transcript was not significantly changed by this repetitive treatment. From these preliminary results it seems that there is no evidence of up-regulation of the pump by the drug. In the animals that overexpress the Pgp protein after acute seizures, we are studying whether there is a difference compared with controls in brain concentrations of anticonvulsant drugs after their systemic administration.

Abbott: Which AEDs did you try?

Vezzani: Only phenytoin. We have done some experiments with carbamazepine, but I don't have the results yet.

Wood: What is the appropriate control for seizures? If you are looking at expression of something in brain tissue after seizure, the assumption is that there is a specific effect of the seizure. But it seems that any kind of trauma might do something: you need some control for the seizure experiment.

Meldrum: This is where our results with the GEPR rats are particularly valuable, because we get the same results as Dr Vezzani does following kainate, and we see the same time-course of increase. With kainate, there is histological damage, but for the GEPR rats we use just a modest sound stimulus that is repeatable and does not cause pathology. It seems reasonable to say that it is a consequence of the local seizure activity and essentially nothing else. I don't think you need some other control.

Kwan: For the GEPR model there was no change in other brain areas that are not involved in the seizure pathway.

Meldrum: We are convinced that it is the local seizure activity, not any systemic effects.

Schmutz: You mentioned that you measured at 3, 6, 24 and 72 h after seizure induction in your kainate model. In between these time points was there ongoing seizure activity?

Vezzani: No. In this kind of model we use transient seizure activity that lasts for 90 min. Then the activity disappears and there are no more seizures.

Ling: The interesting observation here is the fact that MDR1 can be induced under some kind of 'trauma' situation. This is significant. However, what happens in the mouse or rat may not be happening in humans. What we have found, at least in tissue culture, is that in some cell lines using drugs as an insult could induce MRP, other cell lines may not. It could be tissue, cell line or even species specific.

Vezzani: The best thing would be to try different experimental models of seizures. This is just a starting point — a proof of principle.

Sills: You showed that phenytoin doesn't increase MDR1 expression. It would appear from our discussions that phenytoin is a weak Pgp substrate. Do any of the oncologists have evidence which suggests that stronger substrates can induce expression?

Newman: It has been seen in the clinic (Abolhoda et al 1999).

Bates: There is a lot of circumstantial evidence. You see in the clinic that people who have been treated have higher levels. There are the promoter models where we give drugs and we see increased promoter activity for Pgp. Then there is the differentiation model that shows there is inducible Pgp. But it is really hard in a cancer population to sort out induction versus selection. The data are not that strong, but people who do promoter work would say that the drugs can induce Pgp. There is a nice clinical paper showing induction in sarcoma (Abolhoda et al 1999). Patients with lung metastases from sarcoma went to surgery, had doxorubicin administered by isolated perfusion, and had biopsies performed before and after the perfusion. *MDR1*, as measured by RT-PCR, was induced over the course of the 50 min perfusion. This is a good induction model.

Sills: Is the level of induction related to the affinity for the transporter?

Brinkmann: I think the level of induction is more defined by the affinity for the transcription factors.

Ling: The way I read it is that it is possible that these drug transporters can be induced. The challenge now is to determine whether or not this happens in a clinical situation.

Pirmohamed: Is all induction related to transcriptional activation? Is there any post-translational modification going on, such as phosphorylation, which makes the protein more stable and perhaps more active?

Vezzani: We only measured the transcript in our experiments.

Pirmohamed: In oncology studies, have people looked not only at the increase in mRNA but also protein stabilization?

Newman: Serum concentration has been shown to influence Pgp stability in cell culture models.

Varadi: We made mutants knocking out all the phosphorylation sites. We found that there was no difference in ATPase activity stimulated by drugs.

Wood: The fact that rifampin does it would suggest that it is. Rifampin clearly induces Pgp in humans.

Bates: What are the rifampin data?

Wood: There are data with fexofenadine showing an alteration in the kinetics of fexofenadine that is not metabolized. It is a Pgp substrate. It would appear that this is due to the rifampin inducing Pgp.

Pirmohamed: St John's wort also induces Pgp.

Ling: Would it be useful to explore where the experimental models are going in this whole area? In particular, I would like to ask Wolfgang Löscher about whether it will be easy to home in on the relevant molecules or genes using a screening approach like the chip arrays that Peter Atadja described earlier. Or will it be better to characterize responders and non-responders at a physiologoical level, such as by using PET (positron emission tomography) imaging?

Löscher: We have to posit hypotheses which we can test directly. Related to the main topic of this meeting, we have looked for different multidrug transporters at the gene level in different regions of the hippocampus, for example. I am a little frustrated. If it really is the case that overexpression of these transporters is transiently induced by a seizure and then returns to normal, it would have little relevance for pharmacoresistance. In a pharmacoresistant brain the drug is there. If there is no seizure, there cannot be any induction of transporter. If there is a seizure, there must be another reason for it because the drug is already there. Perhaps overexpression of drug transporters is only an epiphenomenon. We are more interested in more permanent alterations. We kindle animals and wait for a week or two before we look at the mRNA levels for different drug transporters. Only then, if there is a stable increase, can we explain something. These transient effects cannot explain pharmacoresistance.

Vezzani: The change we showed is only transient because the model itself is transient. But in spontaneously epileptic rats, perhaps the level of the protein would remain elevated, even if the seizures are subclinical. As long as there is some epileptic activity in the crucial areas, this may be sufficient to increase the pump expression to a level that has functional relevance.

Ruetz: There is an interesting observation in tissue culture where cells are selected under drug pressure. This can result in cells with differing levels of resistance. If the drug pressure is removed, the Pgp levels decrease, but they settle at a slightly higher level than before selection began. If you keep this culture, the levels are permanently elevated. This translates into a slight increase in resistance to anticancer drugs in classical assays. There is the possibility that a cell reaches a higher level of Pgp expression.

References

Abolhoda A, Wilson AE, Ross H, Danenberg PV, Burt M, Scotto KW 1999 Rapid activation of *MDR1* gene expression in human metastatic sarcoma after in vivo exposure to doxorubicin. Clin Cancer Res 5:3352–3356

Schinkel AH, Wagenaar E, Mol CA, van Deemter L 1996 P-glycoprotein in the blood-brain barrier of mice influences the brain penetration and pharmacological activity of many drugs. J Clin Invest 97:2517–2524

Cellular mechanisms of pharmacoresistance in slices from epilepsy surgery

R. A. Deisz

Department of Cell and Neurobiology, Institute of Anatomy, Charité, 10098 Berlin, Germany

Abstract. Slices of human cortical tissue from epilepsy surgery were investigated with intracellular recordings to elucidate the mechanisms contributing to augmented synaptic excitation and to repetitive activity. The analysis of single synaptic potentials revealed, amongst other differences to rodent cortex, a disturbance of $GABA_A$ inhibition, namely depolarizing responses. A tentative ionic mechanism, impaired KCl outward-transport (KCC2), was evaluated in a rat model (0-Mg hyperexcitability). The observed down-regulation of KCC2 mRNA after 0-Mg-ACSF exposure of slices may contribute to the depolarizations by GABA. The factors enabling repetitive activity were addressed with a paired-pulse paradigm. In slices from epilepsy surgery, synaptic responses were virtually constant with interstimulus intervals between 100 and 1000 ms. Tiagabine markedly prolonged the effects of released GABA at $GABA_A$ receptors, but paired-pulse behaviour was only slightly affected. We demonstrate that bicuculline-induced paroxysmal activity of rat cortex is frequency-limited (to about $<1\,Hz$) by presynaptic $GABA_B$ receptors. The lack of frequency limitation of synaptic events suggests an impaired $GABA_B$ receptor function in the human epileptogenic cortex. The data are discussed regarding the pivotal role of KCl transport in epileptic disorders of various origins and the role of $GABA_B$ receptors in the frequency limitation of paroxysmal activity.

2002 Mechanisms of drug resistance in epilepsy: lessons from oncology. Wiley, Chichester (Novartis Foundation Symposium 243) p186–206

GABA, the main inhibitory transmitter in the CNS, activates two distinct families of receptors coined $GABA_A$ and $GABA_B$. The former is a pentameric arrangement of at least 17 different subunits, each with four transmembrane domains (see Möhler et al 1997). The latter are heterodimers of two subunits (Kaupmann et al 1998) and occur pre- and postsynaptically (see Deisz 1997). Numerous studies demonstrated the induction of epileptiform activity by antagonists of $GABA_A$ receptors (for example Gutnick et al 1982) or high frequency stimulation (Ben-Ari et al 1979). These findings fostered the concept that reduced $GABA_A$ receptor-mediated inhibition contributes to the initiation and spread of epileptiform activity. Conversely, several classes of drugs which enhance the action of $GABA_A$ receptors, such as benzodiazepines or barbiturates, are established anticonvulsants (see Upton & Blackburn 1997). The expression of aberrant $GABA_A$ receptors during early phases of epilepsy development in rodents underscores the crucial role of $GABA_A$ receptors (Brooks-Kayal et al 1998). However, in human temporal lobe epilepsy, GABAergic inhibition appears to be normal, at least remote from the focus (McCormick 1989), and $GABA_A$ inhibition compares well with data obtained from adult rat cortex (Gibbs et al 1996). Impairment of $GABA_B$ receptors appears to play a minor role in the induction of epileptiform activity; antagonists do not induce paroxysmal activity (e.g. Deisz et al 1997, Deisz 1999a), yet do prolong paroxysmal activity and increase the frequency (Karlsson et al 1992).

The subtle balance between excitation and inhibition may also be disturbed by an enhancement of excitatory synaptic transmission. Such a mechanism may be inferred from the attenuation of epileptiform activity by the NMDA receptor antagonist D-APV in animal models (Dingledine et al 1986). In human epileptogenic tissue from epilepsy surgery, available data are at odds. Avoli & Olivier (1987) reported a marked attenuation of paroxysmal activity, whereas Köhling et al (1998) found no effects of D-APV on sharp wave activity. Interestingly, comparison of NMDA receptor-mediated currents from the least and most abnormal cortex from epilepsy surgery revealed no significant differences (Wuarin et al 1992).

Thus, the conclusion of Avoli & Williamson (1996), that 'Electrophysiological and pharmacological studies of the human neocortex obtained during surgery have so far been unsuccessful in isolating any definite mechanism that may account for the epileptiform activity *in situ*', still holds. Here, I review some of my ongoing projects on human cortical tissue from epilepsy surgery.

Materials and methods

Human neocortex, resected to cure pharmacoresistant epilepsy, was used. All patients provided informed consent in written form to use the tissue for research. The experiments were approved by the local ethics committee in accord with the Declaration of Helsinki. The methods of preparing neocortical slices were similar to those described previously for rat (Deisz 1999a) and human tissue (Deisz 1999b). Briefly, tissue was collected in the operating theatre and transferred to the laboratory (typically $<30\,min$) in cold modified artificial cerebrospinal fluid (ACSF, 4–8 °C). The tissue was cut in slices of nominally $400\,\mu m$, which were stored in beakers filled with ACSF, containing (in mM): NaCl 124.0, KCl 5.0, $CaCl_2$ 2.0, $MgSO_4$ 2.0, NaH_2PO_4 1.25, $NaHCO_3$ 26.0, and glucose 10.0

(equilibrated with 95% O_2 and 5% CO_2). Intracellular recordings, data acquisition and analysis were as described previously (Deisz 1999b).

Results

Neuronal properties

The properties of human cortical neurons were comparable to those of rodent cortex, membrane potential averaged -71.9 ± 4.5 mV ($n=63$) and depolarizing current steps (usually 600 ms) elicited in all neurons a train of action potentials of fairly regular interval with amplitudes averaging 92.6 ± 8.4 mV (Fig. 1A). The neuronal input resistance (57.7 ± 28.4 MΩ), was about 50% higher compared to neurons from rodents. Moreover, hyperpolarizing current steps revealed typically only a slight anomalous inward rectification, indicating a considerably smaller I_h type current compared to rodent neurons. Bursting neurons (see Deisz 1996) have not been encountered so far.

Properties of synaptic responses

Despite the apparently 'normal' firing behaviour of the individual neurons, synaptic responses were clearly different from those in rodent cortex. Orthodromic stimulation elicited large depolarizations (about 25 mV), consisting of a slow component with action potentials on top. The amplitude increased fairly abruptly with increases in stimulus intensity, resembling the behaviour of paroxysmal depolarization shifts (PDS) in the presence of $GABA_A$ antagonists (e.g. Gutnick et al 1982). The number of action potentials following the depolarization was small (<5), and often the threshold was exceeded without generation of action potentials (Fig. 1A). Therefore, the term PDS does not seem appropriate and I will refer to these synaptic events as depolarization shifts (DS).

Some of the neurons ($<10\%$) exhibited spontaneous postsynaptic potentials (PSP) consisting of individual or trains of partly superimposed PSPs of small amplitude (<10 mV). In a few neurons the amplitudes of spontaneous PSPs were comparable to the evoked DS ($n=8$). The frequencies ranged from 0.22 to 2.8 Hz, on average 1.04 Hz. Interestingly, in slices from two resections, the spontaneous activity was confined to slices from a certain block, whereas in the adjacent block the spontaneous activity was absent, indicating that a heterogeneity of hyperexcitability exists in rather small volumes of tissue.

To elucidate the receptor mechanisms involved in the DS, established blockers of various transmitter receptors were applied. Firstly, we tested the contribution of NMDA receptor-mediated components (Avoli & Olivier 1987). The NMDA receptor antagonist D-APV (usually $20\,\mu$M) caused a slight decrease in the amplitude of the DS (see Fig. 1B), on average, the amplitudes were reduced by

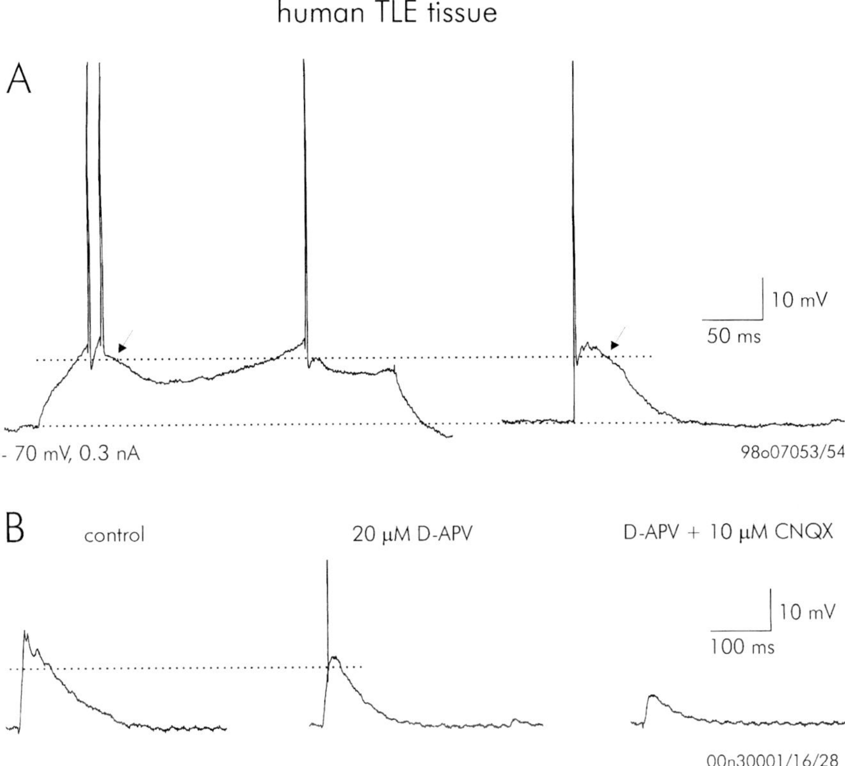

FIG. 1.   Intracellular recordings from human neocortical neurons. (A) Depolarizing current injection elicits action potentials (left panel), orthodromic stimulation evokes a depolarizing response exceeding threshold for about 20 ms without initiating action potentials. (B) Orthodromic stimulation elicits a depolarizing response without action potentials (left). Application of 20 µM D-APV (middle) slightly reduces the amplitude and time integral of the DS, eliciting an action potential, despite the smaller amplitude. After addition of CNQX (10 µM), a considerable depolarization persisted (right). Stimulus artifacts have been digitally removed in these and all subsequent figures.

13% ($P=0.22$). The time integrals of DSs were more consistently reduced, on average by 25% ($n=8$; $P=0.018$). This indicates that NMDA receptor-mediated components do not predominate the synaptic response, as suggested by Avoli & Olivier (1987). These data are also in contrast to the report by Köhling et al (1998) who found no effect of D-APV. The variability observed here, however, may account for both types of observations if the two extremes were found more regularly in a given setting. In any case, a NMDA component on the order of about 20% is also occasionally observed in rat cortical neurons (Deisz et al 1991, cf. Sutor & Hablitz 1989). Application of the AMPA/kainate receptor antagonist CNQX greatly reduced the DS, but, even when added to the D-APV containing solution, a considerable depolarization persisted (Fig. 1B). The reversal potential of the remaining synaptic response (near -50 mV) was inconclusive regarding the ionic mechanism involved. The $GABA_A$ receptor antagonist bicuculline (50 μM) eliminated the synaptic depolarization, indicating that the response is mediated by $GABA_A$ receptors (Deisz et al 1998).

We have tested the possibility that the GABA-mediated depolarization is critically involved in a spontaneous or evoked DS (Schwartzkroin & Haglund 1986). Application of bicuculline (10 μM) invariably induced a marked increase in the amplitude and duration of DSs, comparable to bicuculline-induced PDSs of rodent cortex (Fig. 2). The amplitudes of the synaptic responses increased to 31.5 ± 14.6 mV ($n=6$) in bicuculline (10 μM); membrane potential was not significantly affected by bicuculline. The increase in synaptic excitability with bicuculline at first glance seems at odds with the impaired inhibition due to the depolarizing reversal potential. However, the GABA-mediated inhibition still provides a considerable shunt despite the depolarization, whereas in the presence of bicuculline, the shunt is absent causing a more pronounced hyperexcitability.

The pharmacological isolation further revealed that the efficacy of synaptic inhibition was quite variable between slices and tissues. Judging from the amplitudes at a given driving force in some neurons, the early inhibitory

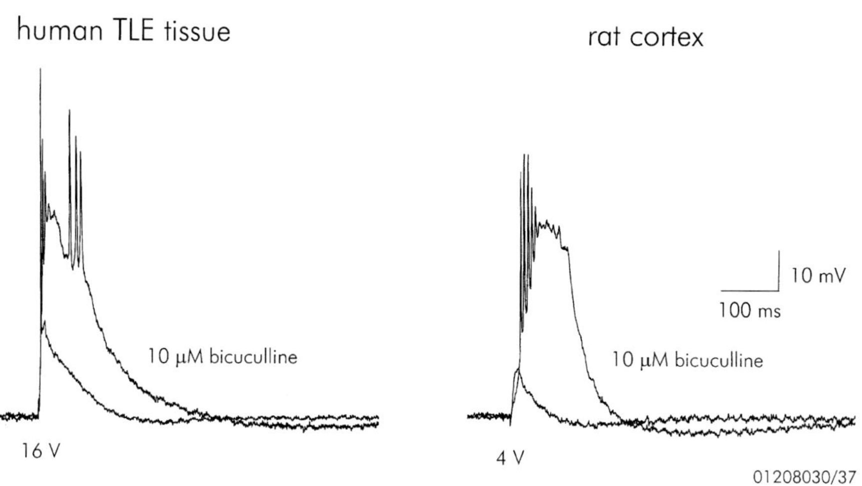

FIG. 2.   Effects of bicuculline on synaptic responses from human and rat cortical neurons. Two traces in control and in the presence of bicuculline (10 μM) have been superimposed. Note the more pronounced after-hyperpolarization of the rat cortical neuron.

postsynaptic potentials mediated by $GABA_A$ receptors ($IPSP_A$s) were almost approaching the reversal potential, whereas in other neurons, the $IPSP_A$ was only about 10% of the driving force. These differences could be due to either differences in the amount of GABA released or differences in the dose–response characteristics of the receptors, perhaps related to altered expression of $GABA_A$ receptor subunits (Brooks-Kayal et al 1998). Also, the $IPSP_B$ was usually small or not detectable (see Figs 1A and 2). Determination of the conductance yielded considerably lower values compared to rats and guinea pigs, on average about 20% (Deisz 1999b). Paired-pulse depression of isolated $IPSP_A$ (reflecting activation of presynaptic $GABA_B$ receptors) was considerably less compared with rat neurons (Deisz 1999b), indicating that presynaptic $GABA_B$ receptors are also less effective.

Frequency dependence of synaptic responses

Considering the recurrent activity occurring in epilepsy *in vivo*, the behaviour of synaptic responses with repetitive activation also needs to be addressed. Interestingly, the PDS induced by penicillin in the neocortex of guinea pigs exhibits a marked failure at interstimulus intervals below about 800 ms (Gutnick et al 1982). DSs in the human tissue, however, display no obvious attenuation at frequencies between 0.05 and 2 Hz (Deisz 1999b). More recently, we further investigated the frequency-dependence using a paired-pulse paradigm with interstimulus intervals between 100 ms and 1.5 sec, revealing almost constant responses at all interstimulus intervals (Fig. 3). This absence of paired-pulse failures of DS may be due to the weak $GABA_B$ responses or due to an insufficient release of GABA. Therefore, the blocker of GABA uptake, tiagabine, was applied to prolong availability of GABA; this should facilitate the diffusion of GABA (Deisz & Dose 1984) and recruitment of $GABA_B$ receptors (Isaacson et al 1993). Tiagabine marginally reduced the amplitudes of the synaptic responses (on average by 3%; $P=0.03$, $n=13$), i.e. not significantly. The time integrals of the synaptic response were slightly more affected and decreased consistently in 10 of 13 neurons by between 6% and 40% (on average by 16%; $P=0.003$, $n=13$). This reduction, however, was only significant at low to intermediate stimulus intensities; at higher stimulus intensities the difference was insignificant.

It may be argued that GABA release is not sufficient to cause detectable effects of tiagabine on the paired-pulse behaviour (see Fig. 4A). We therefore evaluated neuronal excitability by brief (300 ms) current pulses, injected at various intervals after an orthodromic stimulus. Synaptic responses, without an obvious inhibitory component, reduced the number of action potentials by about 60% at a 100 ms delay. The depression of neuronal excitability gradually decayed and was absent at delays of 500 ms (Fig. 4B1 versus B2). In the presence of tiagabine, this

human TLE tissue

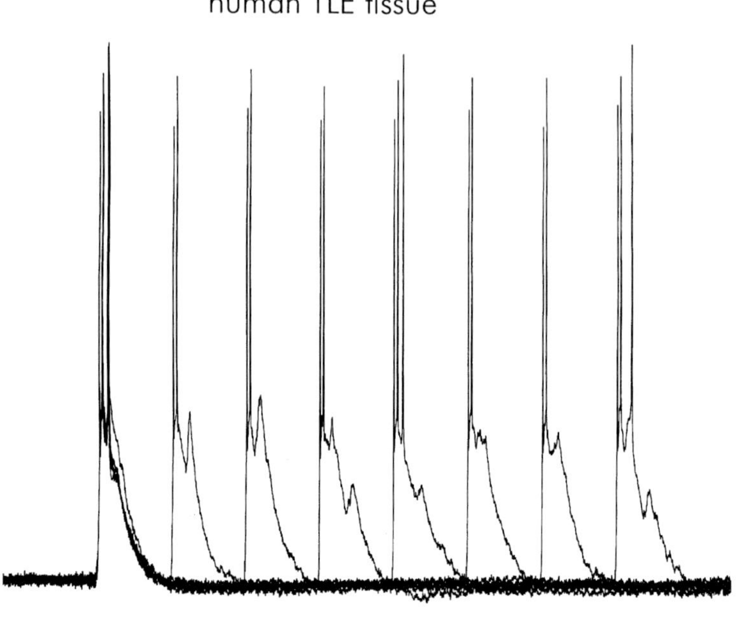

rat cortex with 10 µM Bicuculline

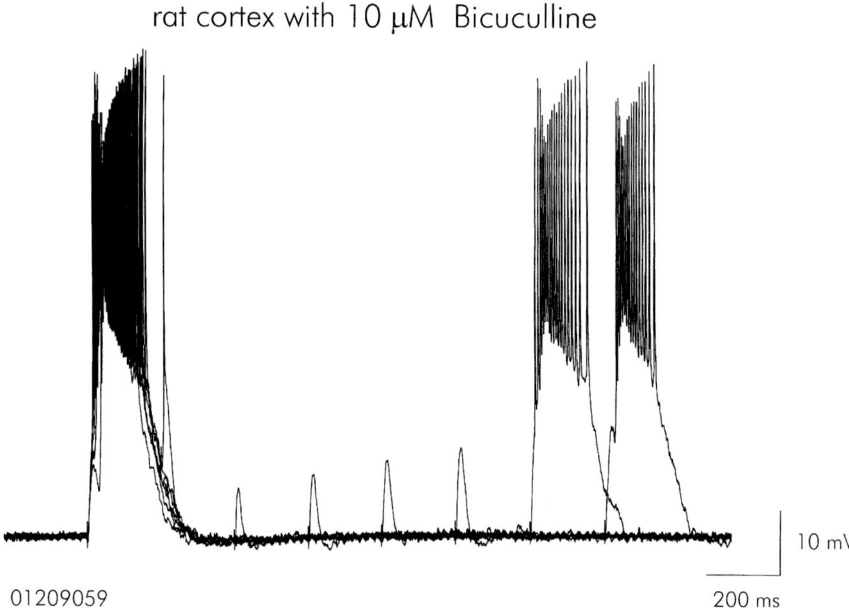

depression was greatly enhanced in magnitude and duration (Fig. 4B). Current pulses typically failed to elicit action potentials for up to 1 s, on average; at this delay the number of action potentials was reduced by 85%. Application of CGP55845A was without effect on the augmented decrease in excitability. These data indicate that a considerable amount of GABA is released to cause depression of excitability through $GABA_A$ receptors.

The constancy of DSs with various interstimulus intervals, even in the presence of sufficient amounts of GABA to decrease the neuronal excitability, was unexpected and prompted us to investigate the mechanisms underlying this failure in an animal model. Two possibilities might account for the failing of PDSs at higher frequencies: either through the depression of excitatory transmission by $GABA_B$ receptors (Howe et al 1987) activated by spill-over of excess GABA, or by a fading of NMDA receptor-mediated components (Sutor & Hablitz 1989). The latter appeared unlikely in view of the small NMDA component; we therefore tested the former possibility directly in the rat cortex treated with bicuculline. Application of $10 \mu M$ bicuculline invariably caused a marked increase in excitability yielding a typical PDS. Paired stimulation revealed a marked depression of PDSs at interstimulus intervals between 100 ms and up to 1 s. Comparable effects were also obtained after 0-Mg exposure (R. A. Deisz & L. Spilker, unpublished results). Application of the $GABA_B$ receptor antagonist CGP 55845A caused a prolongation of the first PDS, but more prominently eliminated the paired-pulse failure of the PDSs (Fig. 5).

Discussion

One key finding is the depolarizing $GABA_A$ response in human epileptogenic tissue. In the rat neocortex, the reversal potential of $GABA_A$ inhibition is governed by a KCl outward transport (Thompson et al 1988) originally described in crayfish stretch receptors (Deisz & Lux 1982, Aickin et al 1982). The $GABA_A$ reversal potential, however, is about 15 mV less negative than the chloride gradient due to the partial bicarbonate permeability of $GABA_A$ channels (Kaila et al 1993). The depolarizing $GABA_A$ response hence may be due to reduced KCl outward transport, equilibrating the chloride gradient with the membrane potential, and the bicarbonate permeability (Deisz et al 1998). Preliminary data with RT-PCR on the 0-Mg model (Mody et al 1987) indicated a marked

---

FIG. 3.   Comparison of paired-pulse stimulation of synaptic responses from human and rat cortical neurons (as indicated). Families of traces with increasing interstimulus intervals have been superimposed. Note the constancy of responses in the human neuron as opposed to the marked depression of the PDS in the rat neuron after the presence of bicuculline.

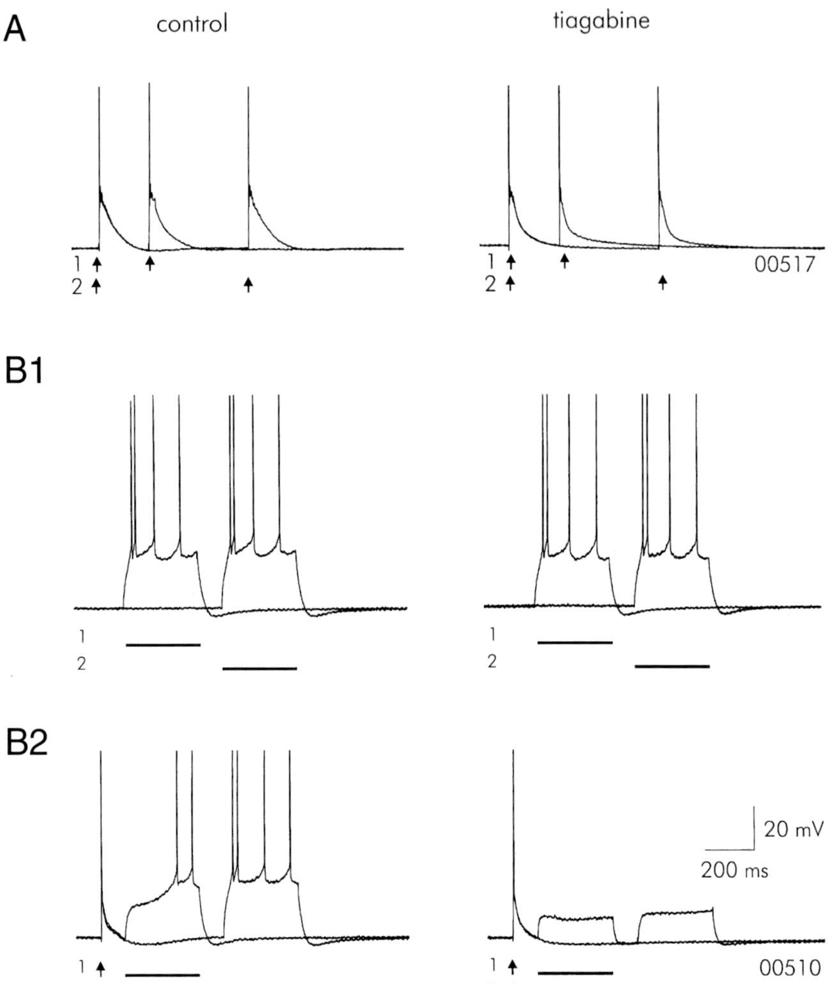

FIG. 4.   Effects of tiagabine on synaptic responses and on neuronal excitability. (A) Traces with two interstimulus intervals (indicated by arrows) have been superimposed. Note the constancy of the responses with and without tiagabine. (B) Superimposed traces of successive current injections (0.7 nA) at various delays with (B2) and without (B1) preceding stimulation. The stimulus pattern is indicated below the traces. Note the marked depression of neuronal excitability in the presence of tiagabine following an orthodromic stimulus.

down-regulation of the mRNA for the neuronal isoform of KCl transporter (KCC2; Payne et al 1996), but not of the KCC1 isoform (A. Klöthing, L. Spilker, O. Ninnemann, R. Nitsch & R. A. Deisz, unpublished results), after 4 h 0-Mg exposure. Also, *in situ* hybridization against KCC2 revealed a decrease in the density of the signal throughout the necortex after 1 h 0-Mg exposure (A. Bräuer, L. Spilker, O. Ninnemann, R. Nitsch & R. A. Deisz, unpublished results). The data obtained so far, if confirmed statistically in further experiments, suggest that during a transient hyperexcitability not only is the expression of $GABA_A$ receptors altered (Vick et al 1996), but also the transporter maintaining the ionic gradient of inhibition is down-regulated.

The data provide some evidence of altered GABAergic function at the level of postsynaptic receptors (from the decreased efficacy of transmission) and for an altered ionic gradient of GABAergic inhibition. Deficits in receptor function could be counteracted by some of the established drugs modulating $GABA_A$ receptors and hence are unlikely to present the crucial component of pharmacoresistance. The depolarizing ionic gradient of $GABA_A$ inhibition, however, causes two problems for therapy. Firstly, enhancing $GABA_A$ receptor function in the presence of a depolarizing gradient is of limited use. Secondly, hypothetical pharmacological strategies to improve the function of the KCl transporter are bound to fail in the absence of the transporter. It is tempting to speculate that impairment of KCl transport may play a pivotal role in pharmacoresistant epilepsy, and this is substantiated by several lines of evidence. Metabolic disorders causing an elevation of cerebral ammonium levels induce seizure activity, which may be due to a reduction of KCl transport (Deisz & Lux 1982, Aickin et al 1982, Thompson et al 1988). Moreover, temporal lobe epilepsy is often associated with a history of febrile convulsion. Interestingly, elevation of temperature or trauma induces a depolarizing shift of the GABA reversal potential of cultured cortical neurons (van den Pol et al 1996), compatible with impaired KCl transport. Considering the highly conserved sequence of the KCC2 protein, defects of the gene or its post-translational processing might contribute to familial forms of epilepsy. The impaired KCl transport might thus present a unifying mechanism for the onset of epilepsy and pharmacoresistance.

With respect to repetitive neuronal discharges, not only individual synaptic events but also the temporal properties are worthy of consideration. In the human tissue, paired stimulation revealed only a small paired-pulse depression (Deisz 1999b) which appears *prima vista* to be at variance with the view that depression of inhibition represents an initial mechanism for the initiation of epileptiform activity (Ben-Ari et al 1979). However, the frequency-dependent depression of inhibition via presynaptic $GABA_B$ receptors (Deisz & Prince 1989) may facilitate spread of focal activity, and within the focus the constancy of depolarizing inhibition would elevate excitability. Our data from rat cortical neurons with bicuculline and CGP 55845A indicate that excessive GABA may spillover (perhaps due to saturation of GABA uptake, Deisz et al 1984) to glutamatergic terminals and sufficiently decreases release via $GABA_B$ receptors to prevent PDS generation for up to 1 s. Therefore, the constant DSs at all stimulus

10 μM Bicuculline

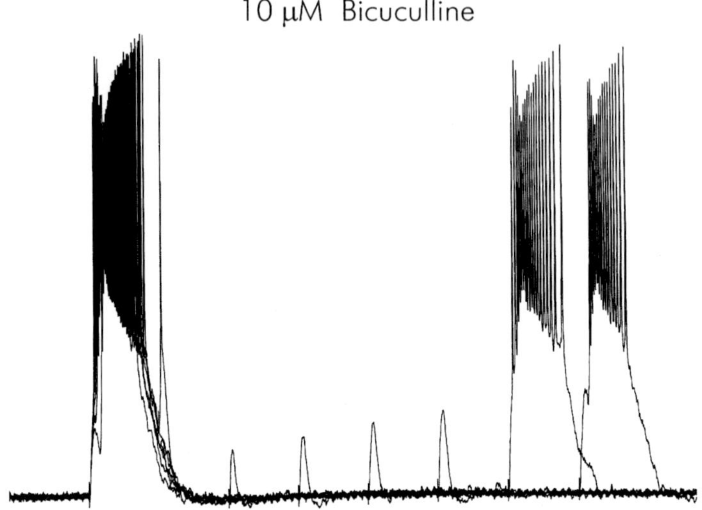

10 μM Bicuculline +2 μM CGP 55845A

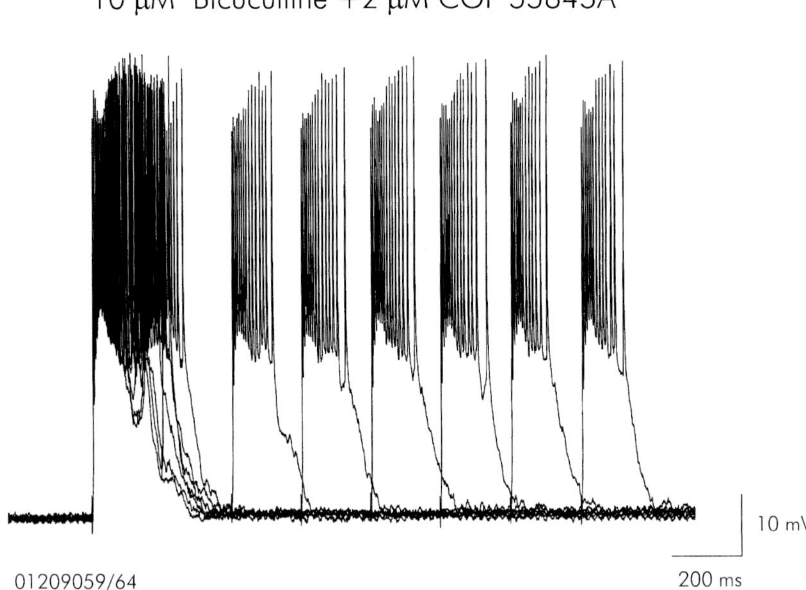

FIG. 5.   Effects of CGP 55845A on paired-pulse behaviour of PDSs following 10 μM bicuculline of a rat cortical neuron. Superimposed traces with incremented interstimulus intervals. Note the elimination of marked paired-pulse failing of PDS in the presence of CGP 55845A.

intervals in the human tissue (even in the presence of tiagabine), strongly suggest that $GABA_B$ receptors on glutamatergic terminals are impaired. The decline in $GABA_B$ receptor function not only eliminates frequency-dependent depression of inhibition, but also the frequency limitation of DSs. Calcium entry during the DSs at higher frequencies may exceed the kinetic constraints of calcium sequestration, the resulting increase of excess intracellular calcium may have cytotoxic effects.

The considerations above are also pertinent to the effects of tiagabine. Our data suggest that tiagabine exerts two beneficial effects in human tissue: (i) a decrease in excitability through a prolonged $GABA_A$ receptor action (evidenced by constant effects after addition of the $GABA_B$ antagonist CGP 55845A), and (ii) a reduction of synaptic responses at low to intermediate stimulus intensities. But, our data also reveal the limitations of tiagabine: firstly, tiagabine fails to attenuate DSs evoked at high stimulus intensities, when depression of excitation is needed most. Secondly, high frequency synaptic activity is not attenuated by tiagabine. The anticipated effect, augmented recruitment of $GABA_B$ receptors (Isaacson et al 1993), was absent due to the impaired $GABA_B$ receptors in the human epileptogenic tissue (see above). On the other hand, if the $GABA_B$ system were functioning, enhancement of the negative feedback of $GABA_B$ on its release (Deisz & Prince 1989) would alter the temporal pattern of inhibition and thus may contribute to initiation of absence-type activity (see Deisz 1999b).

In conclusion, I have presented two findings which may contribute to pharmacoresistance. At the level of single responses an altered ionic gradient of $GABA_A$ inhibition is noteworthy, which has effects approaching those of $GABA_A$ antagonists. The key difference being, however, that under these conditions, conventional strategies to enhance the postsynaptic $GABA_A$ responsiveness are bound to fail. In the time domain, the relatively weak $GABA_B$ effects of human focal tissue may contribute to repetitive DS activity and to the failure of tiagabine to suppress DS. A reduced $GABA_B$ receptor function appears to be a common denominator in most of the intractable epilepsy tissues we have examined so far, despite the various pathologies. Interestingly, this is in accord with the self-sustained limbic status epilepticus model (Mangan & Lothman 1996). Since metabotropic glutamate receptors are also impaired in human temporal lobe epilepsy with ammons horn sclerosis (Dietrich et al 1999), pharmacoresistance may be more a problem of metobotropic than of ionotropic receptors, apart from impaired KCl transport.

Acknowledgements

I am indebted to Professor H. J. Meencke and his team at the Epilepsy Center Berlin for the care and preoperative diagnostics of the patients and to Professor W. R. Lanksch and Dr T. N.

Lehmann who provided the tissue. I am grateful to Professor Nitsch, who provided a stimulating and interactive environment. Supported by the Deutsche Forschungsgemeinschaft (De 419/3-1).

References

Aickin CC, Deisz RA, Lux HD 1982 Ammonium action on post-synaptic inhibition in crayfish neurones: implications for the mechanism of chloride extrusion. J Physiol 329:319–339

Avoli M, Olivier A 1987 Bursting in human epileptogenic neocortex is depressed by an N-methyl-D-aspartate antagonist. Neurosci Lett 76:249–254

Avoli M, Williamson A 1996 Functional and pharmacological properties of human neocortical neurons maintained *in vitro*. Prog Neurobiol 48:519–554

Ben-Ari Y, Krnjevic K, Reinhardt W 1979 Hippocampal seizures and failure of inhibition. Can J Physiol Pharmacol 57:1462–1466

Brooks-Kayal AR, Shumate MD, Jin H, Rikhter TY, Coulter DA 1998 Selective changes in single cell $GABA_A$ receptor expression in temporal lobe epilepsy. Nat Med 4:1166–1172

Deisz RA 1996 A tetrodotoxin-insensitive sodium current initiates burst firing of neocortical neurons. Neuroscience 70:341–351

Deisz RA 1997 Electrophysiology of $GABA_B$ receptors. In: Enna SJ, Bowery N (eds) The GABA receptors, 2nd edn. Humana Press, Clifton, NJ, p 157–207

Deisz RA 1999a The $GABA_B$ receptor antagonist CGP 55845A reduces presynaptic $GABA_B$ actions in neocortical neurons of the rat *in vitro*. Neuroscience 93:1241–1249

Deisz RA 1999b $GABA_B$ receptor-mediated effects in human and rat neocortical neurones *in vitro*. Neuropharmacology 38:1755–1766

Deisz RA, Lux HD 1982 The role of intracellular chloride in post-synaptic inhibition of crayfish stretch receptor neurones. J Physiol 326:123–138

Deisz RA, Prince DA 1989 Frequency-dependent depression of inhibition in guinea-pig neocortex *in vitro* by $GABA_B$ receptor feedback on GABA release. J Physiol 412:513–541

Deisz RA, Fortin G, Zieglgänsberger W 1991 Voltage dependence of excitatory postsynaptic potentials of rat neocortical neurons. J Neurophysiol 65:371–382

Deisz RA, Dose M, Lux HD 1984 The time course of GABA action on the crayfish stretch receptor: evidence for a saturable GABA uptake. Neurosci Lett 47:245–250

Deisz RA, Billard JM, Zieglgänsberger W 1997 Presynaptic and postsynaptic $GABA_B$ receptors of neocortical neurons of the rat *in vitro*: differences in pharmacology and ionic mechanisms. Synapse 25:62–72

Deisz RA, Lehmann TN, Lanksch WR, Meencke HJ, Nitsch R 1998 Receptor mechanisms involved in hyperexcitability of cortical tissue from epilepsy surgery. J Physiol 513:P35–P36

Dietrich D, Kral T, Clusmann H, Friedl M, Schramm J 1999 Reduced function of L-AP4-sensitive metabotropic glutamate receptors in human epileptic sclerotic hippocampus. Eur J Neurosci 11:1109–1113

Dingledine R, Hynes MA, King GL 1986 Involvement of N-methyl-D-aspartate receptors in epileptiform burst firing in the rat hippocampal slice. J Physiol 380:175–189

Gibbs JW III, Zhang YF, Kao CQ, Holloway KL, Oh KS, Coulter DA 1996 Characterization of $GABA_A$ receptor function in human temporal cortical neurons. J Neurophysiol 75:1458–1471

Gutnick MJ, Connors BW, Prince DA 1982 Mechanisms of neocortical epileptogenesis *in vitro*. J Neurophysiol 48: 1321–1335

Howe JR, Sutor B, Zieglgänsberger W 1987 Baclofen reduces post-synaptic potentials of rat cortical neurons by an action other than its hyperpolarizing action. J Physiol 384:539–569

Isaacson JS, Solis, JM, Nicoll RA 1993 Local and diffuse synaptic actions of GABA in the hippocampus. Neuron 10:165–175

Kaila K, Voipio J, Paalasmaa P, Pasternack M, Deisz RA 1993 The role of bicarbonate in GABAA receptor-mediated IPSPs of rat neocortical neurones. J Physiol 464:273–289

Karlsson G, Kolb C, Hausdorf A, Portet C, Schmutz M, Olpe HR 1992 GABA_B receptors in various *in vitro* and *in vivo* models of epilepsy: a study with the GABA_B receptor blocker CGP 35348. Neuroscience 47:63–68

Kaupmann K, Malitschek B, Schuler V et al 1998 GABA_B receptor subtypes assemble into functional heterodimeric complexes. Nature 396:683–687

Köhling R, Lücke A, Straub H et al 1998 Spontaneous sharp waves in human neocortical slices excised from epileptic patients. Brain 121:1073–1087

Mangan PS, Lothman EW 1996 Profound disturbances of pre- and postsynaptic GABAB-receptor-mediated processes in region CA1 in a chronic model of temporal lobe epilepsy. J Neurophysiol 76:1282–1296

McCormick DA 1989 GABA as an inhibitory neurotransmitter in human cerebral cortex. J Neurophysiol 62:1018–1027

Möhler H, Benke D, Benson J, Lüscher B, Rudolph U, Fritschy JM 1997 Diversity in structure, pharmacology and regulation of GABAA receptors. In: Enna SJ, Bowery N (eds) The GABA receptors, 2nd edn. Humana Press, Totowa, NJ, p 11–63

Mody I, Lambert JDC, Heinemann U 1987 Low extracellular magnesium induces epileptiform activity and spreading depression in rat hippocampal slices J Neurophysiol 57:869–888

Payne JA, Stevenson TJ, Donaldson LF 1996 Molecular characterization of a putative K-Cl cotransporter in rat brain. A neuronal specific isoform. J Biol Chem 271:16245–16252

Schwartzkroin PA, Haglund MM 1986 Spontaneous rhythmic synchronous activity in epileptic human and normal monkey temporal lobe. Epilepsia 27:523–533

Sutor B, Hablitz JJ 1989 EPSPs in rat neocortical neurons *in vitro*. I. Electrophysiological evidence for two distinct EPSPs. J Neurophysiol 61:607–620

Thompson SM, Deisz RA, Prince DA 1988 Relative contributions of passive equilibrium and active transport to the distribution of chloride in mammalian cortical neurons. J Neurophysiol 60:105–124

Upton N, Blackburn T 1997 Pharmacology of mammalian GABAA receptors. In: Enna SJ, Bowery N (eds) The GABA receptors, 2nd edn. Humana Press, Clifton, NJ, p 11–63

van den Pol AN, Obrietan K, Chen G 1996 Excitatory actions of GABA after neuronal trauma. J Neuroscience 16:4283–4292

Vick RS, Rafiq A, Coulter DA, Jakoi ER, DeLorenzo RJ 1996 GABA_A α2 mRNA levels are decreased following induction of spontaneous epileptiform discharges in hippocampal-entorhinal cortical slices. Brain Res 721:111–119

Wuarin JP, Peacock WJ, Dudek FE 1992 Single-electrode voltage-clamp analysis of the N-methyl-D-aspartate component of synaptic responses in neocortical slices from children with intractable epilepsy. J Neurophysiol 67:84–93

DISCUSSION

Ling: When you get these tissue slices and put them on a plate, how long is this piece of tissue viable for?

Deisz: The slices are stored in 100 ml beakers with artificial CSF which is equilibrated with carbogen at room temperature. Judging from the electrophysiological properties of the neurons, the slices are viable up to 24 h.

Ling: So 24 h later the tissue is giving the same pattern.

Deisz: Yes, the tissue seems stable for about 24 h. We ascertained the stability of the preparation in the following way: membrane potential and action potential amplitudes were plotted versus the time *in vitro* (27 neurons from 10 resections, each in normal ACSF). Linear regression revealed a slight decline with time, but membrane potential was, on average, better than -70 mV for 22 h.

Ling: Presumably, you could put these slices in very different external medium conditions and then look at the ability of the slices to regulate their internal environment.

Deisz: Yes, and this presents a great potential. Not only can the physiology and pharmacology of synaptic processing of the human neocortex be investigated, but also the cellular mechanisms of ischaemic damage would be accessible. For instance, we were looking at the effects of TRAIL (TNF-related apoptosis inducing ligand) last year and found that TRAIL induces apoptosis in all cells of the CNS — neurons oligodendrocytes and astrocytes alike (Nitsch et al 2000).

Meldrum: I have a question about the $GABA_A$ response inversion. Do you have some specimens that don't show it, and some that do? Or can you differentiate them in terms of whether the specimen is part of an epileptic focus or whether it is relatively normal cortex? Or do you get the same thing in every anterior temporal lobe resection?

Deisz: We do have specimens that don't show $GABA_A$ response inversion. They have a reversal potential of the pharmacologically isolated $IPSP_A$ of approximately -70 mV, which is comparable to rodent cortex (e.g. Deisz & Prince 1989). Regarding a possible correlation of depolarizing $GABA_A$ responses in specimen from focal tissue and relatively normal tissue, this has not been done so far. We are trying to compare tissue samples from tailored resections where the previously implanted subdural grid electrode allows such a distinction. As these grid electrodes are not routinely used we have not enough data yet to attempt making a meaningful correlation. Unfortunately, the data are not consistent from specimen to specimen. Even within a given specimen of, let's say, about $2\,cm^3$, the excitability is quite variable: in one part a pronounced spontaneous activity is obvious and in the adjacent tissue spontaneous activity is absent.

Meldrum: In your 0-Mg experiments in the rat cortex, which after an hour showed a reduction of KCl transporter, do you actually see reversal of the $GABA_A$ effect?

Deisz: We detected a decrease in the mRNA for the KCC2, the neuronal isoform of the KCl transporter. The experiments in which we tried to evaluate possible changes of the $GABA_A$ reversal potential after 0-Mg exposure have not been convincing so far. Despite a clear hyperexcitability after 0-Mg, the reversal potentials of the isolated $GABA_A$ responses were about -60 mV. This is in the right direction but not as dramatic as in some of the human temporal lobe epilepsy (TLE) specimens.

Meldrum: So you haven't got any functional evidence that this change in mRNA is significant.

Deisz: Yes, but this wouldn't be surprising. Firstly, the turnover may not be fast enough to decrease the membrane protein within a few hours of a decrease in the mRNA. Secondly, even if the functional protein would decrease within the first few hours, the reduced protein might still be capable of maintaining the chloride gradient if the influx were small. Therefore, I wonder whether small decreases in KCC2 could be measured in the time available (about 12 h) with acute rat slice preparations. We are trying to approach this in two ways: first, to increase the viability of slices by using slice cultures and second to use an anti-KCC2 antibody to reveal possible decreases in the protein.

Löscher: Of course, in the temporal lobe there are diverse types of neurons. Which type or types are you recording from?

Deisz: Most of the data I presented were obtained with sharp microelectrodes. Using this method, the neurons are recorded without visual control and are therefore not morphologically identified. All I can say is that we choose neurons in the upper layers (layer II, upper layer III) of the temporal lobe, and the majority of the neurons we obtain are more or less regularly spiking neurons, i.e. pyramidal neurons. We have only a few recordings from fast spiking neurons, i.e. interneurons.

Abbott: You are obliged to use the rat tissue as a control. It is difficult to say whether your results show differences between human normal and human pathology, or between human and rat. Is there any way you can look at the edges of your human slice, which are presumably just outside the epileptic focus, and compare those with the centre?

Deisz: We do not consider the rat experiments as controls. They just serve as a comparison. But you are right that it is not certain which of the differences relate to the pathology of TLE and which to species differences. A comparison between different parts of the resected tissue is certainly possible and has been done. Within a given block of tissue we occasionally find marked differences in excitability, as mentioned before. Yet, normally, with standard resection, we don't know which part is focal and which isn't. The best approach is certainly to compare two specimens from a given patient with defined epileptogenicity as documented by the subdural grid electrodes. But even within such a defined focal tissue local differences may exist, once you look at smaller parts of it. Nevertheless, Dave McCormick published a paper in 1989 in which he stressed that he was using tissue far from the focus (McCormick 1989). In this tissue, he found that both GABA$_A$ and GABA$_B$ receptor-mediated inhibition was comparable to that from rodent cortex. Since we also find normal GABA$_A$ responses, at least the depolarizing GABA$_A$ responses are unlikely to be due to a general flaw in our methods. I therefore suspect that the depolarizing GABA$_A$ responses do relate to the pathophysiological activity, although these responses may only be present in a fraction of particularly vulnerable neurons.

Abbott: Have people been recording in slices taken from the kindling model of rat, to see whether something similar occurs?

Löscher: This has been done. There are a lot of similarities to the human situation.

Deisz: One similarity that I would like to emphasize is the impaired GABA$_B$ receptor-mediated inhibition. In the model of self-sustained limbic status epilepticus, Mangan & Lothman reported (1996) the virtual absence of GABA$_B$ receptor mediated components, both presynaptic as well as postsynaptic. They were kind of puzzled by this finding because a constant IPSP without the common frequency-dependent depression (Deisz & Prince 1989) appears to be at variance with the concept that frequency-dependent depression of inhibition through presynaptic GABA$_B$ receptors would facilitate the initiation and spread of epileptiform activity. However, in the TLE tissue, not only is the frequency dependence reduced but also the gradient is reversed. The combination of the two effects may account for hyperexcitability and high frequency discharges, particularly if GABA$_B$ receptors on excitatory terminals were affected as well.

Abbott: In some pathologies including epilepsy, activated glial cells show abnormal ion currents not seen in normal glia, which could contribute to the hyperexcitability. Can you detect glial cells in your recordings, and do they show normal currents?

Deisz: We occasionally get recordings from cells which have membrane potentials of about $-75\,\text{mV}$ and do not generate action potentials on depolarizing current injection. In such cases, we usually just go further into the lobe to get a neuron. H. Kettenmann's group reported that oligodendrocytes from low-grade tumours are capable of generating action potentials (Labrakakis et al 1997). They considered that this might contribute to the epileptogenicity of tumours.

Ling: Has the comparison been done between responding and refractile rats?

Deisz: No, unfortunately, we do not have responsive and pharmacoresistant rats. In addition to the 0-Mg model and the bicuculline model, we are now also using pilocarpine-treated rats, kindly provided by P. Mares, Prag.

Sills: The tissues you study are resected from patients with refractory epilepsy that are, by definition, resistant to AEDs. Do you have any evidence that the abnormal activity in the tissue slice, whether it is spontaneous or evoked, is resistant to treatment with standard AEDs?

Deisz: No, we have not tried standard AEDs so far. We have chosen to start with tiagabine because this is a drug with a well defined mechanism of action. I wonder whether it is sensible to test the established anticonvulsant drugs on this tissue. The patients have usually been treated with several anticonvulsant drugs and are included in the operating programme when these drugs prove not to work.

Sills: You showed some nice physiological evidence for the basis of the abnormal activity in these slices. However, I wonder whether you can really call this pharmacoresistance when, based on the physiological evidence, we are using drugs with the wrong pharmacology. Your results suggest that we should be using GABA antagonists to treat the abnormal activity, whereas clinically we use GABA agonists to treat epilepsy. Can this really be classed as pharmacoresistance if we are using inappropriate pharmacological approaches in the first place?

Deisz: This is a crucial point. The pharmacoresistance is defined by the available drugs. Perhaps the more recent AEDs or novel therapeutic strategies will reduce the number of pharmacoresistant patients.

Ling: It may be worth saying that this is some kind of surrogate marker.

Sander: It's fair to say that often in those samples you might not know exactly what is abnormal and what is not.

Deisz: That is true.

Sander: Within the same piece of tissue that comes from the surgeon you might not know what is normal and what is abnormal. Do you always get the same response?

Deisz: In cases of standard resection, we do not know which part is normal and which isn't. I believe, however, that such spontaneous activity is unlikely to be normal since I have never seen it in the neocortex from guinea pigs or rats. With regard to the second part of your question, we have an interesting finding from two resections that is revealing in this context. In both cases, the spontaneous activity was confined to slices from a certain beaker, i.e. from a certain volume of the tissue. When we recorded neurons in slices from tissue part 1 we noticed marked spontaneous activity. Later in the experiment, we used a slice from tissue part 2 which exhibited no spontaneous activity. Although the neuron was within the acceptable limits, I thought the slices might have deteriorated and lost their spontaneous activity. I then took another slice from the tissue part 1 and the neuron in this slice exhibited a comparable spontaneous activity. I don't know right now how far apart the two tissue parts had been, perhaps 1 cm. We take this difference as an indication of a considerable heterogeneity of excitability in small volumes of tissue.

Sisodiya: What was the pathology you were looking at?

Deisz: A whole range of various pathologies. About 70% of cases are TLEs, with or without hippocampal sclerosis.

Sisodiya: In patients with hippocampal sclerosis, are you only looking at the neocortex?

Deisz: Yes. The tissue used for research purposes is split between two laboratories in Berlin. We arranged for the hippocampal tissue to be used in U. Heinemann's laboratory and my laboratory receives the cortical tissue. Mind you, we have not only used tissue from the temporal lobe, we have also used tissue from the frontal cortex. What I tried to show is not so much the correlation between a certain effect and a given pathology, but rather the common denominator underlying perhaps all of these pharmacoresistant epilepsies. After all, these patients had pharmacoresistant epilepsy, irrespective of the pathology. This is why the tissue had to be removed. The fact that the resected tissue to some extent causes the problem is evident from the clinical outcome: 80–90% of the patients are seizure free after the surgery.

Sander: In someone with hippocampal sclerosis, if you don't get a sample it is unlikely that the tissue you get is going to be diseased. It could be normal.

Deisz: This would account for the huge variability we see. The tissue could be normal, it also could be affected by the ongoing hyperexcitability recruiting the cortex and inducing altered expression of ligand- or voltage-activated channels or transporters.

Sander: When you say you use tiagabine, do you use tiagabine or nipecotic acid? Tiagabine is nipecotic acid with a lipophilic anchor, to go through the blood–brain barrier.

Deisz: Tiagabine.

Sander: If you are using it directly shouldn't you use nipecotic acid rather than tiagabine?

Deisz: No, in addition to reduction of uptake, nipecotic acid was proposed to act as a false transmitter and reduce the release of GABA (Lerma et al 1984). Tiagabine is devoid of these effects and only decreases uptake.

Ling: Are we still in a situation where we do not have the non-pharmacoresistant samples to compare? This is a limitation in the field, I suppose.

Deisz: I would like to have some of Dr Löscher's rats to test.

Löscher: In the rats, phenytoin in slices is efficacious in the non-responders, even though this is a hippocampus from a rat that is non-responding *in vivo*. The same is true for human hippocampal slices. Speckmann's group in Munster is testing anticonvulsant drugs in biopsy samples from pharmacoresistant patients. They induce epileptic-like activity in the slice and then test the effect of different anticonvulsant drugs on this activity. AEDs are clearly efficacious in this situation. You shouldn't forget that you isolate the tissue from the network. I agree with Brian Meldrum's notion yesterday that epilepsy is a network phenomenon. If you take away one part of the network, this may make a patient responsive to treatment. Once again, most of these patients still have to be treated with AEDs after surgery or they will have seizures. It could be that in a dish this part of the network is not pharmacoresistant at all, because it is only one part of the whole system. It is probably more complicated than we think. Data from Speckmann in Germany tell me that this tissue in the dish is responsive to AEDs.

Deisz: I quite agree. All we know is that the patient is not adequately responding. Whether the response of a given tissue *in vitro* relates to the responsiveness *in situ* is debatable. People working on slices usually tacitly imply that within a slice the local circuitry and neuronal properties reflect the *in vivo* situation for a limited time. But, during the slicing, the tissue might be traumatized which, in turn, might unleash entirely different mechanisms from those present *in vivo*.

Löscher: Another argument for this network idea is that the patient *in vivo* has seizures. If you take away one part of this network from this patient, such as the hippocampus, there are no seizures *in vitro*: these slices don't show the spontaneous activity.

Deisz: They do. The spontaneous activity I showed corresponds to the interictal activity.

Löscher: If you ask Uwe Heinemann, he never sees this.

Deisz: Uwe Heinemann and his group are using the hippocampus, whereas we are using the neocortex. According to our neurosurgeon, Dr T. N. Lehmann, who is doing most of the epilepsy surgery, on average the resected the hippocampus of patients with mesiotemporal epilepsy exhibits sclerosis in about half the cases and various other pathologies in a further 30%. Thus, the majority of specimens used by Heinemann and his group may not have a sufficient neuronal density to generate spontaneous activity.

Löscher: That is not always true. There are patients with TLE where there are no injuries in the hippocampus, and some groups use these patients as a control. They have epilepsy, but there is no lesion in the hippocampus. These studies have compared the non-lesioned hippocampus from epileptic patients with the lesioned hippocampus. There is no spontaneous epileptiform activity in either of these hippocampi. It might be a neocortex phenomenon. But at least in the hippocampus, which many people believe is the target for the neurosurgery, there is no spontaneous activity.

Shorvon: The best evidence for epilepsy being a network phenomenon is that many patients have the 'auras' which continue after surgery, even though the seizures have stopped. These are exactly what you would think would disappear if this was of focal origin, spreading out. The aura is the first part of the seizure; this is a paradoxical finding. Furthermore, stimulation experiments in humans, in all parts of the brain, can reproduce the aura in someone with hippocampal sclerosis. It is a remarkable finding that can only be explained by a network phenomenon of a most sophisticated nature. Is it not also true that if you get large limbic slices, rather than just hippocampal slices, then you do see spontaneous activity? Furthermore, this activity can start in various parts of the slice. In fact, in human recording activity can start all over the place, even in a person with a very focal aetiology.

Ling: In parallel with oncology, it has always been a dream that if one takes a tumour sample out, grows it in tissue culture and looks for drug responsiveness, that one might be able to predict the responsiveness of the patient. This approach could have great ramifications for the therapy of patients. It is a huge challenge. It is even more challenging in epilepsy. If one could take a small tissue sample and devise some predictive assays, this could be very beneficial.

References

Deisz RA, Prince DA 1989 Frequency-dependent depression of inhibition in guinea pig neocortex in vitro by $GABA_B$ receptor feedback on GABA release. J Physiol 412:513–541

Labrakakis C, Patt S, Weydt P, Cervos-Navarro J, Meyer R, Kettenmann H 1997 Action potential-generating cells in human glioblastomas. J Neuropathol Exp Neurol 56:243–254

Lerma J, Herreras O, Herranz AS, Munoz D, del Rio RM 1984 In vivo effects of nipecotic acid on levels of extracellular GABA and taurine, and hippocampal excitability. Neuropharmacology 23:595–598

Mangan PS, Lothman EW 1996 Profound disturbances of pre- and postsynaptic GABAB-receptor-mediated processes in region CA1 in a chronic model of temporal lobe epilepsy. J Neurophysiol 76:1282–1296

McCormick DA 1989 GABA as an inhibitory neurotransmitter in human cerebral cortex. J Neurophysiol 62:1018–1027

Nitsch R, Bechmann I, Deisz RA et al 2000 Human brain-cell death induced by tumour-necrosis-factor-related apoptosis-inducing ligand (TRAIL). Lancet 356:827–828

Functional polymorphisms of the human multidrug resistance (*MDR1*) gene: correlation with P glycoprotein expression and activity *in vivo*

Ulrich Brinkmann

Epidauros Biotechnology, Pharmacogenetics Laboratory, Am Neuland 1, 82347 Bernried, Germany

Abstract. The human *MDR1* gene encodes an integral membrane protein, P glycoprotein (Pgp), whose function is the energy dependent export of substances from the inside of cells, and from membranes, to the outside. Its physiological role is the protection of cells from toxic substances or metabolites. Many drugs that have been developed for the treatment of human diseases are substrates of Pgp. Because of that, the degree of expression and the functionality of the *MDR1* gene product can directly affect the therapeutic effectiveness of such agents. This is of particular importance in cancer therapy where high expression and activity of *MDR1* causes cancer cells to become refractory to the treatment with many agents, all of which are Pgp substrates. *MDR1* is also expressed on different non-malignant cells in various organs, e.g. in the intestine and at the blood–brain barrier. Modulation of *MDR1* expression in these normal cell types can also influence the activity and bioavailability of drugs. In the intestine, modulation of *MDR1* may control the degree of drug uptake following drug ingestion. At the blood–brain barrier, Pgp may influence the uptake of substrates into the brain: high Pgp levels may limit the uptake of sufficient amounts of desired drugs into the brain, and reduced Pgp activity could lead to abnormally increased accumulation in the brain and undesired side effects of drugs.

2002 Mechanisms of drug resistance in epilepsy: lessons from oncology. Wiley, Chichester (Novartis Foundation Symposium 243) p 207–212

The overall human multidrug resistance (*MDR1*) gene activity controlling P glycoprotein (Pgp)-dependent drug transport, is dependent on two parameters. First, the level of expression of the *MDR1* gene controls the amount of protein that is synthesized in the cells and, second, the functionality of the *MDR1*-encoded Pgp, which determines which substrates are recognized and transported with what effectiveness. The first parameter, level of expression of *MDR1*, has been intensively analysed, particularly because the sensitivity of

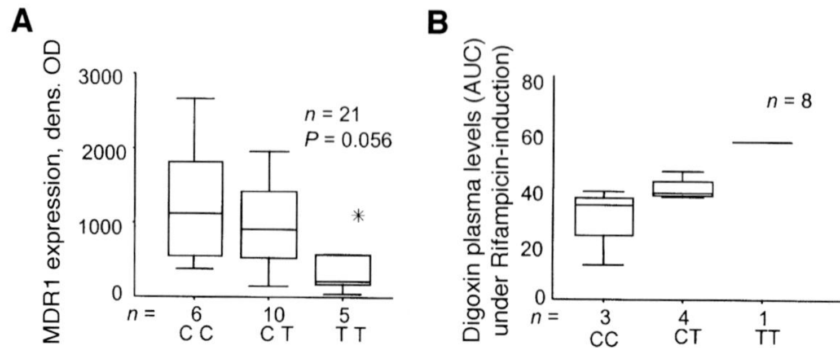

FIG. 1. *MDR1* expression and Pgp *in vivo* activity after rifampicin induction. (A) *MDR1* genotype in exon 26 and distribution of rifampicin-induced Pgp protein expression in the duodenum. (B) Distribution of plasma levels of digoxin after rifampicin induction. The plasma levels of digoxin (AUC) are inverse proportional to Pgp activity in the duodenum.

tumour cells towards chemotherapy often correlates inversely with increased *MDR1* expression. *MDR1* overexpression can partially be attributed to gene amplifications, but it is known that other factors must also exist. Allelic differences in individual *MDR1* gene sequences may be associated with or even causative for different expression levels.

The first evidence for the presence of polymorphisms in the human *MDR1* gene was reported by Mickley et al (1998). They identified single nucleotide polymorphisms (SNPs) in exons 21 and 24 (G2677T and G2995A) in a population of tumour patients, in drug-selected cell lines, in cells from refractory malignant malignomas and in healthy volunteers. A screen of the entire *MDR1* gene for the presence of additional SNPs was undertaken by Hoffmeyer and co-workers (Hoffmeyer et al 2000), in which 15 SNPs were detected in the human *MDR1* gene in a Caucasian population.

Although the likelihood of SNPs to be of functional consequence can be predicted to some degree from their position within the gene and protein (e.g. SNPs that lead to amino acid changes may account for altered activity), for the three polymorphisms (located in exons 2, 5 and 11) that changed the amino acid sequence, no correlation of protein–SNPs with altered function or Pgp activity has been reported to date. In contrast, for one non-coding SNP, a C3435T change at a wobble position in exon 26, pharmacological consequences such as a significant correlation with *MDR1* expression levels and Pgp activity *in vivo*, could be observed. Genotype–phenotype correlations, performed in volunteers whose Pgp expression and function in the duodenum had been determined by Western blots or by plasma concentrations after orally administered digoxin, revealed a significant correlation of a polymorphism in intron 26 (C3435T) of *MDR1* with expression levels of the *MDR1* gene and function of *MDR1* (Fig. 1). The C3435T

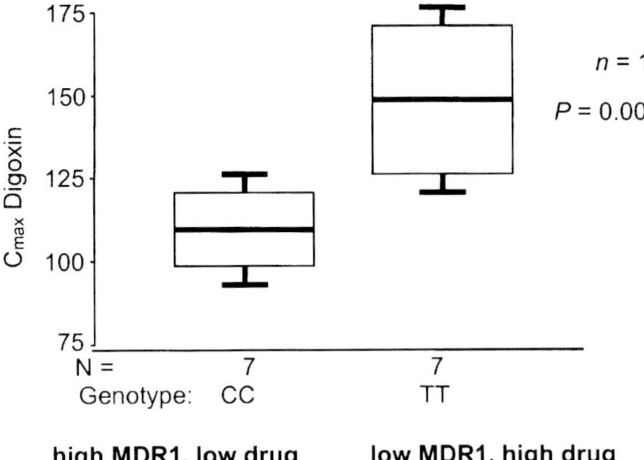

FIG. 2.   Correlation of *MDR1* genotype and digoxin uptake *in vivo*. The *MDR1* genotype in exon 26 was analysed in human volunteers who participated in an experimental clinical study that addresses blood levels of digoxin after oral application. The digoxin blood levels of seven probands that each harboured the relevant T/T and C/C genotype in exon 26 show a correlation of *MDR1* genotype and digoxin blood levels, with the T/T genotype that correlates with low levels of intestinal Pgp showing significantly higher blood levels than the C/C genotype (high levels of intestinal Pgp).

position correlates with Pgp expression in the intestine. This in turn influences the uptake of orally administered Pgp substrates. The T allele is associated with low intestinal expression and the corresponding C allele with elevated expression. Individuals that homozygously carry the low expressor (T) allele, show increased digoxin plasma levels due to increased uptake (Fig. 2). Homozygosity for this variant was observed in 25% of our sample population. The same polymorphism is also associated with increased (C allele) or decreased (T allele) expression in tubular cells of the kidney and in CD56$^+$ lymphocytes. It is also possible (and likely), that variable expression of *MDR1* at the blood–brain barrier is associated with these different alleles.

Transporter pharmacogenetics may play a significant role in drug therapy. Absorption, distribution, metabolism and elimination are the factors that affect the efficacy of compounds. Pgp and other ABC transporters significantly contribute to these processes. They act as a barrier against the entry of compounds into the body and can control their transfer between tissues and compartments. Because of that, genetic variations that influence the function or expression of Pgp can directly influence intestinal absorption or elimination of compounds. One important parameter that is affected by *MDR1* is the transport of substances across the blood–brain barrier. Limitations in the ability of compounds to enter the brain may well be a crucial factor in determining the therapeutic efficacy of CNS drugs, such as those that are applied to treat epilepsy.

Acknowledgements

This work was prepared in cooperation with the Institute of Clinical Pharmacology, Charite Berlin (Professor I. Roots), and the Dr Margarete Fischer-Bosch Institute of Clinical Pharmacology, Stuttgart (Professor M. Eichelbaum).

References

Hoffmeyer S, Burk O, von Richter O et al 2000 Functional polymorphisms of the human multidrug-resistance gene: multiple sequence variations and correlation of one allele with P-glycoprotein expression and activity in vivo. Proc Natl Acad Sci USA 97:3473–3478

Mickley LA, Lee JS, Weng Z et al 1998 Genetic polymorphism in MDR-1: a tool for examining allelic expression in normal cells, unselected and drug-selected cell lines, and human tumors. Blood 91:1749–1756

DISCUSSION

Ling: How do you think this polymorphism works? Clearly, mRNA is at a higher level.

Brinkmann: Yes, this is very interesting. We are a bit lost with this. The SNP is not changing the protein. In recombinant expression experiments we didn't see any change in mRNA stability, although these experiments are pretty unreliable, so this doesn't tell us much. Our hypothesis is that it is linked to some other SNP in a regulatory region that is important. This is something that is seen quite often: this SNP is just an indicator, like *Escherichia coli* in drinking water. *E. coli* doesn't make you sick but if it is there it indicates there's a problem. We have screened over 20 kb of the whole promoter region. Initially we had only the co-promoter, which is 2.5 kb, but we figured that there might be some other element somewhere. There is nothing there. These experiments are quite easy to do. You just take five samples of each genotype and then see what other SNP is 100% linked. We have sequenced a couple of introns and found nothing. In my opinion it is something that is in some of the larger introns that affects splicing efficiency.

Pirmohamed: I am curious about the wobble polymorphism and its functional effects. If you took a group of low expressors plus high expressors and exposed them to rifampicin, would you get differences in induction, or would inducibility come up to a high expression level?

Brinkmann: It is a parallel shift. It is not about inducibility. We had a big programme going to try to find promoter SNPs and other SNPs which would predict inducibility. We have been unsuccessful so far. If you have induced patients or non-induced patients it is a parallel shift.

Shorvon: Did you look at different tissues in the same people? Is there a marked tissue variation?

Brinkmann: We have not looked in other tissues. These are tumour patients, so we can't take samples of different tissues.

Shorvon: Would you expect that in the high expressors that this expression would be high in all the different tissues?

Brinkmann: Yes, because it is the same correlation with genotype in all tissues. I think that this polymorphism would also be predictive for the blood–brain barrier.

Sander: Have you only looked at this one polymorphism?

Brinkmann: We have many more polymorphisms. Our first experiment involved using a computer to associate all genotypes with phenotypes. The only one that correlates is this one.

Kwan: What are the functional consequences of this polymorphism? You first identified this in a Caucasian population and then you tested it in a Japanese population to see its frequency. Have you thought of doing a similar functional analysis in a non-Caucasian population?

Brinkmann: We have done this, and there are clearly other polymorphisms there. Our problem is that we don't have access to clinical centres in order to phenotype them. We have a list of polymorphisms which are specific for Asians and African Americans, but we have problems obtaining a clear phenotype correlation for these. Without a phenotype a SNP is not worth anything.

Kwan: So you haven't been able to do a functional analysis of these SNPs.

Brinkmann: Not yet.

Newman: The results that Dr Brinkmann presented with the CD56$^+$ lymphocytes demonstrate that what you get in a Pgp inhibitor assay is highly dependent on the amount of Pgp present and the type of assay. There is a disconnect between what is seen in a Pgp assay and what might be relevant *in vivo*. You may see only a small effect in an assay, but in oncology all we may need to do is increase the amount of chemotherapeutic agent that stays in a tumour cell by a relatively small amount. There is a difference between the ultimate physiology and the assays we use.

Brinkmann: The usefulness could be shown if we can prove that this is true in the blood–brain barrier. If you do therapeutic drug monitoring, any severe effects of liver enzymes are being levelled out by dose adjustment. There is still the same dose in the blood and more or less of the dose penetrates the blood–brain barrier. There we have a situation where even if the liver enzymes are a greater factor, this factor can be eliminated by measuring drug concentration in the blood. But we can't eliminate the effect of Pgp on the blood–brain barrier.

Bates: Did you have any polymorphisms at the amino acid sequence level?

Brinkmann: Originally we had three or four, and now we are looking for the different ethnic sub groups. It might be argued that some of these are mutations rather than polymorphisms because their frequency is less than 5% or so.

Bates: Do you know whether these have functional correlates?

Brinkmann: A couple have been tested by Michael Gottesman. All he found was that they were present on the membrane in a delayed manner, indicating some misfolding or less efficient processing.

Bates: In our CD56$^+$ assays we have seen occasional outliers that didn't have inhibition or rhodamine efflux, despite adequate blood concentrations of modulator, but we haven't seen any that didn't have efflux (Robey et al 1999).

Brinkmann: In our assays the inhibitor was given directly to the cells.

Reference

Robey R, Bakke S, Stein W et al 1999 Efflux of rhodamine from CD56+ cells as a surrogate marker for reversal of P-glycoprotein-mediated drug efflux by PSC 833. Blood 93:306–314

OC144-093, a novel P glycoprotein inhibitor for the enhancement of anti-epileptic therapy

Michael J. Newman, Ross Dixon and Barry Toyonaga

Ontogen Corporation, 6451 El Camino Real, Carlsbad, CA 92009, USA

Abstract. Inhibitors of P glycoprotein (Pgp) may be useful for the enhancement of blood–brain barrier penetration of anti-epileptic drugs (AEDs). Due to polypharmacy and the need for chronic treatment, Pgp inhibitors used in epilepsy should be highly specific and non-toxic. In particular, it may be essential to use compounds that produce minimal inhibition of enzymes involved in metabolism of AEDs and other drugs used by epilepsy patients. OC144-093 is a novel substituted diarylimidazole generated using the OntoBLOCK® system, a solid-phase combinatorial chemistry technology, in combination with high-throughput cell-based screening. The compound is an extremely potent inhibitor of Pgp-mediated multidrug resistance (MDR) in cancer with an average EC_{50} of 32 nM, but does not inhibit multidrug resistance-associated protein (MRP1). OC144-093 is the least non-specifically toxic Pgp inhibitor described to date, with an average cytostatic IC_{50} of $>60\,\mu$M in 15 cell types. It is not metabolized by cytochrome P450s CYP3A4, 2C8 or 2C9 enzymes involved in AED metabolism. OC144-093 does not produce a pharmacokinetic (PK) interaction with paclitaxel and has exhibited an excellent PK and safety profile in phase I clinical trials. Our results suggest that OC144-093 may represent an ideal candidate for use in enhancement of AED blood–brain barrier penetration.

2002 Mechanisms of drug resistance in epilepsy: lessons from oncology. Wiley, Chichester (Novartis Foundation Symposium 243) p 213–230

Ontogen is a chemical drug discovery and development company that is integrating modern tools of biology, chemistry, engineering, and information technologies to discover and optimize novel, small molecules for a variety of therapeutic indications. The company's technology is based on the application of state-of-the art engineering approaches to the evolving needs of biology and chemistry. As a consequence of these efforts Ontogen has developed and patented the OntoBLOCK® System, a comprehensive array of software and hardware modules to plan, conduct and track the high-speed synthesis of small molecule libraries. Such parallel syntheses on solid support have provided large, proprietary, spatially diverse combinatorial libraries, in milligram quantities per compound, which have been used in a variety of drug discovery and lead optimization programmes.

Recent engineering efforts have been focused on instrumentation for high-throughput chromatographic purification. This technology, called OntoCHROM®, is now used in our laboratories for the practical and efficient high-throughput purification of moderately large libraries (10 000–40 000 compounds). OntoCHROM® not only produces high quality, purified libraries with minimal amounts of solvent, but allows, for the first time, the realization of one of the original promises of combinatorial libraries, that is, high quality structure–activity relationships from the high-throughput biological screening of the libraries. The OntoCHROM® system is a roboticized instrument employing multichannel super critical fluid chromatography, in which target compounds are identified in real time by mass spectrometry and directly collected in a 96-well microtitre plate with well-to-well mapping from the original plate. The development and use of novel high throughput combinatorial chemistry technologies has been validated at Ontogen as a result of the discovery and early development of OC144-093, an inhibitor of P glycoprotein (Pgp).

Currently, over 75% of cancer chemotherapy patients exhibit intrinsic or develop acquired resistance to treatment. Multidrug resistance (MDR) is now recognized as the most common cause of failure of cancer chemotherapy. The MDR phenotype results from cross-resistance to a variety of structurally and functionally unrelated natural products used for cytotoxic anti-tumour therapy. These include anthracyclines, vinca alkaloids, epipodophyllotoxins and taxanes. Ling and co-workers identified a 170 kDa membrane glycoprotein (Pgp), which was subsequently found to mediate ATP-dependent efflux of each of these cancer therapeutics from multidrug-resistant tumour cells (Sikic 1997, van Zuylen et al 2000, for reviews). Additional mechanisms contributing to MDR have been described, including expression of the multidrug resistance-associated protein (MRP) class of transporters. MRP-related proteins appear to be able to transport certain anthracyclines, vinca alkaloids and epipodophyllotoxins, but not taxanes. Members of this family are also involved in normal biliary transport (Borst et al 2000, for review).

Significant progress has been made on determination of the role of Pgp and related proteins in normal physiology. One Pgp gene (*MDR1*) in human and two genes (*Mdr1a*, *Mdr1b*) in rodents have been shown to play a significant role in drug resistance. Additional members of the Pgp gene family are involved in phospholipid and bile salt transport. While simultaneous genetic knockout of *Mdr1a* and *Mdr1b* resulted in healthy mice, indicating that Pgp is not essential for basic physiological functions, the mice exhibited significant alterations in the pharmacological handling of drugs. Blood–brain barrier (BBB) function was decreased and intestinal absorption of drugs was increased (Schinkel 1998, for review). The involvement of Pgp in BBB function suggests that it may play a role in resistance to drugs targeting the CNS. For example, a significant percentage of epilepsy patients fail to respond to conventional anti-epileptic drug (AED) therapy. Several studies have demonstrated elevated levels of Pgp in brain tissue obtained from patients with drug-resistant epilepsy (Tishler et al 1995, Lazarowski et al 1999, Sisodiya et al 1999). In addition, at least one widely prescribed AED, phenytoin, has been shown to be a Pgp substrate (Schinkel et al 1996).

Studies carried out over the last several years have demonstrated that intrinsic and acquired expression of Pgp play a major role in clinical MDR. Tumour types that frequently express Pgp in the absence of exposure to chemotherapy include colorectal, renal cell, hepatocellular, and adrenocortical cancers, as well as chronic leukaemia. Several additional tumour types express Pgp at diagnosis in approximately 10–30% of cases. Examples include breast carcinoma, acute myelogenous leukaemia and ovarian carcinoma (Ramachandran & Melnick 1999, van Zuylen et al 2000, Newman et al 2000, for reviews). Pgp expression at diagnosis in these tumour types can play a significant role in treatment outcome. For example, patients with breast carcinomas expressing Pgp are three times more likely to fail to respond to chemotherapy than patients whose tumours are Pgp negative (Trock et al 1997).

Chemotherapy can induce Pgp expression and/or select for expansion of Pgp-expressing MDR tumour cells. In addition, Pgp inhibitors have been found to decrease the mutation rate for resistance to doxorubicin, and suppress activation of *Mdr1* and the appearance of MDR mutants in tissue culture models. In light of these findings, it appears that the most effective way to use chemotherapeutic agents that are Pgp substrates will be in conjunction with a Pgp inhibitor at the time of tumour diagnosis (Sikic 1997, van Zuylen et al 2000, Bates 1999, for reviews).

The first attempts to reverse Pgp-mediated MDR in cell lines, tumour-bearing animals, and in the clinic, took advantage of the observation by Tsuruo and coworkers that Ca^{2+} channel blockers such as verapamil are inhibitors of MDR. Similar observations were subsequently made with cyclosporin A (Sikic 1997, van Zuylen et al 2000, for reviews). While having some efficacy, these agents are relatively weak Pgp inhibitors ($EC_{50}s = 2–10\ \mu M$), are often substrates for Pgp, and exhibit dose-limiting side effects that severely restrict their clinical utility. To address the problems described above there has been considerable interest in second-generation Pgp inhibitors. PSC 833 (Atadja et al 1998), VX-710 (Germann et al 1997) and XR9051 (Dale et al 1998) are 3–100-fold more potent than the first generation compounds and typically do not elicit significant toxicity at doses required for Pgp inhibition. Common dose-limiting toxicities for these types of compounds are ataxia and hyperbilirubinaemia, which are reversible upon cessation of drug treatment.

An additional problem with many Pgp inhibitors is that they are metabolized by enzymes, such as cytochromes P450 CYP3A4 and CYP2C8, involved in the metabolism of a wide variety of therapeutics, including anticancer drugs (Sonnichsen et al 1995, Desai et al 1998) and AEDs (Kerr et al 1994, Komatsu et al 2000). This can result in significant pharmacokinetic (PK) interactions, necessitating close monitoring and reductions in the dose of the co-administered therapeutic agent. For example, PSC 833 and VX-710 have been reported to produce significant PK interactions with agents such as paclitaxel (Sikic 1997, van Zuylen et al 2000, for reviews). Although dose reduction in cancer therapy is feasible, interpatient variability in PK interaction makes this approach problematic, particularly in the 'up-front' therapy setting, designed to kill cancer cells already expressing Pgp and prevent the appearance of MDR before multiple resistance mechanisms evolve. In epilepsy, where chronic treatment and polypharmacy must be considered, it may not be possible to adequately anticipate potential drug interactions when using a Pgp inhibitor that is metabolized by the most abundant and broadly acting P450, CYP3A4. These considerations have led to a search for third generation Pgp inhibitors, which combine high potency with minimal potential for PK interactions.

The Pgp inhibitor properties likely to be required for safe and effective MDR cancer therapy and enhancement of AED CNS penetration are low nanomolar potency, Pgp specificity, lack of non-specific toxicity, relatively long duration of action with reversibility, good oral bioavailability, and lack of PK interaction via metabolism by major P450s. OC144-093 appears to be one of the first inhibitors to meet all of these requirements.

Results and conclusion

Discovery and characterization of OC144-093

A high-throughput, cell-based screen for inhibitors of Pgp was initiated at Ontogen. The assay was based on restoration of vinblastine-mediated cytotoxicity in Pgp-expressing multidrug resistant human lymphoma cells (CEM/VLB1000). Screening resulted in initial leads from a diarylimidazole library and these compounds formed the basis for further optimization. The clinical development compound, OC144-093, was the result of structure-activity studies guided by *in vitro* potency, pharmacokinetic, and metabolic data (Fig. 1) (Newman et al 2000, Sarshar et al 2000, Zhang et al 2000).

OC144-093 blocks the binding of [^{3}H]azidopine to Pgp and inhibits Pgp ATPase activity in the nanomolar concentration range. OC144-093 reverses multidrug resistance to doxorubicin, paclitaxel and vinblastine in human lymphoma, breast, ovarian, uterine and colorectal carcinoma cell lines expressing

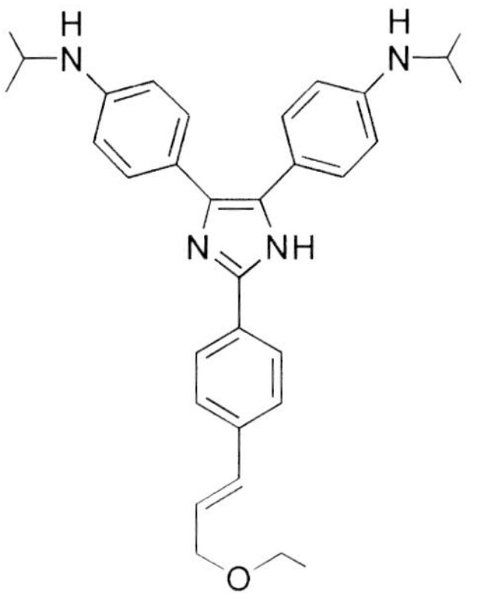

OC144-093

FIG. 1.   Structure of OC144-093.

Pgp, with an average EC_{50} of 32 nM (Table 1). Full reversal of MDR is observed at doses between 0.25 and 1.0 μM (Newman et al 2000). OC144-093 is at least as potent as other third generation Pgp inhibitors currently in development, such as LY335979 (Dantzig et al 1996, Starling et al 1997) and XR9576 (Roe et al 1999, Mistry et al 1999).

OC144-093 is not cytotoxic by itself against 15 normal, non-transformed or tumour cell lines, regardless of Pgp status, with an average cytostatic IC_{50} of $>60\,\mu$M, demonstrating less non-specific cytotoxicity than any previously

TABLE 1   Reversal of MDR by OC144-093 in Pgp-expressing cell lines[a]

| | $OC144\text{-}093\ EC_{50}\ (\mu M \pm SD)$ | | |
Cell Line	Doxorubicin	Vinblastine	Paclitaxel
CEM/VLB1000[b]	0.09 ± 0.06	0.07 ± 0.01	
MES-SA/DX5[c]	0.024 ± 0.006	0.034 ± 0.007	0.027 ± 0.007
SK/VLB1000[d]	0.025 ± 0.008	0.015	0.033
MCF-7/ADR[e]	0.038 ± 0.006	0.02 ± 0.01	0.031 ± 0.004
MDA/LCC6[MDR1e]	0.013		0.009
HCT-15[f]			0.016

[a]The IC_{50}s for the indicated antitumour agents were determined in the presence of various concentrations of OC144-093. The OC144-093 EC_{50} is the concentration that produced half-maximal reversal of antitumour agent resistance. Each experiment was carried out two to four times. Reprinted from Newman et al 2000. [b]lymphoma, [c]uterine, [d]ovarian, [e]breast, [f]colorectal carcinoma.

TABLE 2   Effect of OC144-093 on the proliferation of various cell lines[a]

Human cell type/line	Pgp expression[b]	OC144-093 IC$_{50}$ (µM)
Primary fibroblast		
CCD-986SK		>100
Smooth muscle		
HISM		>100
Lymphoma		
CEM	Neg	38
CEM/VLB1000	Pos	32
Ovarian carcinoma		
SKOV3	Neg	48
SK/VLB1000	Pos	15
Uterine carcinoma		
MES-SA	Neg	51
Breast carcinoma		
MCF-7	Neg	30
MCF-7/ADR	Pos	68
MDA/LCC6	Neg	>100
MDA/LCC6^{MDR1}	Pos	>100
Colorectal carcinoma		
SW480	Pos	>100
SW620	Neg	>100
HT-29	Neg	12
HCT-15	Pos	6

[a]The IC$_{50}$ for inhibition of the growth of cell lines by OC144-093 was determined. Each experiment was carried out at least two times with similar results. Reprinted from Newman et al 2000.
[b]Direct analysis and (or) from literature.

described Pgp inhibitor (Table 2). OC144-093 has no effect *in vitro* on the response to cytotoxic agents by cells that do not express Pgp (Fig. 2, Newman et al 2000), or that express MRP1 (Newman et al 2000), further demonstrating the specificity of this inhibitor.

Inhibition of MDR in tissue culture by OC144-093 is reversible, but the effect persists for at least 12 hours after removal of the compound from the culture medium (Newman et al 2000). Taken together with our observation that the non-specific cytotoxicity of OC144-093 is similar for Pgp-expressing and non-expressing cell lines (Table 2), our studies suggest that OC144-093 may not be a transport substrate of Pgp. This can also be assessed indirectly by loading

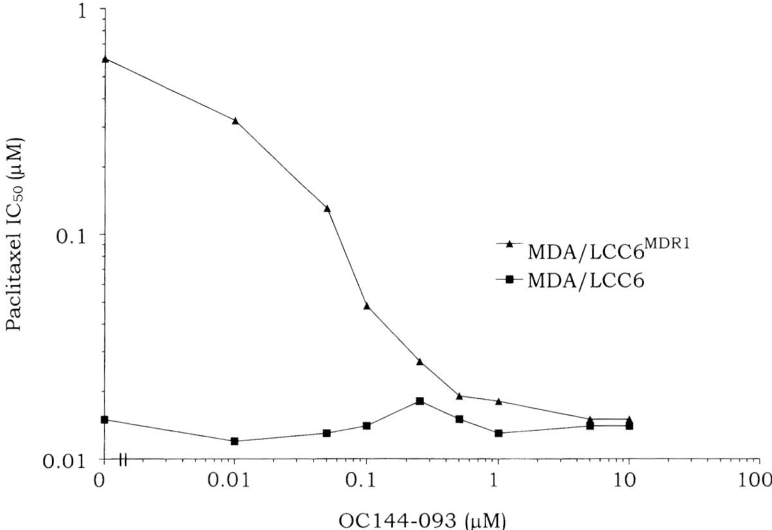

FIG. 2.   Effect of OC144-093 on paclitaxel IC_{50} in Pgp-negative and Pgp-transduced MDA/ LCC6 human breast carcinoma cells. Cell proliferation IC_{50}s were determined from 3 day dose–response curves carried out in triplicate. The figure is reprinted from Newman et al (2000). Pgp expression or lack thereof was confirmed by antibody staining and RT-PCR analysis.

Pgp-expressing cells with daunomycin in the presence of an energy poison such as azide, washing away the azide and exogenous daunomycin, and then monitoring Pgp-mediated daunomycin efflux by fluorescence-activated cell sorting (FACS) analysis. Inclusion of a Pgp inhibitor in the loading and efflux buffers can prevent daunomycin efflux. If the inhibitor is not a Pgp substrate, daunomycin efflux is prevented for a significant period of time after washing the cells, even if the inhibitor is not included in the efflux buffer. If the inhibitor is a Pgp substrate, it must be added to the efflux buffer in order to prevent rapid loss of both the inhibitor and daunomycin from the washed cells. The potential for the major AEDs carbamazepine and phenytoin to act as Pgp inhibitors was assessed by this technique. Therapeutically relevant concentrations of carbamazepine or phenytoin inhibited daunomycin efflux from Pgp-expressing CEM/VLB1000 cells, but only when they were included in both loading and efflux buffers, suggesting that they are Pgp substrates (Fig. 3). Significant inhibition of daunomycin efflux by OC144-093 persisted for up to 8 h, even when the compound was not included in the efflux buffer, suggesting that this compound is not an efficient substrate for Pgp-mediated transport (Fig. 3, Newman et al 2000).

OC144-093 is > 50% orally bioavailable in rodents and dogs and does not alter the plasma PK of i.v. administered paclitaxel in rodents (Newman et al 2000). Our

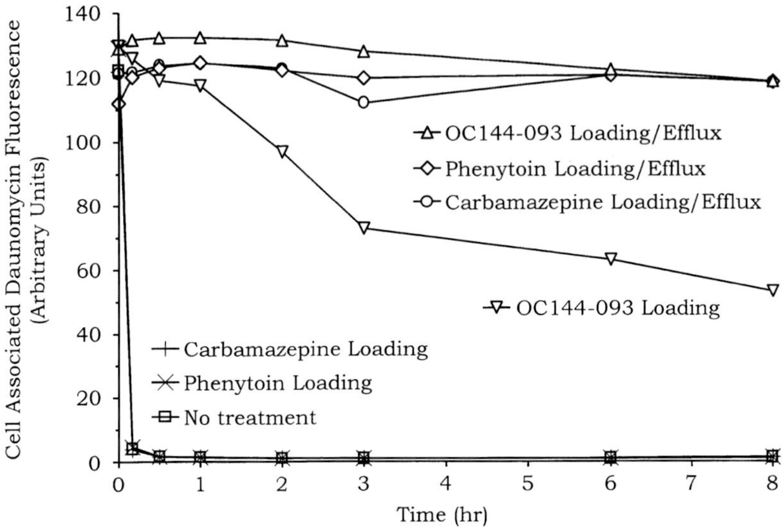

FIG. 3. Effects of phenytoin, carbamazepine, and OC144-093 on daunomycin efflux in Pgp-expressing CEM/VLB1000 lymphoma cells. Cells were pre-incubated in glucose-free loading medium containing 17.7 μM daunomycin, 10 mM NaN_3 and phenytoin (50 μM) or carbamazepine (50 μM) or OC144-093 (2 μM). The cells were washed and resuspended in efflux medium with or without the putative Pgp substrate/inhibitor. Daunomycin retention at various time points was determined by FACS analysis as described in Newman et al (2000). Similar results were obtained in two independent experiments.

studies indicate that OC144-093 is metabolized by P450 CYP2E1 and not by P450s CYP 1A2, 2B6, 2C8, 2C9, 2D6 or 3A4 (Tomlinson et al 1998). P450s CYP 2C8, 2C9, 2C19 and 3A4 mediate metabolism of the major AEDs carbamazepine and phenytoin (Kerr et al 1994, Komatsu et al 2000). Our results suggest that OC144-093 is unlikely to exhibit a PK interaction with carbamazepine or phenytoin, other than what might occur as a result of Pgp inhibition. In addition, we predict that OC144-093 will exhibit a relatively low propensity for drug interactions with other therapeutics, in light of its restricted cytochrome metabolism profile.

OC144-093 restores doxorubicin and paclitaxel sensitivity in mice engrafted with multidrug-resistant P388 leukaemia and MDA/LCC6[MDR1] human breast carcinoma cells, without a significant increase in doxorubicin or paclitaxel toxicity. The compound also enhances paclitaxel efficacy against intrinsically Pgp-expressing human colorectal carcinoma xenografts (Newman et al 2000).

OC144-093 does not enhance paclitaxel efficacy against MDA/LCC6 human breast carcinoma cells in monolayer culture (Fig. 2). This result was expected, because of the lack of Pgp expression by these cells. Thus, we were surprised to observe that OC144-093 enhanced paclitaxel anti-tumour efficacy against these cells *in vivo*. In this orthotopic model, a non-toxic dose of paclitaxel administered once per week was able to delay tumour growth for 3–4 weeks, but the tumours then started to regrow, even with continued paclitaxel treatment. When OC144-093 was added to the paclitaxel regimen, the tumour growth delay was maintained during the entire treatment course, producing a significant improvement in paclitaxel efficacy (Fig. 4) (Newman et al 1999). Rapid loss of paclitaxel sensitivity under monotherapy *in vivo* may result from induction of Pgp in the tumour, tumour stroma or vasculature. Chemotherapy-mediated Pgp induction has been observed in humans (Abolhoda et al 1999). It is possible that this phenomenon does not occur under tissue culture conditions, explaining the difference between our *in vitro* and *in vivo* results. Regardless of the mechanism, our results indicate that OC144-093 should be administered at the initiation of chemotherapy, where it may both enhance killing of Pgp-expressing tumour cells and prevent the rapid emergence of resistance.

As a result of intrinsic cytotoxicity and PK interactions, many Pgp inhibitors enhance paclitaxel toxicity, both *in vitro* and *in vivo*. Our studies have

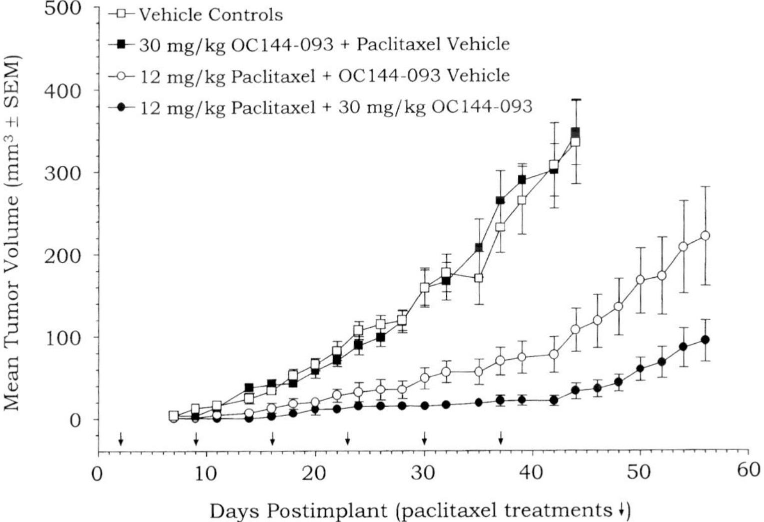

FIG. 4.   Effect of OC144-093 on the *in vivo* antitumour activity of paclitaxel against Pgp-negative MDA/LCC6 human breast carcinoma cells. Tumour cells were implanted in the mammary fat pads (2 sites per mouse, 6 mice per group) of RAG-2 SCID mice on day 0. Oral OC144-093 treatment was initiated on day 1 and i.v. paclitaxel on day 2, with three OC144-093 treatments per paclitaxel treatment, as described in the legend to Table 3. Paclitaxel treatments were once per week. All other aspects of the study were carried out as described for MDA/LCC6[MDR1] cells in Newman et al (2000). Similar results were obtained in three independent studies, including the initiation of treatment with established tumours.

demonstrated that therapeutically relevant doses of OC144-093 do not enhance paclitaxel toxicity *in vitro* or *in vivo* (Newman et al 2000). We made a second unexpected observation when titrating paclitaxel in the presence of OC144-093 *in vivo*. OC144-093 protected the mice from paclitaxel toxicity, preventing death under LD_{100} conditions (Table 3). This prompted us to investigate whether we could enhance paclitaxel efficacy against non-Pgp expressing tumours by using toxic doses of the compound in the presence of OC144-093. A paclitaxel dose of 20 mg/kg was added to a repeat of the experiment described in Fig. 4. This dose of paclitaxel produced an LD_{50} (three drug toxicity-related deaths out of six mice within 16 days). In the presence of 20 mg/kg paclitaxel plus OC144-093, only one possible drug toxicity-related death was observed on day 30. Tumour growth was almost completely suppressed, with three of 12 tumour implantation sites free of palpable tumour (Fig. 5) (Newman et al 1999). No tumour-free sites were observed with 20 mg/kg paclitaxel alone and all of the tumours started to regrow after cessation of treatment, as indicated in Fig. 5. The mechanisms by which OC144-093 enhances the anti-tumour efficacy of paclitaxel against non-Pgp expressing tumours and protects against paclitaxel toxicity are currently under investigation. If OC144-093 protects humans against paclitaxel toxicity, it may be possible to administer more effective paclitaxel doses for longer periods of time.

Clinical Development of OC144-093

Preclinical toxicology studies have been conducted in the rat and the dog in accordance with FDA guidelines under Good Laboratory Practice (GLP) conditions. Following continuous intravenous infusion over 24 h, the maximum

TABLE 3   Effect of OC144-093 on paclitaxel toxicity in athymic mice[a]

Treatment	Survival
OC144-093 + paclitaxel vehicle	4/4
Paclitaxel + OC144-093 vehicle	0/4
Paclitaxel + OC144-093	4/4

[a]OC144-093 (30 mg/kg p.o.) or OC144-093 vehicle was administered the afternoon before, two hours before and six hours after each paclitaxel or paclitaxel vehicle treatment. Paclitaxel or paclitaxel vehicle was administered once every five days at 10 a.m. (six i.v. treatments at 24 mg/kg followed by two treatments at 36 mg/kg). All of the mice treated with paclitaxel alone died within three days of the last treatment, without exhibiting mean group weight loss. Mice treated with paclitaxel and OC144-093 gained weight and appeared healthy when observed for thirteen days after cessation of treatment. Compounds were administered as described in Newman et al (2000). The experiment was carried out at the Southern Research Institute, Birmingham, Alabama. Protection from paclitaxel toxicity by OC144-093 has been observed in three independent experiments.

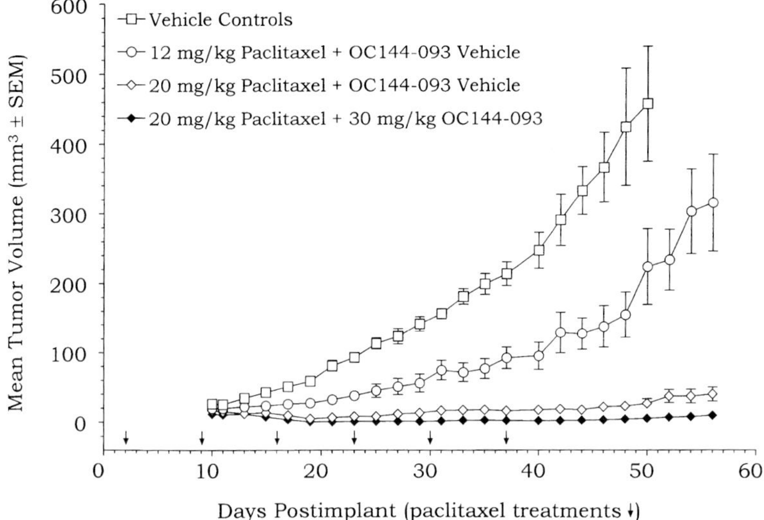

FIG. 5. Effect of OC144-093 on the *in vivo* anti-tumour activity and toxicity of 20 mg/kg paclitaxel. The experiment was carried out with non-Pgp-expressing MDA/LCC6 cells as described in the legend to Fig. 4. Treatment with 12 mg/kg paclitaxel plus OC144-093 resulted in enhanced anti-tumour efficacy, compared to paclitaxel alone, as demonstrated in Figure 4 (data not shown). Treatment with 20 mg/kg paclitaxel resulted in 3 drug-related deaths out of 6 mice within 16 days and did not completely suppress tumour growth at any of the implantation sites. Treatment with 20 mg/kg paclitaxel plus OC144-093 resulted in one possible drug-related death after 30 days and produced three implantation sites without palpable tumours.

tolerated doses (MTD) of OC144-093 were 75 mg/kg in the rat and 30 mg/kg in the dog, with complete recovery within 24 h. In the dog, the most sensitive species, ataxia and CNS depression were observed at a dose of 50 mg/kg. No target organ for toxicity was identified during histopathological evaluation and the only treatment-related finding was thrombo-phlebitis at the infusion site (vena cava). These findings were attributed to the low pH of the infusion solution of the drug. Following oral administration in aqueous solution to the dog, the MTD was 20 mg/kg given every 8 h over 24 h (60 mg/kg/day). Ataxia was the only effect observed at this dose with complete recovery within 24 h. The no-effect oral dose was 15 mg/kg t.i.d. (45 mg/kg/day). No histopathological changes were noted at any dose, including the MTD (Dixon & Toyonaga 1998).

A Phase 1, single-blind, placebo-controlled, ascending dose study of the intravenous safety, tolerability and PK of OC144-093 mesylate salt in healthy male volunteers was completed in the UK (Dixon & Toyonaga 2000). Escalating doses of 1.0, 2.5, 5.0 and 7.5 mg/kg (free base equivalents) were given by intravenous infusion over 6 h and 10.0 mg/kg over 24 h. No systemic effects, such as ataxia, were observed even at plasma levels in excess of 2000 ng/ml (4 μM). The only adverse effects were mild to moderate thrombo-phlebitis at the infusion site with the higher doses. The latter is not surprising in view of the previous infusion toxicology findings. As expected, there was transitory increase in direct and total serum bilirubin at the higher doses (5.0, 7.5 and 10.0 mg/kg).

Non-compartmental PK analysis of the plasma concentration data indicated linear kinetics of OC144-093 at these dose levels. The mean total plasma clearance (CL) was 0.48 l/h/kg, which suggested that OC144-093 should be orally bioavailable in humans if it was absorbed from the gut. As expected from preclinical studies and its high lipophilicity, OC144-093 was extensively distributed with a mean volume of distribution at steady-state (Vss) of 3.6 l/kg. The 'apparent' half-life was about 5.5 h, but this was probably an underestimate of the true terminal elimination half-life due to the limited blood sampling in the post-infusion phase.

A study to determine the relative oral bioavailability of a single oral dose of OC144-093 with and without food has also been completed in healthy male volunteers (Dixon & Toyonaga 2000). A single 400 mg dose, which is approximately 5 mg/kg for an 80 kg male, was chosen for this study. It was administered in a randomized crossover fashion to six subjects following an overnight fast and a high-fat breakfast with a 1 week wash-out period between treatments. Blood samples were taken at selected intervals over 48 h post-dose and the plasma assayed for intact OC144-093 by a validated HPLC method. As anticipated, there was a significant 'food effect' with an almost twofold increase in relative oral bioavailability when given with food compared to the fasted state. The absolute oral bioavailability was estimated to be greater than 60% by comparison with the mean area under the curve (AUC) obtained for OC144-093 following the 5 mg/kg intravenous dose in the previous study. Plasma levels in excess of 500 ng/ml (1 μM) were achieved over 12 h with food and in some subjects the peak levels were over 2000 ng/ml. The terminal half-life following oral dosing was about 22 h, suggesting that once or twice-a-day oral dosing might be appropriate in the clinic.

A limited multidose oral evaluation of the PK and safety of OC144-093 was recently completed in healthy male volunteers. The study was placebo controlled in parallel groups ($n=6$) of men. In each group, one subject got placebo and five were administered OC144-093 with food. The dosing schedule consisted of three sequential doses of 200, 300 or 400 mg of OC144-093 at 6, 12 or 24 h intervals, respectively, as might be used in a clinical oncology setting. Blood samples were taken for PK analysis following the first and third doses. In most subjects, OC144-093 was well tolerated and there were no serious adverse events. One subject experienced drowsiness and two others experienced dizziness. One additional subject exhibited mild ataxia. This observation was probably due to the high plasma level of OC144-093 ($>4\,\mu$M). As expected, transient increases in serum bilirubin were observed in some of the volunteers but these increases were not dose limiting. The PK data indicated that 200–300 mg of OC144-093 given twice a day might be a suitable dosing schedule prior to and during chemotherapy or AED drug therapy to maintain plasma levels of the modulator in excess of 500 ng/ml ($1\,\mu$M). At this concentration, complete reversal of MDR has been demonstrated in preclinical models.

Our results demonstrate that OC144-093 is an orally active, potent and non-toxic inhibitor of Pgp that exhibits all of the desired properties for prevention and treatment of Pgp-mediated MDR, as well as for the enhancement of the BBB penetration of CNS therapeutics that are Pgp substrates.

References

Abolhoda A, Wilson AE, Ross H, Danenberg PV, Burt M, Scotto KW 1999 Rapid activation of *MDR1* gene expression in human metastatic sarcoma after *in vivo* exposure to doxorubicin. Clin Cancer Res 5:3352–3356

Atadja P, Watanabe T, Xu H, Cohen D 1998 PSC-833, a frontier in modulation of P-glycoprotein mediated multidrug resistance. Cancer Metastasis Rev 17:163–168

Bates SE 1999 Drug resistance: Still on the learning curve. Clin Cancer Res 5:3346–3348

Borst P, Evers R, Kool M, Wijnholds J 2000 A family of drug transporters: the multidrug resistance-associated proteins. J Natl Cancer Inst 92:1295–1302

Dale I, Tuffley W, Callaghan R et al 1998 Reversal of P-glycoprotein-mediated multidrug resistance by XR9051, a novel diketopiperazine derivative. Br J Cancer 78:885–892

Dantzig AH, Shepard RL, Cao J et al 1996 Reversal of P-glycoprotein-mediated multidrug resistance by a potent cyclopropyldibenzosuberane modulator, LY335979. Cancer Res 56:4171–4179

Desai PB, Duan JZ, Zhu YW, Kouzi S 1998 Human liver microsomal metabolism of paclitaxel and drug interactions. Eur J Drug Metab Pharmacokinet 23:417–424

Dixon R, Toyonaga B 1998 P-glycoprotein inhibitor OC144-093; pharmacokinetics of a novel MDR modulator derived via solid-phase combinatorial chemistry. Ninth Annual Japanese–American Conference on Pharmacokinetics & Biopharmaceutics, Nagoya, Japan, July 1998

Dixon R, Toyonaga B 2000 P-glycoprotein inhibitor OC144-093: Phase 1 intravenous and oral pharmacokinetics of a novel mltidrug resistance modulator. Proc Amer Assoc Cancer Res 41:607 (Abstr 3863)

Germann UA, Shlyakhter D, Mason VS et al 1997 Cellular and biochemical characterization of VX-710 as a chemosensitizer: reversal of P-glycoprotein-mediated multidrug resistance *in vitro*. Anticancer Drugs 8:125–140

Kerr BM, Thummel KE, Wurden CJ et al 1994 Human liver carbamazepine metabolism. Role of CYP3A4 and CYP2C8 in 10,11-epoxide formation. Biochem Pharmacol 47:1969–1979

Komatsu T, Yamazaki H, Asahi S et al 2000 Formation of a dihydroxy metabolite of phenytoin in human liver microsomes/cytosol: roles of cytochromes P450 2c9, 2c19, and 3a4. Drug Metab Dispos 28:1361–1368

Lazarowski A, Sevlever G, Taratuto A, Massaro M, Rabinowicz A 1999 Tuberous sclerosis associated with MDR1 gene expression and drug-resistant epilepsy. Pediatr Neurol 21: 731–734

Mistry P, Stewart A, Plumb J et al 1999 *In vitro* and *in vivo* evaluation of XR9576, a novel potent modulator of P-glycoprotein (Pgp) mediated multidrug resistance (MDR). Proc Am Assoc Cancer Res 40:313 (Abstr 2079)

Newman M J, Rodarte JC, Benbatoul KD et al 2000 Discovery and characterization of OC144-093, a novel inhibitor of P-glycoprotein-mediated multidrug resistance. Cancer Res 60: 2964–2972

Newman M J, Rodarte JC, Benbatoul KD et al 1999 Preclinical characterization and clinical safety/pharmacokinetics of OC144-093, a novel inhibitor of P-glycoprotein-mediated multidrug resistance. Amer Assoc for Cancer Res/Nat Cancer Inst/Eur Org for Res and Treat of Cancer, International Conference on Molecular Targets and Cancer Therapeutics: Discovery, Development and Clinical Validation, Nov 1999, Washington DC (Abstr #0731)

Ramachandran C, Melnick S J 1999 Multidrug resistance in human tumors-molecular diagnosis and clinical significance. Mol Diagn 4:81–94

Roe M, Folkes A, Ashworth P et al 1999 Reversal of P-glycoprotein mediated multidrug resistance by novel anthranilamide derivatives. Bioorg Med Chem Lett 9:595–600

Sarshar S, Zhang C, Moran EJ et al 2000 2,4,5-Trisubstituted imidazoles: novel nontoxic modulators of P-glycoprotein mediated multidrug resistance. Part 1. Bioorg Med Chem Lett 10:2599–2601

Schinkel AH 1998 Pharmacological insights from P-glycoprotein knockout mice. Int J Clin Pharmacol Ther 36:9–13

Schinkel AH, Wagenaar E, Mol CA, van Deemter L 1996 P-glycoprotein in the blood–brain barrier of mice influences the brain penetration and pharmacological activity of many drugs. J Clin Invest 97:2517–2524

Sikic BI 1997 Pharmacologic approaches to reversing multidrug resistance. Semin Hematol 34:40–47

Sisodiya SM, Heffernan J, Squier MV 1999 Over-expression of P-glycoprotein in malformations of cortical development. Neuroreport 10:3437–3441

Sonnichsen DS, Liu Q, Schuetz EG, Schuetz JD, Pappo A, Relling MV 1995 Variability in human cytochrome P450 paclitaxel metabolism. J Pharmacol Exp Ther 275:566–575

Starling J J, Shepard RL, Cao J et al 1997 Pharmacological characterization of LY335979: a potent cyclopropyldibenzosuberane modulator of P-glycoprotein. Adv Enzyme Regul 37:335–347

Tishler DM, Weinberg KI, Hinton DR, Barbaro N, Annett GM, Raffel C 1995 MDR1 gene expression in brain of patients with medically intractable epilepsy. Epilepsia 36:1–6

Tomlinson ES, Bullock PL, Reimer M, Dixon R, Mayer LD 1998 Identification of metabolites and cytochrome P450's involved in the metabolism of OC144-093 — A new modulator of MDR in cancer chemotherapy. Amer Assoc Pharma Sci Annual Meeting 1:s50 (Abstr 1162)

Trock B J, Leonessa F, Clarke R 1997 Multidrug resistance in breast cancer: a meta-analysis of MDR1/gp170 expression and its possible functional significance. J Natl Cancer Inst 89:917–931

van Zuylen L, Nooter K, Sparreboom A, Verweij J 2000 Development of multidrug-resistance convertors: sense or nonsense? Investig New Drugs 18:205–220

Zhang C, Sarshar S, Moran EJ et al 2000 2,4,5-Trisubstituted imidazoles: novel nontoxic modulators of P-glycoprotein mediated multidrug resistance. Part 2. Bioorg Med Chem Lett 10:2603–2605

DISCUSSION

Löscher: Are there any data showing that your compounds penetrate the BBB?

Newman: Nothing that I would call definitive.

Shorvon: For the epilepsy field, we need long-term treatment. Is there a long-term toxicity issue with your drug?

Newman: Any time you move out of the oncology area to anything else, you have to ask this question. In oncology toxicity is much less of an issue. We don't know the chronic toxicity profile of the compound. If it were going to be used in epilepsy, we would need to look at this more carefully. It might be possible (and advisable) to get a proof of principle first.

Shorvon: The obvious model is stasis.

Ling: I find the protection against toxicity fascinating, but I don't understand it. Will it protect against more than just Taxol?

Newman: We have looked at a couple of other cytotoxic chemotherapeutic agents. This is not a general phenomenon. The compound did not protect against cisplatin and doxorubicin toxicity. It may be something particular to paclitaxel.

Wood: In pursuing the protection against toxicity, it seems to me that this must be a metabolic effect (which you are saying it is not) or it must be a transporter effect on something other than Pgp, because it goes in the wrong direction. Alternatively, it could be a non-specific effect that is hard to understand. The thing to pursue first would be the metabolic and transport effects. But I gather from what you said that you are fairly confident that it is not an inhibitor of other transporters. Is that right?

Newman: We have only looked at MRP1, so we don't know about other transporters. If we go back to what Taxol does from a toxicity point of view, we are talking about myelosuppression or peripheral neuropathy in terms of dose-limiting toxicities in animals or in the clinic. We can now look in animals, at least, to see if we are protecting against these. We need to find a dose of Taxol that doesn't quite kill the animals and then a dose of OC144-093 that protects well in that setting. I would want to do this first and look at blood counts and CNS tests before we look at lots of other potential transporters.

Wood: The other possibility is that the drug itself is being metabolized. This was an *in vivo* experiment. Although you might be confident that the parent drug is not an inhibitor of metabolism, or an inhibitor of some other transporter, in an *in vivo* setting you need to be sure that it is not a metabolite that is having an effect.

Newman: That is an excellent point. We are looking at the metabolites. We know that the major metabolite has no Pgp inhibitory activity.

Wood: If you know which pathway is producing this, a simple experiment would be to inhibit this pathway and see whether you still get the protection. If it is all P450 CYP2E1 you could just inhibit this.

Newman: The other thing we want to do is just take the metabolite and see whether it gives the same protection.

Bates: We recently demonstrated that PSC 833 shifted the metabolites of Taxol. Some of them may be less toxic than others (Kang et al 2001).

Newman: We see no effect on the levels of the parent compound.

Wood: This is an important point: just because you don't see a difference in the parent compound, it doesn't mean that there might not be a major shift in some metabolite that is a relatively trivial contributor to the overall excretion of the drug.

Varadi: Have you tried to demonstrate direct interaction of this compound with MDR1?

Newman: Yes, we did the standard tritiated azidopine photoaffinity labelling protection study. We completely blocked azidopine photoaffinity labelling at submicromolar concentrations of OC144-093. It also inhibits Pgp ATPase at nanomolar concentrations. We don't know were it binds. The binding sites are very complicated. It may bind competitively with respect to transport substrates, but all of our data support the notion that it is not itself transported. One other piece of evidence for this is that when you look at non-specific cytotoxicity with a Pgp inhibitor, across a lot of cell lines that both do and don't express Pgp, if your compound is a substrate you would expect to see a differential in the non-specific cytotoxicity. We don't see this.

Sander: Would you envisage this compound being given with carbamezipine or phenytoin?

Newman: You would either give it at the same time orally, or you might give it a little earlier than the AED in order to get it to the blood–brain barrier (BBB) first.

Wood: There is a fundamental issue that relates to that question. If we were going to use a Pgp inhibitor to enhance carbamazepine efficacy, there are three things to consider. First we need to demonstrate that it works independently of increasing oral absorption. Second, it would need to decrease seizures. Third, and most importantly, it would need to work selectively in the seizure-inducing area, in contrast to increasing brain penetration of the drug to produce adverse CNS effects.

Löscher: When there is a localized overexpression of some of those transporters, for instance in the focal area, then there is a chance this approach will work. In this case it might be that you need only a relatively low level of the inhibitor to cut down the overexpression to a normal expression level. Otherwise, you would increase everything, including the undesirable effects of the drug.

Ling: Presumably one would treat the responding rat with the same dose. You would adjust the dose that would give the responding rat an effect, and see whether the same dose would have an effect on the non-responder.

Löscher: I showed you data from only one dose of phenytoin. The first thing we tried was to see whether the non-response could be overcome just by increasing the dose. This was not possible. It was an all-or-none phenomenon. I cannot see how just increasing the brain penetration by Pgp inhibitors should resolve this.

Shorvon: Sanjay Sisodiya's work should make one slightly more optimistic about this. The abnormal cells in epilepsy seem to express these proteins more.

Wood: There is another approach, which is to ask the question of whether there are drugs that have been shown to be effective *in vitro* which for one reason or another haven't been effective *in vivo*. In this subset of drugs there might be some that were Pgp substrates and would have been very effective anti-epileptics, but which didn't make it because of either oral bioavailability or brain access. This might be the most productive area to proceed with rapidly: it might open a whole new spectrum of AEDs that can be developed fairly quickly.

Sander: For every drug that has been launched, thousands have been thrown away. Many drugs have looked exactly how you describe: they got into phase II/III trials but were abandoned because of a lack of *in vivo* efficacy in patients, even though they worked in animal models. I could tell you of several AEDs that have been thrown out in the last two or three years.

Sills: If it is Pgp that is preventing these drugs working in patients, it should also prevent them from working in animal models, assuming that the model is appropriate and the pattern of Pgp expression is similar.

Löscher: The problem here is that because industry has to test thousands of compounds, simple screening-like animal models are called for. Models such as the maximal electroshock seizure (MES) test are used, where many compounds can be tested in a short time. This is a model in which the common AEDs work. Then you go to the clinic and test these compounds in pharmacoresistant patients. It is naïve to believe that then there is any predictive ability. It surprises me that the prediction is as good as it is.

Shorvon: They are selecting the wrong drugs.

Sisodiya: The regionalization of overexpression of the drug resistance proteins is an important issue that has been brought up a number of times. I am not aware of the distribution of overexpression having been looked at in models. It is not just the BBB that we are talking about; it is an issue of local penetration to the area that is causing the epilepsy. For human epilepsy there is local overexpression.

Wood: There are strategies. Terfenadine (Seldane®), the commonly used antihistamine, was successful initially as a drug because it was metabolized to a Pgp substrate: it was well absorbed and because the metabolite was a Pgp substrate it didn't enter the brain and produce a central antihistamine effect.

Ruetz: There is a widely used assay involving Caco-2 cells which can be grown in monolayers with tight junctions. There is an apical and basolateral side. Caco-2 cells have MDR1. The neat thing about this system is that it is not necessary to use labelled compounds to measure conduction across the cell barrier.

Newman: We need to be cautious about what drugs and what settings we go into. They may not be the ideal ones and then we will probably fail. It would be helpful if in our discussions we can come to some consensus about the best cell and animal models, both to test whether a Pgp inhibitor can do what we would like it to do and also what would be the most predictive model to test it in.

Meldrum: I may be missing something important, but I can't understand the relationship between Pgp and AEDs. The problem is that there is Pgp in the gut and Pgp in the BBB, but all the AEDs we use have good oral bioavailability. They also penetrate the BBB extremely well. Therefore, Pgp doesn't seem to be a terribly big issue when discussing their movement, bioavailability and biological actions. This hypothesis that Pgp is somehow critical at the epileptic focus is all well and good, but there is no evidence for it.

Bates: We are using Pgp as a model for all these other transporters. Your field needs to look at whether the MRPs 1–7 or ABC2 or MXR/BCRP are also playing a role here. The idea that there could be localized overexpression of Pgp or other transporters is still very plausible.

Wood: Instead of doing surgery in patients with epilepsy, what about trying to transfect the focus with the transporter? I'm only being somewhat facetious. I agree with Brian Meldrum's point. We could step back and say that things don't look too terrific, but on the other hand it would be nice to have some way to manipulate drug entry into specific cells of the brain. What appears to me to make epilepsy somewhat different is that there may be foci that you could attack with gene therapy, and then target delivery to these specific tissues. The attraction to me is that this is an experiment that you could do in animals relatively quickly. You could design a carrier that took drugs and got them in and out, and demonstrate the proof of principle fairly quickly.

Sander: This has been done. Valproate has been put around a phosphoglycoprotein and delivered locally.

Wood: You want to have it in a format that would not be delivered normally, so it wouldn't get into the brain except when Pgp is inhibited.

Newman: I don't think any of us are completely convinced that there is a direct connection between Pgp and drug resistance in epilepsy. We have some suggestive evidence. It is a hypothesis that might be worth testing, if we can come up with reasonably easy and cost-effective ways of testing it.

Reference

Kang MH, Figg WD, Ando Y et al 2001 The P-glycoprotein antagonist PSC 833 increases the plasma concentrations of 6α-hydroxypaclitaxel, a major metabolite of paclitaxel. Clin Cancer Res 7:1610–1617

Final general discussion

Pirmohamed: Our interest in epilepsy resistance started with the paper by Tishler et al (1995). We wanted to look at carbamazepine initially, to see whether this was a substrate for P glycoprotein (Pgp). We were already interested in carbamazepine with respect to other issues such as hypersensitivity and we had well developed assays. It is also a cytochrome P450 CYP3A4 substrate, and there is an overlap between CYP3A4 and Pgp substrates, although it is not a complete overlap. There is also a well known interaction between verapamil and carbamazepine which results in carbamazepine neurotoxicity. We used three systems: an *in vivo* system as well as two *in vitro* systems. The first problem that we ran into was the fact that we only had cold compound, and not radiolabelled. We had to develop another HPLC assay in order to analyse carbamazepine in brain, despite the fact that we had previously developed and well-validated HPLC assays for plasma and buffers. When we initially used carbamazepine, extraction efficiency wasn't very good from the brains, so we had to develop a more reliable extraction procedure from these transgenic mice as well as a new HPLC assay (Owen et al 2001a). The precision and accuracy of this assay is very good after extraction from murine brain, with values well above 90% (Table 1 [*Pirmohamed*]). We used *Mdr1a/Mdr1b* knockout mice. Wild-type and knockout mice were given two doses of carbamazepine, the mice were sacrificed at 1 h and 4 h, brain and blood were removed and carbamazepine was quantified by HPLC with UV detection. The results showed that at all doses and time points we couldn't find any difference in the drug concentration within the brain between wild-type and knockouts (Owen et al 2001b). This suggested that Pgp was not affecting entry of carbamazepine into the brain. In blood we found similar results. The problem is that we were looking at the whole brain, so we could have missed specific regional variation in brain levels. We concluded that in terms of the whole blood–brain barrier, Pgp wasn't affecting transport of carbamazepine in this model.

We then went on to look at Caco-2 cells, where there is vectorial transport. There is very high expression of Pgp at one apical border. We used apparent permeability. This was done in the presence and absence of PSC 833. We didn't get a ratio above one, which is what you would expect if there was vectorial transport, and PSC 833 had no effect. We did RT-PCR on these cells in comparison with our primary cell line, and we also did Western blotting. We found very high levels of Pgp in these cells. We also used indinavir as a positive control in the same experiments, and this

TABLE 1 (*Pirmohamed*) **Intra-day precision, inter-day precision and accuracy of analysis of carbamazepine in murine brain at specified concentrations**

Concentrations (μg/ml)	Intra-day precision	Inter-day precision	Accuracy
0.2	92.4, 94.1, 96.3, 96.5, 99.4	95.7 ± 2.6	$92.0 \pm 0\,6.1$
0.8	92.1, 93.8, 95.6, 98.8, 98.3	95.6 ± 2.7	103.4 ± 2.6
1.6	97.3, 98.5, 98.9, 99.1, 99.6	98.7 ± 0.9	99.3 ± 0.6

Values for intra-day precision are RSDs of quadruplicate determinations of five different samples at the stated concentration. Values for inter-day precision and accuracy are mean $\pm$ SD ($n = 4$).

showed very good vectorial transport in this system, in contrast to carbamazepine. Lastly, we used a rhodamine efflux assay. Again, we didn't use CD56[+] cells here; we just used whole peripheral blood lymphocyte populations. But we used verapamil as a positive control. We got increased fluorescence with verapamil, suggesting that it was acting as a Pgp inhibitor in this system. When we used both low and high doses of carbamazepine (10 and 100 μM) we saw no increase in fluorescence. This suggests that carbamazepine was not affecting rhodamine efflux within the assay. This is consistent with our results *in vivo* and with the Caco-2 cells. This contradicts some of the results we have seen during this meeting, and I am slightly confused about whether these drugs are substrates for Pgp. A crucial point before we begin using Pgp inhibitors in epilepsy is to determine for certain that the anti-epileptic drugs (AEDs) are substrates for Pgp. I understand that there are other transporters that may be important, and I agree with Professor Meldrum's point that these drugs do have good bioavailability and cross the blood–brain barrier. Therefore one has to wonder whether Pgp is important. I agree that there is Pgp overexpression in certain areas of the brain, but one has to determine why it is being overexpressed in that particular area. It may be a result of disease, or even therapy. Some of the studies we are currently doing are looking at whether carbamazepine, phenytoin and phenobarbitone can induce Pgp in different model cell systems. Other experiments we have in mind involve using a well characterized DNA bank of patients who have undergone surgery. When Dr Brinkmann's paper (Hoffmeyer et al 2000) was published last year one of the things we wanted to do is to test whether the exon 26 genotype is associated with pharmacoresistance in this patient group. This may be a fishing expedition, but we have the potential for catching a big fish.

Vezzani: How much is the protein overexpressed in your cell lines that overexpress Pgp?

Pirmohamed: I can't remember the exact figure, but it was an order of magnitude higher.

Vezzani: I am just wondering whether it is possible to set up an *in vitro* experiment in which you overexpress the transport pumps to different extents, to see whether there is a level at which you can affect the anticonvulsant drug transport. The issue is, how much do you need to increase the pump to have a functional effect?

Pirmohamed: One of the things we found is that Western blotting is semi-quantitative at best, and so is conventional RT-PCR. We are now doing real-time PCR, which works very well. Hopefully we can then see what the different levels of Pgp expression are.

Kwan: One of the things we struggled with in our experiments on *Mdr1* knockout mice is how to administer the drug. I noticed that you gave the drug intraperitoneally. We chose the subcutaneous route in order to avoid any gut absorption problems. In addition, with hindsight, we thought we could have looked at the 10,11 epoxide of carbamazepine. Have you had any chance to look at this?

Pirmohamed: We haven't done this, but we did try to measure 10,11 epoxide in the brain tissue using our HPLC assay. We didn't see any metabolism in the brain tissue. Although this was a highly sensitive assay, it still is not as good as using radiolabelled compounds.

Newman: Whether or not one is going to see Pgp-mediated transport is highly dependent on the amount of Pgp and the type of assay that is chosen. This may be related to the different results that we are all seeing. It may turn out to be necessary to pick the best one — the one that has the best evidence for being transported by Pgp. Then we need to try to get the drug into some convenient animal model and see what happens.

Sills: I agree that one of the most important things is to determine which drugs are substrates. If none of the drugs are substrates, we may be wasting our time. Unfortunately, as we have heard, there is no gold standard for determining substrate specificity. We may have to employ a number of different models to ascertain which AEDs are substrates for Pgp. In my opinion, the first assumption we are making, in terms of the role of multidrug resistance (MDR) in epilepsy, is that some, if not all, AEDs are substrates. The second assumption concerns the expression of the protein in the brain as a whole. The theory is that there is localized overexpression. If there isn't, again, we may be wasting our time. Thus, there are two principle issues: are the drugs substrates, and is the overexpression localized?

Löscher: There is a third issue: there are other transporters than just Pgp. There is good evidence that valproate is a substrate for MRP2. We found more than 20 years ago in dogs that probenecid markedly increases the brain concentrations of valproate. At that time, these multidrug transporters had not yet been described. Our idea at the time was that because valproate is a simple fatty acid, it uses a transporter for such acids. Years later, these results were reproduced in primates and a number of other species. Three years ago it was shown that valproate is a good substrate for MRP2 (Huai-Yun et al 1998). The Cleveland group have recent data that MRP2 is highly overexpressed in epileptic tissue from human patients (Abbott et al 2002, this volume).

Pirmohamed: This might be a shot in the dark, but MRP2 is the transporter that is deficient in Dubin–Johnson syndrome; is there any evidence that patients with this syndrome are also more liable to get valproate toxicity or require lower doses of valproate?

Sander: For some reason, valproate is not used for people with liver problems.

Varadi: There is a knockout rat for MRP2.

Newman: Does valproate cause hyperbilirubinaemia?

Pirmohamed: It causes mild transaminitis, but in rare cases it can cause microvesicular steatosis, which can be associated with hepatic failure.

Löscher: In addition to this there are recent data showing that gabapentin is a substrate for active transport. The two drugs, valproate and gabapentin, have one thing in common: there is no linear relationship between dosing, plasma concentration and brain concentration. There is a saturable transport, which is not the case for all the other AEDs, which have a relatively linear relationship between dose and CSF or brain drug level. This is an argument against Brian Meldrum's hypothesis: for these two drugs (valproate and gabapentin) at least, it is not as simple.

Oza: Is it valid to assume that the knockout mice experiment is the functional opposite of selective overexpression? Can you assume that if it works in one way in knockout mice it has to be the opposite in either tumours or in brain tissue that overexpresses Pgp?

Newman: One of the hypotheses is that Pgp only becomes important in drug resistance in epilepsy when it starts to become overexpressed. That is, it is not playing a role in the normal state. If this is the case, you won't expect to see anything in the knockout mouse. At normal levels, Pgp is not playing a role. You will only see something if you go to localized over-expression.

Oza: That is my point: are there any animal models where we should be looking at overexpression?

Wijnhold: We don't have mice overexpressing Pgp or MRP1 in the brain.

Vezzani: We have seen that seizures lead to the overexpression of the Pgp proteins. This could be an experimental approach.

Newman: Schinkel et al (1996) showed that phenytoin is a weak Pgp substrate.

Wijnholds: Some other Pgp substrates such as etoposide do not penetrate the blood–brain barrier well.

Newman: Etoposide is also an MRP1 substrate, so this gets complicated.

Wood: With regard to the question of whether the knockout is the mirror image of the over-expression, the whole cancer field was built on the over-expression system. Right now, it hasn't worked. On the other hand, we do know that for drugs that are substrates, inhibiting Pgp increases brain effects. I am not sure where this comes into the question, but it does raise a certain amount of caution about jumping to define overexpression as being fundamentally different from the knockout, in that ivermectin clearly produced a profound effect in knockout but not in wild-type, and loperamide is lethal in knockout and not in wild-type. I would be careful about going too far down the road of saying that overexpression is fundamentally different from the mirror image of a knockout.

References

Abbott J, Khan EU, Rollinson CMS et al 2002 Drug resistance in epilepsy: the role of the blood–brain barrier. In: Mechanisms of drug resistance in epilepsy: lessons from oncology. Wiley, Chichester (Novartis Found Symp 243) p 38–53

Hoffmeyer S, Burk O, von Richter O et al 2000 Functional polymorphisms of the human multidrug-resistance gene: multiple sequence variations and correlation of one allele with P-glycoprotein expression and activity in vivo. Proc Natl Acad Sci USA 97:3473–3478

Huai-Yun H, Secrest DT, Mark KS et al 1998 Expression of multidrug resistance-associated protein (MRP) in brain microvessel endothelial cells. Biochem Biophys Res Commun 243:816–820

Owen A, Tettey JN, Morgan P, Pirmohamed M, Park BK 2001a LC determination of carbamazepine in murine brain. J Pharm Biomed Anal 26:573–577

Owen A, Pirmohamed M, Tettey JN, Morgan P, Chadwick D, Park BK 2001b Carbamazepine is not a substrate for P-glycoprotein. Br J Clin Pharmacol 51:345–349

Schinkel AH, Wagenaar E, Mol CA, van Deemter L 1996 P-glycoprotein in the blood–brain barrier of mice influences the brain penetration and pharmacological activity of many drugs. J Clin Invest 97:2517–2524

Tishler DM, Weinberg KI, Hinton DR, Barbaro N, Annett GM, Raffel C 1995 MDR1 gene expression in brain of patients with medically intractable epilepsy. Epilepsia 36:1–6

Closing remarks

Victor Ling

BC Cancer Agency, 600 West 10th Avenue, Vancouver, BC, Canada V5Z 4E6

The purpose of this meeting was to see whether there are lessons that have been learned from the understanding of drug resistance in oncology that can be applied to refractile epilepsy. From this perspective the last three days have been extremely successful. Many issues have been brought to light. Cynics might suggest that we are now confused at a much more sophisticated level than we were previously! At least we are better off than before.

The second point that is clear is that whether or not Pgp has anything to do with epilepsy, it is a model on which we can base our understanding of the role of transporters allowing movement of molecules from one compartment to another. In the long run, I believe these kinds of fundamental studies will have an impact in our understanding of epilepsy therapies.

The third point is that we now have increasingly sophisticated tools to look at the whole question of heterogeneity. It would be advantageous to use these tools in both epilepsy and oncology. The genome project has identified some 50 transporters that might be relevant. There are polymorphisms that are probably significant. There will be many opportunities to exploit these tools in a systematic, logical way.

When I came to this meeting I wasn't sure that we have good models for epilepsy, but now I think we have at least the beginnings of these models. With these models we can build a rational approach to understanding the disease and looking for better drugs.

Finally, we want to move towards the design of clinical studies. In this context I was particularly impressed by the work that Susan Bates and Amit Oza have presented. We have the tools to identify the drug transporters in CNS. Then we can ask the question as to whether anti-epileptic drugs (AEDs) are substrates for these. We have various strategies for developing AEDs that are not substrates, or to develop AEDs that are substrates but whose entry can be modulated. Then there is the whole question of the mechanism of resistance. Trial design is also extremely important, as we have learned from oncology. Surrogate markers are important. Finally, we need to avoid overly high expectations, so we can progress logically towards a systematic and rational and understanding of what is happening.

Index of contributors

Subject index